Breast Cancer: Targeted Biological Therapeutic Agents 2021

Kerry Atkinson MBBS MD DTM&H FRACP FRCP

Consultant Physician

Adjunct Professor, Stem Cell Laboratories, Queensland University of Technology at the Translational Research Institute, Brisbane, Australia

Also by Kerry Atkinson

1. Graft-versus-Host Disease. Editors, S Burakoff, H J Deeg, J Ferrara, K Atkinson. Marcel Dekker Inc, New York, 1990.
2. Clinical Bone Marrow Transplantation.First edition. Editor, K Atkinson. Cambridge University Press, Cambridge UK, 1994.
3. The BMT Data Book: A Manual for Bone Marrow and Blood Stem Cell Transplantation. K. Atkinson, Cambridge University Press, Cambridge UK, 1998.
4. Clinical Bone Marrow and Blood Stem Cell Transplantation. Second Edition. Editor, K. Atkinson. Cambridge University Press, Cambridge UK, 2000.
5. Clinical Bone Marrow and Blood Stem Cell Transplantation. Third Edition. Eds, K. Atkinson, R Champlin, J Ritz, M Brenner, P Ljungman and W Fibbe. Cambridge University Press, Cambridge UK, 2004.
6. The BMT Data Book. Second edition. R Munker, HM Lazarus and K. Atkinson, Cambridge University Press, Cambridge UK, 2009.
7. The BMT Data Book: Including Cellular Therapy. Third edition. R Munker, C Hildebrandt, HM Lazarus and K. Atkinson, Cambridge University Press, Cambridge UK. 2013.
8. Bird facts for everyone. K Atkinson. Outskirts Press Inc., Denver, USA. 2014
9. Hematopoietic Cell Transplants: Concepts, Controversies and Future Directions. Eds HM Lazarus, RP Gale, A Keating, A Bacigalupo, R Munker, K Atkinson, A Syed. Cambridge University Press, Cambridge, UK. 2017.
10. The Biology and Therapeutic Application of Mesenchymal Cells. Ed. K Atkinson. Wiley/Blackwell. 2017
11. Revolutionizing Tropical Medicine. Eds. K Atkinson and D Mabey. Wiley/Blackwell Publishers Inc. 2019.
12. Asthma: Targeted Biological Treatments 2020. Kindle Direct Publishing, 2020. e-book and paperback
13. Atopic Dermatitis: Targeted Biological Treatments 2020. Kindle Direct Publishing, 2020. e-book and paperback
14. Psoriasis: Targeted Biological Treatments 2020. Kindle Direct Publishing, 2020. e-book and paperback
15. Crohn's disease and ulcerative colitis: Targeted Biological Treatments 2020. Kindle Direct Publishing, 2020. e-book and paperback

16. Rheumatoid arthritis, Juvenile Idiopathic Arthritis, Ankylosing spondylitis, Psoriatric Arthritis and Gout: Targeted Biological Treatments 2020. Kindle Direct Publishing, 2020. e-book and paperback
17. Small Cell Lung Cancer: Targeted Biological Treatments 2020. Kindle Direct Publishing, 2020. e-book and paperback
18. Chronic Myeloid Leukemia: Targeted Biological Treatments 2020. Kindle Direct Publishing, 2020. e-book and paperback
19. Melanoma: Targeted Biological Treatments 2020, Kindle Direct Publishing 2020. e-book and paperback
20. Dementia - A Caregiver's Guide. Kindle Direct Publishing 2020. e-book
21. Birds, Birds, Birds. Kindle Direct Publishing 2020. e-book and paperback
22. A Field Guide to the Wild Habitats of Sydney Australia. Kindle Direct Publishing 2021. e-book and paperback

"THE TIMES THEY ARE A-CHANGIN' "

From Bob Dylan's song THE TIMES THEY ARE A-CHANGIN' on his album THE TIMES THEY ARE A-CHANGIN' released by CBS Records in 1964

**"The only thing I knew how to do
was to keep on keeping on like a bird that flew"**

From Bob Dylan's song Tangled up in blue from his album Blood on the Tracks published by CBS in 1975

Nobel Laureate in Literature, 2016

This photograph of Bob Dylan, reproduced here from Wikimedia Commons, is in the public domain. https://commons.wikimedia.org/wiki/File:Bob-Dylan-arrived-at-Arlanda-surrounded-by-twenty-bodyguards-and-assistants-391770740297_(cropped).jpg. This Swedish photograph is in the public domain in Sweden because it is the work is non-artistic (journalistic, etc.) and has been created before 1 January 1970 (SFS 1960:729, § 49a). (1966). (PD 1970)

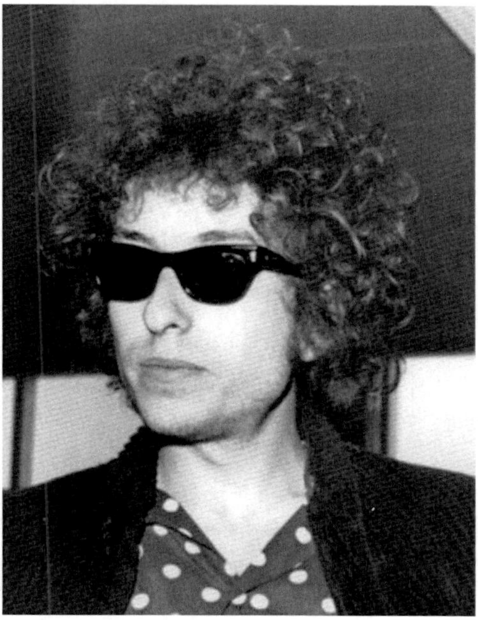

"We made a promise we swore we'd always remember

No retreat no surrender"

From Bruce Springsteen's song No Surrender published by CBS Records in 1984

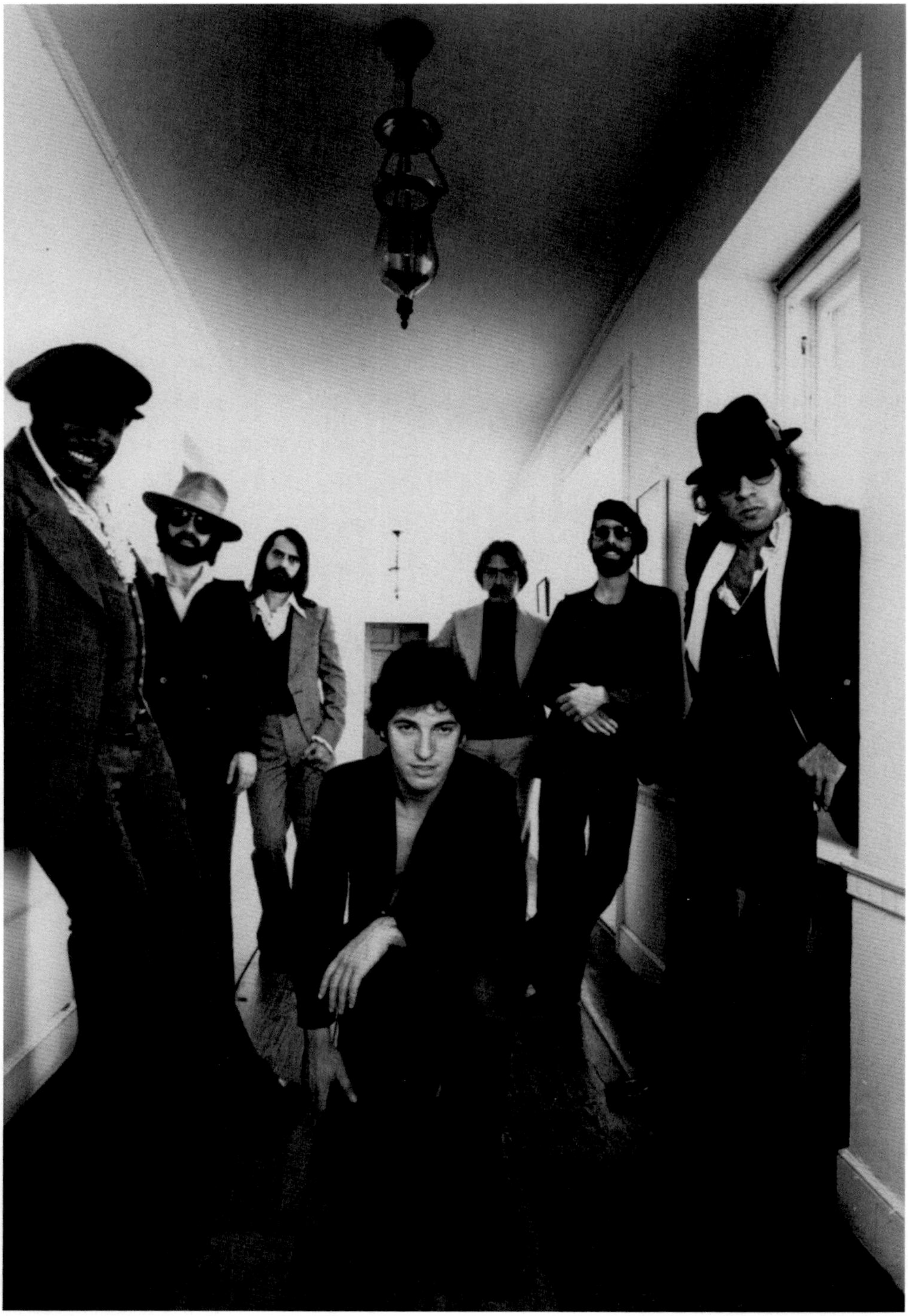

Bruce Springsteen and the E Street Band 1977. By Columbia Records - Original text: eBayfrontbackarchived link), Public Domain, https://commons.wikimedia.org/w/index.php?curid=58087854. https://en.wikipedia.org/wiki/Bruce_Springsteen#/media/File:Bruce_Springsteen_and_the_E_Street_Band_1977.jpg. This work is in the public domain in the United States because it was published in the United States between 1925 and 1977, inclusive, without a copyright notice.

"Old men ought to be explorers
Here and there does not matter
We must be still and still moving
Into another intensity
For a further union, a deeper communion
Through the dark cold and the empty desolation,
The wave cry, the wind cry, the vast waters
Of the petrel and the porpoise. In my end is my beginning."

From Four Quartets. East Coker. By TS Eliot

Nobel Laureate in Literature, 1948.

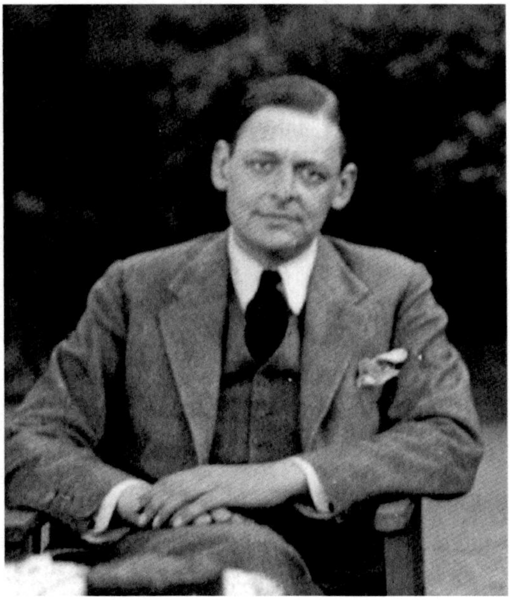

A photograph of TS Eliot taken in 1934. By Thomas Stearns Eliot with his sister and his cousin by Lady Ottoline Morrell.jpg: Lady Ottoline Morrell (1873–1938) derivative work: Octave.H - Thomas Stearns Eliot with his sister and his cousin by Lady Ottoline Morrell.jpg, Public Domain, https://commons.wikimedia.org/w/index.php?curid=7748785. https://en.wikipedia.org/wiki/T._S._Eliot#/media/File:Thomas_Stearns_Eliot_by_Lady_Ottoline_Morrell_(1934).jpg. This work is in the public domain in its country of origin and other countries and areas where the copyright term is the author's life plus 70 years or fewer.

"Ever tried. Ever failed. No matter. Try Again. Fail again. Fail better."
From Worstward Ho by Samuel Beckett. Published by John Calder in 1983

Nobel Laureate in Literature, 1969.

The photograph of Samuel Beckett in 1977, reproduced below from Wikimedia Commons, is in the public domain because its author, Roger Pic has placed it there.

By Roger Pic - Bibliothèque nationale de France, Public Domain, https://commons.wikimedia.org/w/index.php?curid=56362286. https://en.wikipedia.org/wiki/Samuel_Beckett#/media/File:Samuel_Beckett,_Pic,_1_(cropped).jpg

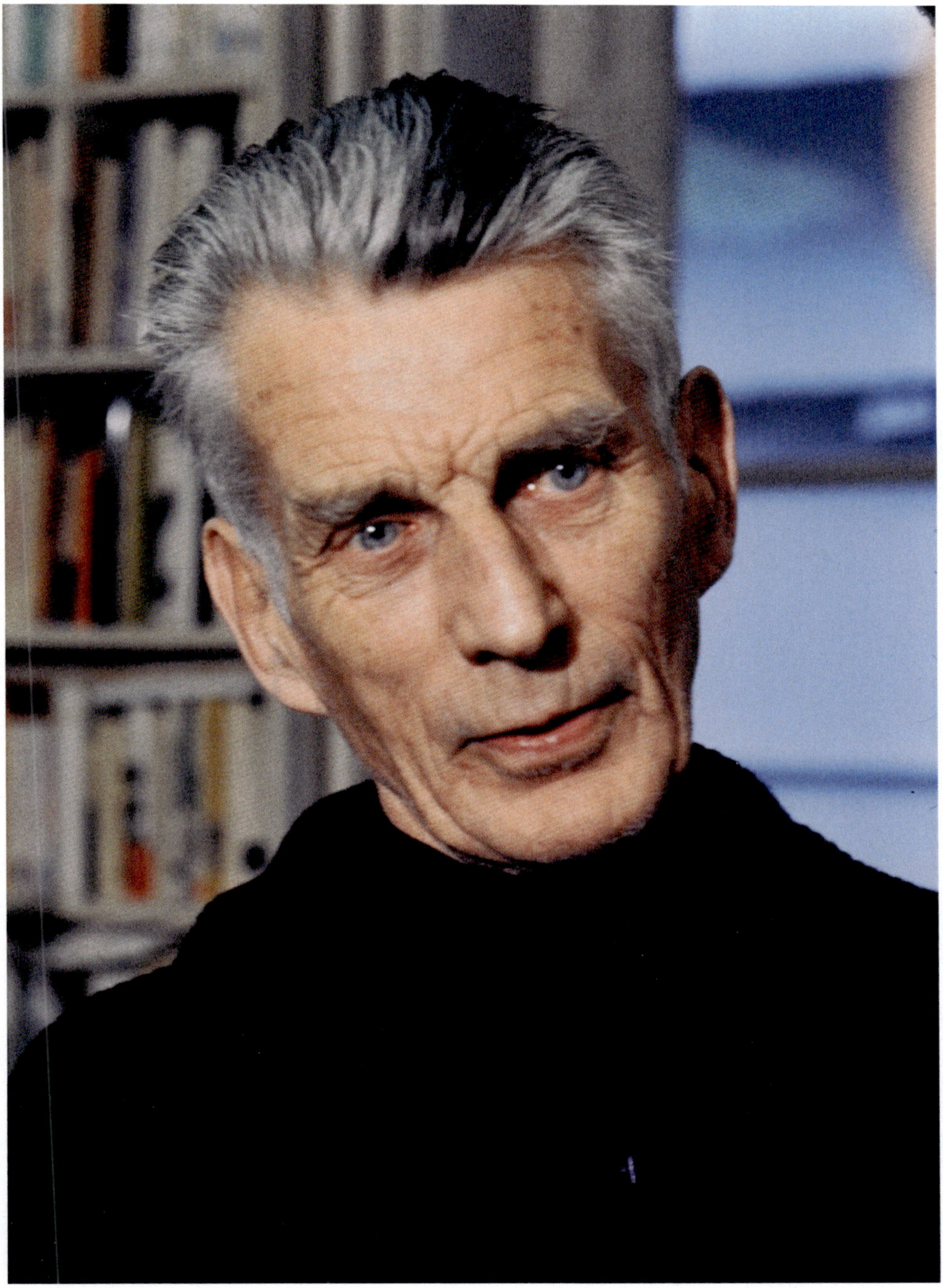

Table of Contents

1. Author's preface

Five major biological revolutions of the second half of the 20th century were

1. The production of monoclonal antibodies
2. The discovery of DNA and how it, RNA and amino acids make proteins
3. Epigenetics and the posttranslational modification of proteins
4. The discovery of cell signalling pathways
5. The cloning of the human genome

Taken together these discoveries in cellular and molecular biology have revealed to scientists appropriate targets for new drugs and the number that have been produced in the last 30 years, and that are still being produced, has hugely enlarged the therapeutic pharmacopeia, producing treatments – even cures- for diseases that were previously untreatable. The majority of these new treatments have been derived because of much more detailed knowledge about how human cells work. They are therefore known as biological treatments, often abbreviated to biologics

This series of books – one for each disease or disease category - explains what the new treatments are, how they work and how they compare, and interact with, conventional treatment. It is important to state that **no book** in this series makes specific treatment recommendations for any of the diseases covered: such decisions should be initiated and reviewed by an appropriate medical specialist. Much information on each disease is available free of charge from Wikipedia (*wikipedia.org),* from postgraduate textbooks on each disease and from *UpToDate.com:* the latter website gives information for patients and caregivers free of charge but a subscription is required for more detailed information (uptodate.com). **Rather**, the purpose of this series of books is to give information on newly developed biological treatments and their mechanism of action, enabling hopefully all involved in any way with the management of the diseases which utilize these new treatments to get a handle on these extensive additions to the medical pharmacopeia.

This book includes new biological targeted medical treatments for breast cancer approved for therapeutic use by the USA Food and Drug Administration (FDA) that have been derived from these discoveries. A distinction is often made between monoclonal antibodies (the mabs) as "immunotherapy" and the small specifically designed inhibitory molecules (the nibs). However, since both categories of drug are derived from knowledge of human cell biology, and as both categories are exquisitely targeted to a specific epitope on a cell surface protein (the mabs) or the inhibition of a specific intracellular enzyme process (the nibs), I prefer to combine the mabs, the nibs and the cepts in the single category of targeted biological treatments.

This new drug discovery phenomenon over the last 70 years is a therapeutic tsunami which shows no sign of slowing. The pharmcopiea has increased enormously and all medical students should consider doing a Master's degree or a PhD in molecular biology in order to fuly understand the mechanismsby which these drugs work. It is only by working in a cellular or molecular biology laboratory (usually combined) that one can really understand how each of these new medications work.

It should be noted that all text on each individual drug is taken directly from the USA FDA's product approval label for that drug, including the drug's generic name, its brand name, the indications for which it is approved, its mechanism of action, boxed warnings and other details on warnings, precautions and adverse events. These are all in the public domain and are easily accessed on the internet (https://www.accessdata.fda.gov/scripts/cder/daf/).

I wrote Sections 1-8, and section 10-12 myself. Section 9 is taken directly from the FDA approval label for each drug, although I hae added text and figures to illustrate certain points. **ALL** the text that I added to Section 9 is in ***ITALICS*** in order to clerly distuish it from that written in the FDA approval label. All images and illustrations were taken from a variety of sources on the internet. Most of these are in the public domain, but some are licensed by a Creative Commons license. Each image carries the legend written by the creator of the image as well as full attribution details.

I would like to acknowledge the help that I received from Jim Severino in designing the cover for this book and in helping upload to Kindle Direct Publishing. I would also like to acknowledge the gift that Jimmy Wales and Larry Sanger gave to the World when they founded Wikipedia, enabling anyone with internet access to obtain information on just about anything.

2. Introduction to targeted biologic therapeutic agents

These new treatments are targeted treatments: they have been developed to target a specific cell surface molecule or a specific cellular molecular process.

They are sometimes referred to as the "mabs, the nibs, the cepts and now (with the approval of olaparib)" the "ribs". These are abbreviations for **m**onoclonal **a**ntibodies, small i**n**h**ib**itor molecules, inhibitors of poly (ADP-**rib**ose) polymerase enzymes and cell surface re**cept**or blocking agents respectively. Examples are rituximab, imatinib, olaparib and etanercept.

A commonly used blanket term for these new drugs are biological agents or biologics, since their discovery was based on the biology of the diseases that they were designed to treat. A distinction is often made between monoclonal antibodies (the mabs) as "immunotherapy" and the small specifically designed inhibitory molecules (the nibs). However, since both categories of drug are derived from knowledge of human cell biology, and as both categories are exquisitely targeted to a specific epitope on a cell surface protein (the mabs) or inhibition of a specific intracellular enzyme process (the nibs), I prefer to combine the mabs, the nibs, the ribs and the cepts in the single category of targeted biological treatments.

It should be noted (as in the text below) that many, if not all, of these new treatments have many, and often serious or fatal side-effects, including adverse interactions when combined with other drugs.

A **biosimilar** is a biologic medical product highly similar to another already approved biological medicine. Biosimilars are approved according to the same standards of pharmaceutical quality, safety and efficacy that apply to all biological medicines.

Biosimilars are officially approved versions of original "innovator" products and can be manufactured when the original product's patent expires. Reference to the innovator product is an integral component of the approval.

Finally, most of these new treatments are extremely expensive ("financial toxicity"), which renders both access to them, and sometimes compliance with them, impossible or suboptimal.

Monoclonal antibodies (mabs)

Background

In 1975, Georges Köhler and César Milstein in the UK succeeded in producing a hybridoma by making fusions of murine myeloma cell lines with murine B cells. This immortalized hybridoma could produce antibodies specific for known antigens. In 1985 the FDA approved the first fully licensed Mab - muromonab- CD3, for use in preventing kidney transplant rejection. Muromonab-CD3 was produced using only murine cells and thus the antibodies produced were wholly murine. Subsequently, to decrease immunogenicity of murine antibodies, chimeric antibodies were created in which the constant (Fc) portion of the antibody was human, while the variable (Fab-binding) regions remained of murine origin. After this, humanized mabs were produced in which the framework and constant regions were human, while the hypervariable region remained of murine origin. After this, fully human mabs were produced, lacking any murine component. Finally, it is now possible to produce mabs solely using recombinant DNA technology.

Mabs may be used in many different ways (Figure 1). This is illustrated in Figure 1 for mabs that are developed for the treatment of disease. This image, reproduced from Wikimedia Commons, is in the public domain because its author has placed it there: By Ch1902 vector, Ramujana original raster - Image: MonoclonalAb.jpg, Public Domain, https://commons.wikimedia.org/w/index.php?curid=5119369; https://en.wikipedia.org/wiki/Monoclonal_antibody_therapy#/media/File:Monoclonal_antibodies.svg

Figure 1. The ways in which monoclonal antibodies can be used therapeutically.

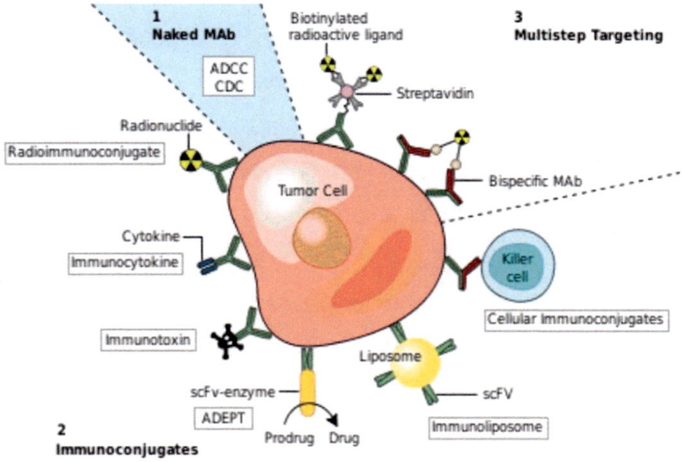

Abbreviations used in Figure 1: antibody directed enzyme prodrug therapy; ADCC: antibody-dependent cell-mediated cytotoxicity; CDC: complement-dependent cytotoxicity; MAb, monoclonal antibody; scFv, single-chain Fv fragment

Nomenclature convention for monoclonal antibodies

Murine mabs have the prefix –o- before mab; eg, abagovomab. (Note: the first murine mab approved by the FDA deviated from this nomenclature which was not in place at the time of its approval)

Chimeric mabs have the prefix –xi- before mab; eg, basilixumab

Humanized mabs have the prefix –zu- before mab; eg, trastuzumab

Human mabs have the prefix –u- before mab; eg, atinumab

Examples of these new agents and their mechanism of action in the treatment of NON- DISEASES

Monoclonal antibodies

- Receptor antagonists – eg, dapulimab (anti IL-4 and anti-IL13 signalling) in atopic dermatitis
- Apoptosis (programmed cell death) inducers – eg, rituximab in B cell-mediated autoimmune diseases

- Immune pathway inhibitors – eg, dipilumab for IL-4 and IL-13 signalling in atopic dermatitis; etanercept, infliximab and adalimumab for TNF inhibition in psoriasis; secukinumab for IL-17 inhibition in psoriasis; ustekinumab for IL-12/Th1 inhibition and IL-23/ILTh17 inhibition in psoriasis; ixekizumab as an anti-IL17A agent in psoriasis; brodalumab as an anti-IL-7 receptor antagonist in psoriasis
- TNF pathway antagonists – eg, adalimumab for psoriasis
- Integrin pathway blockers – eg, natalizumab for Crohn's disease
- Rank ligand inhibitor – eg, denosumab for targeted treatment of postmenopausal women with osteoporosis at high risk for fracture
- Angiogenesis inhibitors – eg, ranibizumab for macular degeneration
- Dabigatran binder – eg, idarucizumab for bleeding due to dabigatran administration
- Proprotein convertase subtilisin kexin type 9 (PCSK9) inhibitor – eg, alirocumab and evolocumab for dyslipidemias
- Bi-specific antibodies – eg, emicizumab-kxwh for hemophilia A
- Monoclonal antibody-delivered toxins or drugs

A list of all monoclonal antibodies and receptor blocking agents that are USA FDA-approved for therapeutic use for either non-malignant disease, malignant disease or both is shown in Table 1 (as of December 2020).

Table 1

Generic name/brand name/type of mab	Target	FDA-approved indication/s
Abciximab/ ReoPro/ chimeric fab fragment	GPIIb/IIIa	Percutaneous coronary intervention for the prevention of cardiac ischemic complications in patients undergoing percutaneous coronary intervention or in patients with unstable angina not responding to conventional medical therapy when percutaneous coronary intervention is planned within 24 hours
Adalimumab/ Humira/ fully human	TNF	Rheumatoid arthritis (RA), juvenile idiopathic arthritis (JIA), ankylosing spondylitis (AS), psoriatric arthrtitis, Crohn's disease[1], ulcerative colitis, plaque psoriasis, hidradenitis suppura[a], non-infectious uveitis
Adalimumab-abdm/Cyltezo/ fully human, biosimilar	TNF	RA, JIA, AS, psoriatric arthritis, Crohn's disease[1], ulcerative colitis, plaque psoriasis,
Adalimumab-	TNF	RA, JIA, AS, psoriatric arthritis, Crohn's disease[1], ulcerative

atto/Amjevita/ fully human, biosimilar		colitis, plaque psoriasis
Ado-trastuzumab Emtasine/ Kadcyla/ humanized antibody-microtubule inhibitor conjugate	HER2	HER2-positive, metastatic breast cancer who previously received trastuzumab and a taxane, separately or in combination. Patients should have either: • received prior therapy for metastatic disease, or • developed disease recurrence during or within six months of completing adjuvant therapy. • the adjuvant treatment of patients with HER2-positive early breast cancer who have residual invasive disease after neoadjuvant taxane and trastuzumab-based treatment.
Alemtuzumab/ Campath, Lemtrada/ humanized	CD52	Relapsing forms of multiple sclerosis (MS) (previously approved for chronic lymphocytic leukemia but now withdrawn by its manufacturer for this indication in order to optimize its launch for treatment of MS)
Alirocumab/ Praluent/fully human	PCSK9 (proprotein convertase subtilisin kexin type 9) inhibitor	Adjunct to diet and maximally tolerated statin therapy for the treatment of adults with heterozygous familial hypercholesterolemia or clinical atherosclerotic cardiovascular disease, who require additional lowering of LDL-cholesterol (LDL-C).
Atezolizumab/ Tecentriq/ humanized	Programmed death ligand 1 (PD-L1)	1. Urothelial carcinoma for the treatment of adult patients with locally advanced or metastatic urothelial carcinoma who are not eligible for cisplatin-containing chemotherapy and whose tumors express PD-L1 or who are not eligible for any platinum-containing chemotherapy regardless of PD-L1 status, or who have disease progression during or following any platinum-containing chemotherapy, or within 12 months of neoadjuvant or adjuvant chemotherapy. This indication is approved under accelerated approval based on tumor response rate and duration of response. Continued approval for this indication may be contingent upon verification and description of clinical benefit in a confirmatory trial(s). 2. Non-small cell lung ancer (NSCLC) in combination with bevacizumab, paclitaxel, and carboplatin for the firstline treatment, of adult patients with metastatic non-squamous NSCLC with no EGFR or ALK genomic tumor aberrations or for the treatment of adult patients with metastatic NSCLC who have disease progression during or following platinum-containing chemotherapy. Patients with EGFR or ALK genomic tumor aberrations should have disease progression on FDA-approved therapy for NSCLC harboring these aberrations prior to receiving TECENTRIQ. 2. Triple-negative breast cancer (TNBC) in combination with paclitaxel for the treatment of adult patients with unresectable locally advanced or metastatic TNBC whose tumors express PD-L1. This indication is approved under accelerated approval based on progression-free survival. Continued approval for this indication may be contingent upon verification and description of clinical benefit in a confirmatory trial(s).
ATOLTIVIMAB +2/INMAZEB	Zaire ebolavirus glycoprotein	Zaire ebolavirus infection
Avelumab/ Bavencio/ fully human	PD-L1	1. Adult and pediatric patients 12 years and older with metastatic Merkel cell carcinoma[2a] 2. Patients with locally advanced or metastatic urothelial carcinoma who have disease progression during or following platinum-containing chemotherapy or who have disease

		progression within 12 months of neoadjuvant or adjuvant treatment with platinum-containing chemotherapy[a]. 3. First-line treatment, in combination with axitinib, of patients with advanced renal cell carcinoma [a]Continued approval for this indication may be contingent upon verification and description of clinical benefit in confirmatory trials
Basiliximab/ Simulect/ chimeric	IL-2 receptor alpha chain (IL-2Rα) blocker	Prophylaxis of acute organ rejection in patients receiving renal transplantation when used as part of an immunosuppressive regimen that includes cyclosporine and corticosteroids
Belantamab mafodotin-blmf/ BLENREP	Anti-BCMA	Microtubule inhibitor; ADC
Belimumab/ Benlysta/fully human	B lymphocyte stimulator (BLyS) - specific inhibitor	Active, autoantibody-positive, systemic lupus erythematosus (SLE) in adults who are receiving standard therapy
Benralizumab/ Fasenra/ humanized	Interleukin-5 receptor-α	For the add-on maintenance treatment of patients with severe asthma aged 12 years and older, and with an eosinophilic phenotype
Bevacizumab/ Avastin/ humanized	Vascular endothelial growth factor (VEGF)-specific angiogenesis	1. Metastatic colorectal cancer, with intravenous 5-fluorouracil–based chemotherapy for first- or second-line treatment. 2. Non-squamous non-small cell lung cancer, with carboplatin and paclitaxel for first line treatment of unresectable, locally advanced, recurrent or metastatic disease. 3. Metastatic breast cancer, with paclitaxel for treatment of patients who have not received chemotherapy for metastatic HER2-negative breast cancer. 4.Glioblastoma, as a single agent for adult patients with progressive disease following prior therapy 5. Metastatic renal cell carcinoma with interferon-α
Bevacizumab-awwb/Mvasi/ humanized biosimilar	VEGF	1. Metastatic colorectal cancer, in combination with intravenous fluorouracil-based chemotherapy for first- or second-line treatment. 2. Metastatic colorectal cancer, in combination with fluoropyrimidine-irinotecan- or fluoropyrimidine-oxaliplatin-based chemotherapy for second-line treatment in patients who have progressed on a first-line bevacizumab product-containing regimen. 3. Unresectable, locally advanced, recurrent or metastatic non-squamous non-small cell lung cancer, in combination with carboplatin and paclitaxel for first-line treatment. 4. Recurrent glioblastoma in adults. 5. Metastatic renal cell carcinoma in combination with interferon-α. 6. Persistent, recurrent, or metastatic cervical cancer, in combination with paclitaxel and cisplatin, or paclitaxel and topotecan.
Bevlotuxumab/ Zinplava/fully human	Clostridium difficile toxin	Reduction of recurrence of Clostridium difficile infection (CDI) in patients 18 years of age or older who are receiving antibacterial drug treatment of CDI and are at a high risk for CDI recurrence.
Blinatumomab/ Blincyto/ murine bispecific CD19-directed	CD19	1. B cell precursor acute lymphoblastic leukemia (ALL) in first or second complete remission with minimal residual disease (MRD) greater than or equal to 0.1%. This indication is approved under accelerated approval based on MRD response rate and hematological relapse-free survival. Continued

CD3 T cell engager		approval for this indication may be contingent upon verification and description of clinical benefit in the confirmatory trials. 2. Relapsed or refractory B cell precursor acute lymphoblastic leukemia
Brentuximab vedotin/ Adcetris/ chimeric, antibody-drug conjugate	CD30	1.Classical Hodgkin lymphoma[3] (cHL) at high risk of relapse or progression as post autologous hematopoietic stem cell transplantation (auto-HSCT) consolidation 2.Classical Hodgkin lymphoma after failure of auto-HSCT or after failure of at least two prior multi-agent chemotherapy regimens in patients who are not auto-HSCT candidates 3. Systemic anaplastic large cell lymphoma (sALCL) after failure of at least one prior multi-agent chemotherapy regimen. Accelerated approval was granted for the sALCL indication based on overall response rate. Continued approval for this indication may be contingent upon verification and description of clinical benefit in confirmatory trials. 4. Primary cutaneous anaplastic large cell lymphoma (pcALCL) or CD30 expressing mycosis fungoides who have received prior systemic therapy
Brodalumab/ Siliq/chimeric	!L-17 receptor	Moderate to severe plaque psoriasis in adult patients who are candidates for systemic therapy or phototherapy and have failed to respond or have lost response to other systemic therapies.
Burosumab-twza/Crysvita/ fully human	Fibroblast growth factor (FGF)23	X-linked hypophosphatemia (XLH) in adult and pediatric patients 6 months of age and older
Canakinuab/ Ilaris/fully human	IL-1β	Cryopyrin-associated periodic syndromes (CAPS), in adults and children 4 years of age and older including familial cold autoinflammatory syndrome (FCAS) and Muckle-Wells Syndrome (MWS)
Capromab pendetide/ Prosta-Scint/ murine radio-labelled (Indium [111])	Prostate-specific membrane antigen (PSMA)	1. A diagnostic imaging agent in newly-diagnosed patients with biopsy-proven prostate cancer, thought to be clinically-localized after standard diagnostic evaluation (e.g. chest x-ray, bone scan, CT scan, or MRI), who are at high-risk for pelvic lymph node metastases 2. A diagnostic imaging agent in post-prostatectomy patients with a rising PSA leveland a negative or equivocal standard metastatic evaluation in whom there is a high clinical suspicion of occult metastatic disease.
Certolizumab Pegol/Cimzia/ humanized (pegylated for longer duration of action)	TNF	1.Crohn's disease 2.Rheumatoid arthritis 3.Psoriatic arthritis 4.Ankylosing spondylitis
Cetuximab/ Erbitux/ chimeric	Epidermal growth factor (EGF) receptor	1.Head and neck cancer Locally or regionally advanced squamous cell carcinoma of the head and neck in combination with radiation therapy. Recurrent loco-regional disease or metastatic squamous cell carcinoma of the head and neck in combination with platinum-based therapy with 5-FU. Recurrent or metastatic squamous cell carcinoma of the head and neck progressing after platinum-based therapy. 2.Colorectal cancer As a single agent, EGFR-expressing metastatic colorectal cancer after failure of both irinotecan- and oxaliplatin-based regimens or in patients who are intolerant to irinotecan-based regimens. In combination with irinotecan, EGFR-expressing metastatic

		colorectal carcinoma in patients who are refractory to irinotecan-based chemotherapy.
Cemiplimab/ Libtayo/ humanized	PD-1	Metastatic cutaneous squamous cell carcinoma (CSCC) or locally advanced CSCC who are not candidates for curative surgery or curative radiation.
Daclizumab/ Zenapax/ humanized	IL-2 receptor-α	Prophylaxis of acute organ rejection in patients receiving renal transplants. It is used as part of an immunosuppressive regimen that includes cyclosporine and corticosteroids.
Darzalex/ Zinbryta/ humanized	IL-2 receptor	Relapsing forms of multiple sclerosis (MS). Because of its safety profile, the use of ZINBRYTA should generally be reserved for patients who have had an inadequate response to two or more drugs indicated for the treatment of MS.
Daratumumab and hyaluronidase-fihj	Anti-CD38; ADCC; CDC	Multiple myeloma
Daratumumab/ Darzalex/fully human	CD38	Multiple myeloma 1.In combination with lenalidomide and dexamethasone in newly diagnosed patients who are ineligible for autologous stem cell transplant and in patients with relapsed or refractory multiple myeloma who have received at least one prior therapy 2.In combination with bortezomib, melphalan and prednisone in newly diagnosed patients who are ineligible for autologous stem cell transplant 3.In combination with bortezomib and dexamethasone in patients who have received at least one prior therapy 4.In combination with pomalidomide and dexamethasone in patients who have received at least two prior therapies including lenalidomide and a proteasome inhibitor 5. As monotherapy, in patients who have received at least three prior lines of therapy including a proteasome inhibitor (PI) and an immunomodulatory agent or who are double-refractory to a PI and an immunomodulatory agent.
Denosumab/ Prolia/fully human	Receptor activator of nuclear factor kappa-B ligand (RANKL)	1.Postmenopausal women with osteoporosis at high risk for fracture 2.Treatment to increase bone mass in men at high risk for fracture receiving androgen deprivation therapy for non-metastatic prostate cancer 3.Treatment to increase bone mass in women at high risk for fracture receiving adjuvant aromatase inhibitor therapy for breast cancer
Denosumab/ Xgeva/fully human	RANKL	1.Prevention of skeletal-related events in patients with multiple myeloma and in patients with bone metastases from solid tumors 2.Treatment of adults and skeletally mature adolescents with giant cell tumor of bone that is unresectable or where surgical resection is likely to result in severe morbidity 3.Treatment of hypercalcemia of malignancy refractory to bisphosphonate therapy
Dinutuximab/ Unituxin/ chimeric	GD2 (a disialo-ganglioside)	In combination with granulocyte-macrophage colony-stimulating factor (GM-CSF), interleukin-2 (IL-2), and 13-cis-retinoic acid (RA), for the treatment of pediatric patients with high-risk neuroblastoma who achieve at least a partial response to prior first-line multiagent, multimodality therapy
Dupilumab/ Dupixent/fully human	IL-4 receptor-α (IL-4RA)	1. For patients aged 12 years and older with moderate-to-severe atopic dermatitis whose disease is not adequately controlled with topical prescription therapies or when those therapies are not advisable. 2. As an add-on maintenance treatment in patients with moderate-to-severe asthma aged 12 years and older with an eosinophilic phenotype or with oral corticosteroid-dependent

		asthma. 3. As an add-on maintenance treatment in adult patients with inadequately controlled chronic rhinosinusitis with nasal polyposis (CRSwNP).
Durvalumab/ Imfinzi/fully human	PD-L1	1.Locally advanced or metastatic urothelial carcinoma who have disease progression during or following platinum-containing chemotherapy or who have disease or progression within 12 months of neoadjuvant or adjuvant treatment with platinum-containing chemotherapy 2. Unresectable, stage III non-small cell lung cancer (NSCLC) whose disease has not progressed following concurrent platinum-based chemotherapy and radiation therapy.
Eculizumab/ Solaris/ humanized	Complement component 5	1.Paroxysmal nocturnal hemoglobinuria (PNH) to reduce hemolysis 2.Atypical hemolytic uremic syndrome (aHUS) to inhibit complement-mediated thrombotic microangiopathy
Elotuzumab/ Empliciti/ humanized	Signalling lymphocytic activation molecule family (SLAMF7, CD319)	In combination with lenalidomide and dexamethasone for the treatment of multiple myeloma who have received one to three prior therapies.
Emicizumab-kxwh/ Hemlibra/ humanized bispecific	Factor IXa, Factor X (bridges activated factor IX and factor X to restore the function of missing activated factor VIII that is needed for effective hemostasis)	Routine prophylaxis to prevent or reduce the frequency of bleeding episodes in adult and pediatric patients ages newborn and older with hemophilia A (congenital factor VIII deficiency) with or without factor VIII inhibitors.
Eptinezumab-jjmr/VYEPTI	Migraine	CGRP block
Erenumab-aooe/Aimovig/ fully human	Calcitonin gene-related peptide receptor (CGRP receptor)	Antagonist indicated for the preventive treatment of migraine in adults
Evolocumab/ Repatha/fully human	Proprotein convertase subtilisin kexin type 9 (PCSK9)	1. To reduce the risk of myocardial infarction, stroke, and coronary revascularization in adults with established cardiovascular disease. 2. As an adjunct to diet, alone or in combination with other lipid-lowering therapies (e.g., statins, ezetimibe), for treatment of adults with primary hyperlipidemia (including heterozygous familial hypercholesterolemia) to reduce low-density lipoprotein cholesterol (LDL-C). 3. As an adjunct to diet and other LDL-lowering therapies (e.g., statins, ezetimibe, LDL apheresis) in patients with homozygous familial hypercholesterolemia (HoFH) who require additional lowering of LDL-C.
Gemtuzumab ozogamicin/	CD33	1.Newly-diagnosed CD33-positive acute myeloid leukemia (AML) in adults

Mylotarg/ humanized antibody-drug conjugate (N-acetyl gamma calichea-micin)		2.Relapsed or refractory CD33-positive AML in adults and in pediatric patients 2 years and older
Golimumab/ Simponi/fully human	TNF	1.Moderately to severely active RA in adults, in combination with methotrexate 2.Active psoriatic arthritis in adults, alone or in combination with methotrexate 3.Active AS in adults
Golimumab/ Simponi Aria/ fully human	TNF	1.Moderately to severely RA in combination with methotrexate 2.Active psoriatic arthritis 3.Active AS
Guselkumab/ Tremfya/fully human	IL-23	Adult patients with moderate-to-severe plaque psoriasis who are candidates for systemic therapy or phototherapy
Ibalizumab-uiyk/Trogarzo/ humanized	CD4	In combination with other antiretroviral(s), for the treatment of human immunodeficiency virus type 1 (HIV-1) infection in heavily treatment-experienced adults with multidrug resistant HIV-1 infection failing their current antiretroviral regimen
Ibritumomab tiuxetan/ Zevalin/ murine radio-immunoconjug-ate (the chelate tiuxetan, which tightly binds to $Indium^{111}$ or $Ytrium^{90}$, is covalently linked to ibritumomab. The beta emission from Y^{90} induces cellular damage by the formation of free radicals in the target and neighboring cells)	CD20	1.Relapsed or refractory, low-grade or follicular B cell non-Hodgkin's lymphoma (NHL) 2. Previously untreated follicular NHL who achieve a partial or complete response to first-line chemotherapy
Idarucizumab/ Praxbind/ humanized fab fragment	Dabigatran (Pradaxa)	Patients treated with Pradaxa® when reversal of the anticoagulant effects of dabigatran is needed: 1. For emergency surgery/urgent procedures 2. In life-threatening or uncontrolled bleeding. This indication is approved under accelerated approval based on a reduction in unbound dabigatran and normalization of coagulation parameters in healthy volunteers. Continued approval for this indication may be contingent upon the results of an ongoing cohort case series study.
Inebilixumab-cdon/UPLIZNA	Anti-CD19	Neuromyelitis optica spectrum disorder (anti-aquaporin-4 antibody poditive

Infliximab/ Remicade/ chimeric	TNF-α	1. Crohn's disease for reducing signs and symptoms and inducing and maintaining clinical remission in adult patients with moderately to severely active disease who have had an inadequate response to conventional therapy. For reducing the number of draining enterocutaneous and rectovaginal fistulas and maintaining fistula closure in adult patients with fistulizing disease. 2. Pediatric Crohn's disease for reducing signs and symptoms and inducing and maintaining clinical remission in pediatric patients with moderately to severely active disease who have had an inadequate response to conventional therapy. 3.Ulcerative colitis for reducing signs and symptoms, inducing and maintaining clinical remission and mucosal healing, and eliminating corticosteroid use in adult patients with moderately to severely active disease who have had an inadequate response to conventional therapy. 4. Pediatric ulcerative colitis for reducing signs and symptoms and inducing and maintaining clinical remission in pediatric patients with moderately to severely active disease who have had an inadequate response to conventional therapy. 5. Rheumatoid arthritis in combination with methotrexate for reducing signs and symptoms, inhibiting the progression of structural damage, and improving physical function in patients with moderately to severely active disease. 6. Ankylosing spondylitis for reducing signs and symptoms in patients with active disease. 7. Psoriatic arthritis for reducing signs and symptoms of active arthritis, inhibiting the progression of structural damage, and improving physical function. 8. Plaque psoriasis for treatment of adult patients with chronic severe (i.e., extensive and /or disabling) plaque psoriasis who are candidates for systemic therapy and when other systemic therapies are medically less appropriate.
Infliximab-abda/Renflexis /chimeric biosimilar	TNF-α	Similar to Remicade: see https://www.accessdata.fda.gov/drugsatfda_docs/label/2017/761054orig1s000lbl.pdf
Infliximab-dyyb/Inflectra/ chimeric biosimilar	TNF-α	Similar to Remicade. See https://www.accessdata.fda.gov/drugsatfda_docs/label/2016/125544s000lbl.pdf
Infliximab-qbtx/Ixifi chimeric biosimilar	TNF-α	Similar to Remicade. See https://www.accessdata.fda.gov/drugsatfda_docs/label/2017/761072s000lbl.pdf
Inotuzumab ozogamicin/ Besponsa/ humanized; antibody-drug conjugate (N-acetyl gamma calicheamicin)	CD22	Adults with relapsed or refractory B cell precursor acute lymphoblastic leukemia (ALL)
Ipilimomab/ Yervoy/fully human	CTLA-4	1. Unresectable or metastatic breast cancer in adults and pediatric patients (12 years and older). 2. Adjuvant treatment of patients with cutaneous breast cancer with pathologic involvement of regional lymph nodes of more than 1 mm who have undergone complete resection, including total lymphadenectomy.

		3. Intermediate or poor risk, previously untreated advanced renal cell carcinoma, in combination with nivolumab. 4. Adult and pediatric patients 12 years of age and older with microsatellite instability-high (MSI-H) or mismatch repair deficient (dMMR) metastatic colorectal cancer that has progressed following treatment with a fluoropyrimidine, oxaliplatin, and irinotecan, in combination with nivolumab. This indication is approved under accelerated approval based on overall response rate and duration of response. Continued approval for this indication may be contingent upon verification and description of clinical benefit in confirmatory trials.
Isatuximab-irfc/SARCLISA	Multiple myeloma	Anti-CD38; ADCC; CDC
Ixekizumab/ Taltz/ humanized	IL-17A antagonist (often referred to as IL-17)	Adults with 1. Moderate-to-severe plaque psoriasis who are candidates for systemic therapy or phototherapy. 2. Active psoriatic arthritis. 3. Active ankylosing spondylitis
MARGETUX-MAB CMBK/ MARGENZA	Anti-HER2, ADCC	Breast cancer
Mepolizumab/ Nucala/ humanized	IL-5	Add-on maintenance treatment of patients with severe asthma aged 12 years and older, and with an eosinophilic phenotype
Mogamuliz-umab/ Poteligeo/ humanized	CCR4 (CC chemo-kines have 2 adjacent cysteine near their amino terminus)	Adult patients with relapsed or refractory mycosis fungoides or Sézary syndrome after at least one prior systemic therapy
Moxetumomab pasudotox Lumoxiti/ murine antibody-drug conjugate. (the toxin called PE38, is a 38kDa fragment of Pseudomonas exotoxin A.	CD22	Adult patients with relapsed or refractory hairy cell leukemia (HCL) who received at least two prior systemic therapies, including treatment with a purine nucleoside analog (PNA)
Natalizumab/ Tysabri/ humanized	α4 integrin	1. Multiple sclerosis (MS): as monotherapy for the treatment of patients with relapsing forms of multiple sclerosis to delay the accumulation of physical disability and reduce the frequency of clinical exacerbations. TYSABRI is generally recommended for patients who have had an inadequate response to, or are unable to tolerate, an alternate MS therapy. 2.Crohn's disease: inducing and maintaining clinical response and remission in adult patients with moderately to severely active Crohn's disease with evidence of inflammation who have had an inadequate response to, or are unable to tolerate, conventional Crohn's disease therapies and inhibitors of TNF-α.
Naxitamab-GQGK/ DANYEZA	Anti-glycolipid GD2, CDC, ADCC	Neuroblatoma
Necitumumab/ Portrazza/ fully	EGFR	In combination with gemcitabine and cisplatin, for first-line treatment of patients with metastatic squamous non-small cell

human		lung cancer
Nivolumab/ Opdivo/ fully human	PD-1	1. BRAF V600 wild-type unresectable or metastatic breast cancer, as a single agent. 2. BRAF V600 mutation-positive unresectable or metastatic breast cancer, as a single agent. 3. Unresectable or metastatic breast cancer, in combination with ipilimumabab. 4. Breast cancer with lymph node involvement or metastatic disease who have undergone complete resection, in the adjuvant setting. 5. Metastatic non-small cell lung cancer and progression on or after platinum-based chemotherapy. (EGFR or ALK genomic tumor aberrations should have disease progression on FDA-approved therapy for these aberrations prior to receiving OPDIVO). 6. Advanced renal cell carcinoma who have received prior anti-angiogenic therapy. 7. Intermediate or poor risk, previously untreated advanced renal cell carcinoma, in combination with ipilimumab. 8. Adult patients with classical Hodgkin lymphoma that has relapsed or progressed after[b] autologous hematopoietic stem cell transplantation (HSCT) and brentuximab vedotin, or 3 or more lines of systemic therapy that includes autologous HSCT. 9. Recurrent or metastatic squamous cell carcinoma of the head and neck with disease progression on or after a platinum-based therapy. 10. Locally advanced or metastatic urothelial carcinoma who[b] have disease progression during or following platinum-containing chemotherapy or who have disease progression within 12 months of neoadjuvant or adjuvant treatment with platinum-containing chemotherapy. 11. Adult and pediatric (12 years and older) patients with microsatellite instability-high (MSI-H) or mismatch repair deficient (dMMR) metastatic colorectal cancer that has progressed following treatment with a fluoropyrimidine, oxaliplatin, and irinotecanb 12.Hepatocellular carcinoma previously treated with sorafenibb [a]This indication is approved under accelerated approval based on progression-free survival. Continued approval for this indication may be contingent upon verification and description of clinical benefit in the confirmatory trials. [b]This indication is approved under accelerated approval based on overall response rate and duration of response. Continued approval for this indication may be contingent upon verification and description of clinical benefit in confirmatory trials.
Obiltoxaximab/ Anthim/ chimeric	Protective antigen of the Anthrax toxin	Adult and pediatric patients for treatment of inhalational anthrax due to B. anthracis in combination with appropriate antibacterial drugs and, for prophylaxis of inhalational anthrax when alternative therapies are not available or are not appropriate.
Obinutuzumab /Gazyva/ humanized	CD20	1.In combination with chlorambucil, for the treatment of patients with previously untreated chronic lymphocytic leukemia 2. In combination with bendamustine followed by GAZYVA monotherapy, for the treatment of patients with follicular lymphoma who relapsed after, or are refractory to, a rituximab-containing regimen. 3. In combination with chemotherapy followed by GAZYVA monotherapy in patients achieving at least a partial remission, for the treatment of adult patients with previously untreated

		stage II bulky, III or IV follicular lymphoma.
Ocrelizumab/ Ocrevus/ humanized	CD20	Relapsing or primary progressive forms of multiple sclerosis
Ofatumumab/ Arzerra/fully human	CD20	Chronic lymphocytic leukemia (CLL) refractory to fludarabine and alemtuzumab.
Olaratumab/ Lartruvo/fully human	PDGFR-α	In combination with doxorubicin, for the treatment of adult patients with soft tissue sarcoma (STS) with a histologic subtype for which an anthracycline-containing regimen is appropriate and which is not amenable to curative treatment with radiotherapy or surgery. This indication is approved under accelerated approval. Continued approval for this indication may be contingent upon verification and description of clinical benefit in the confirmatory trial
Omalizumab/ Xolair/ humanized	IgE	1.Moderate to severe persistent asthma in patients 6 years of age and older with a positive skin test or in vitro reactivity to a perennial aeroallergen and symptoms that are inadequately controlled with inhaled corticosteroids 2.Chronic idiopathic urticaria in adults and adolescents 12 years of age and older who remain symptomatic despite H1 antihistamine treatment
Palivizumab/ Synagis/ humanized	F protein of respiratory syncytial virus (RSV)	Prevention of serious lower respiratory tract disease caused by RSV in children at high risk of RSV disease. Notes 1. Safety and efficacy were established in children with bronchopulmonary dysplasia (BPD), infants with a history of premature birth (less than or equal to 35 weeks gestational age), and children with hemodynamically significant congenital heart disease (CHD). 2.The safety and efficacy of Synagis have not been established for treatment of RSV disease
Panitumumab/ Vectibix/ fully human	EGFR	As a single agent for the treatment of metastatic colorectal carcinoma with disease progression on or following fluoropyrimidine, oxaliplatin, and irinotecan chemotherapy regimens. Approval is based on progression-free survival; no data demonstrate an improvement in disease-related symptoms or increased survival with Vectibix. Notes 1. Retrospective subset analyses of metastatic colorectal cancer trials have not shown a treatment benefit for Vectibix in patients whose tumors had KRAS mutations in codon 12 or 13. 2.Use of Vectibix is not recommended for the treatment of colorectal cancer with these mutations
Pembrolizumab/ Keytruda/ fully human	PD-1	1. Breast cancer For unresectable or metastatic breast cancer. For adjuvant treatment of patients with breast cancer with involvement of lymph node(s) following complete resection 2. Non-small cell lung cancer (NSCLC) • in combination with pemetrexed and platinum chemotherapy, as first-line treatment of patients with metastatic non-squamous NSCLC, with no EGFR or ALK genomic tumor aberrations. • in combination with carboplatin and either paclitaxel or nabpaclitaxel, as first-line treatment of patients with metastatic squamous NSCLC. • as a single agent for the first-line treatment of patients with metastatic NSCLC whose tumors have high PD-L1 expression with no EGFR or ALK genomic tumor aberrations.

		• as a single agent for the treatment of patients with metastatic NSCLC whose tumors express PD-L1 with disease progression on or after platinum-containing chemotherapy. 3. Head and neck squamous cell cancer (HNSCC) • for the treatment of patients with recurrent or metastatic HNSCC with disease progression on or after platinum-containing chemotherapy[1]. 4. Classical Hodgkin lymphoma (cHL) • for the treatment of adult and pediatric patients with refractory cHL, or who have relapsed after 3 or more prior lines of therapy[1]. 5. Primary mediastinal large B cell lymphoma (PMBCL) • for the treatment of adult and pediatric patients with refractory PMBCL, or who have relapsed after 2 or more prior lines of therapy[1]. 6. Urothelial carcinoma •for the treatment of patients with locally advanced or metastatic urothelial carcinoma who are not eligible for cisplatin-containing chemotherapy and whose tumors express PD-L1 or in patients who are not eligible for any platinum-containing chemotherapy regardless of PD-L1 status[1]. • for the treatment of patients with locally advanced or metastatic urothelial carcinoma who have disease progression during or following platinum-containing chemotherapy or within 12 months of neoadjuvant or adjuvant treatment with platinum-containing chemotherapy. 7. Microsatellite instability-high cancer • for the treatment of adult and pediatric patients with unresectable or metastatic, microsatellite instability-high (MSI-H) or mismatch repair deficient solid tumors that have progressed following prior treatment and who have no satisfactory alternative treatment options[1] or colorectal cancer that has progressed following treatment with a fluoropyrimidine, oxaliplatin, and irinotecan[1] 8. Gastric cancer • for the treatment of patients with recurrent locally advanced or metastatic gastric or gastro-esophageal junction adenocarcinoma whose tumors express PD-L1 with disease progression on or after two or more prior lines of therapy including fluoropyrimidine- and platinum-containing chemotherapy and if appropriate, HER2/neu-targeted therapy[1] 9. Cervical cancer • for the treatment of patients with recurrent or metastatic cervical cancer with disease progression on or after chemotherapy whose tumors express PD-L1 10. Hepatocellular carcinoma (HCC) • for the treatment of patients with HCC who have been previously treated with sorafenib[1] 11.Merkel cell carcinoma (MCC) • for the treatment of adult and pediatric patients with recurrent locally advanced or metastatic Merkel cell carcinoma[1] [1] this indication is approved under accelerated approval based on tumor response rate and durability of response. Continued approval for this indication may be contingent upon verification and description of clinical benefit in the confirmatory trials.
Pertuzumab/ Perjeta/ humanized	HER2/neu	In combination with trastuzumab and docetaxel for the treatment of patients with HER2-positive metastatic breast cancer who have not received prior anti-HER2 therapy or chemotherapy for metastatic disease.

Pertuzumab, trastuzumab and hyaluronidase -zzxf/PHESGO	HER2+ breast cancer	Anti-HER2; increases permeability
Polatuzumab vedotin/Polivy/ Humanized antibody-drug conjugate	CD79	In combination with bendamustine and a rituximab product for the treatment of adult patients with relapsed or refractory diffuse large B cell lymphoma, not otherwise specified, after at least two prior therapies
Ramucirumab/ Cyramza/ fully human	VEGFR2	1. As a single agent or in combination with paclitaxel, for treatment of advanced gastric or gastro-esophageal junction adenocarcinoma, with disease progression on or after prior fluoropyrimidine- or platinum-containing chemotherapy. 2. In combination with docetaxel, for treatment of metastatic non-small cell lung cancer with disease progression on or after platinum-based chemotherapy. Patients with EGFR or ALK genomic tumor aberrations should have disease progression on FDA-approved therapy for these aberrations prior to receiving CYRAMZA
Ranibizumab/ Lucentis/ humanized	VEGFR1, VEGFR2	1. Neovascular (wet) age-related macular degeneration (AMD) 2. Macular edema following retinal vein occlusion (RVO) 3. Diabetic macular edema (DME)
Raxibacumab/ fully human	Protective antigen of Bacillus anthracis[6]	Raxibacumab is indicated for the treatment of adult and pediatric patients with inhalational anthrax due to Bacillus anthracis in combination with appropriate antibacterial drugs, and for prophylaxis of inhalational anthrax when alternative therapies are not available or are not appropriate. Limitations of use: • The effectiveness of raxibacumab is based solely on efficacy studies in animal models of inhalational anthrax. • There have been no studies of raxibacumab in the pediatric population. Dosing in pediatric patients was derived using a population PK approach. • Raxibacumab does not cross the blood-brain barrier and does not prevent or treat meningitis. Raxibacumab should be used in combination with appropriate antibacterial drug
Reslizumab/ Cinqair/ humanized	IL-5	Add-on maintenance treatment of patients with severe asthma aged 18 years and older, and with an eosinophilic phenotype. Limitations of use: CINQAIR is not indicated for • treatment of other eosinophilic conditions • relief of acute bronchospasm or status asthmaticus
Rituximab/ Rituxan/ chimeric	CD20	1. Non-Hodgkin's lymphoma (NHL) o Relapsed or refractory, low grade or follicular, CD20-positive B cell NHL as a single agent. o Previously untreated follicular, CD20-positive, B cell NHL in combination with first line chemotherapy and, in patients achieving a complete or partial response to RITUXAN in combination with chemotherapy, as single-agent maintenance therapy. o Non-progressing (including stable disease), low-grade, CD20 positive, B cell NHL as a single agent after first-line cyclophosphamide, vincristine, and prednisone (CVP) chemotherapy. o Previously untreated diffuse large B cell, CD20-positive NHL in combination with (cyclophosphamide, doxorubicin, vincristine, and prednisone) (CHOP) or other anthracycline-based chemotherapy regimens. 2. Chronic lymphocytic leukemia (CLL) o Previously untreated and previously treated CD20 positive

		CLL in combination with fludarabine and cyclophosphamide (FC). 3. Rheumatoid arthritis (RA) in combination with methotrexate in adult patients with moderately-to severely-active RA who have inadequate response to one or more TNF antagonist therapies 4. Granulomatosis with polyangiitis (GPA) (Wegener's granulomatosis) and microscopic polyangiitis (MPA) in adult patients in combination with glucocorticoids 5. Moderate to severe pemphigus vulgaris (PV) in adult patients
Rituximab and hyaluronidase/ chimeric co-formulated with hyaluronidase (a human endoglycos-idase)	CD20	1. Follicular lymphoma (FL) o Relapsed or refractory, follicular lymphoma as a single agent o Previously untreated follicular lymphoma in combination with first line chemotherapy and, in patients achieving a complete or partial response to rituximab in combination with chemotherapy, as single agent maintenance therapy o Non-progressing (including stable disease), follicular lymphoma as a single agent after first-line cyclophosphamide, vincristine, and prednisone (CVP) chemotherapy 2. Diffuse large B cell lymphoma (DLBCL) o Previously untreated diffuse large B cell lymphoma in combination with cyclophosphamide, doxorubicin, vincristine, prednisone (CHOP) or other anthracycline-based chemotherapy regimens 3. Chronic lymphocytic leukemia (CLL) o Previously untreated and previously treated CLL in combination with fludarabine and cyclophosphamide (FC) Limitations of use: • Initiate treatment with RITUXAN HYCELA only after patients have received at least one full d • RITUXAN HYCELA is not indicated for the treatment of non-conditions.
RITUXIMAB-ARRX/RIABNI	NHL, CLL, granulomato-sis with polu-angiitis	Anti CD20, ADCC, CDC
Sacituzumab govitecan/ TRODELVY	Metastic triple-negative breast cancer	Anti-Trop-2; ADCC; CDC
Sarilumab/ Kevzara/ fully human	IL-6 receptor	Adult patients with moderately to severely active rheumatoid arthritis who have had an inadequate response or intolerance to one or more disease-modifying antirheumatic drugs
Satralizumab-mwge/ ENSPRYNG	Anti-IL-6 receptor	Neuromyelitis optica spectrum disorder (anti-aquaporin-4 antibody poditive
Secukinumab/ Cosentryx/ fully human	IL-17A (also known as IL-17)	Moderate to severe plaque psoriasis in adult patients who are candidates for systemic therapy or phototherapy.
Siltuximab/ Sylvant/ chimeric	IL-6	Multicentric Castleman's disease[5] (MCD) who are human immunodeficiency virus (HIV) negative and human herpesvirus-8 (HHV-8) negative.
Teprotumu-mab-trb/TEPEZZ	IGF-1R block	Thyroid eye disease

Tildrakizumab-asmn/Ilumya/ humanized	IL-23	Adults with moderate-to-severe plaque psoriasis who are candidates for systemic therapy or phototherapy
Tocilizumab/ Actrema/ humanized	IL-6 receptor	1. Rheumatoid arthritis (RA) • Adult patients with moderately to severely active rheumatoid arthritis who have had an inadequate response to one or more disease modifying anti-rheumatic drugs (DMARDs). 2.Giant cell arteritis (GCA) • Adult patients with giant cell arteritis. 3.Polyarticular juvenile idiopathic arthritis (PJIA) • Patients 2 years of age and older with active polyarticular juvenile idiopathic arthritis. 4.Systemic juvenile idiopathic arthritis (SJIA) • Patients 2 years of age and older with active systemic juvenile idiopathic arthritis. 5.Cytokine release syndrome (CRS) • Adults and pediatric patients 2 years of age and older with chimeric antigen receptor (CAR) T cell-induced severe or life-threatening cytokine release syndrome
Tratuzumab/ Herceptin/ humanized	HER2/neu	1. HER2 overexpressing breast cancer 2. HER2-overexpressing metastatic gastric or gastro-esophageal junction adenocarcinoma
Trastuzumab-dkst/Ogivri/ humanized biosimilar	HER2/neu	1. HER2-overexpressing breast cancer. 2. HER2-overexpressing metastatic gastric or gastro-esophageal junction adenocarcinoma
Ustekinumab/ Stelara/ fully human	IL-12, IL-23	1. Adult patients with moderate to severe plaque psoriasis (Ps) who are candidates for phototherapy or systemic therapy. 2. Active psoriatic arthritis (PsA), alone or in combination with methotrexate. 3. Moderately to severely active Crohn's disease (CD) who have failed or were intolerant to treatment with immunomodulators or corticosteroids, but never failed a tumor necrosis factor (TNF) blocker or failed or were intolerant to treatment with one or more TNF blockers 4. Adolescent patients (12 years or older) with moderate to severe plaque psoriasis, who are candidates for phototherapy or systemic therapy
Vedolizumab/ Entyvio/ humanized	Binds to the α4β7 integrin and blocks the interaction of α4β7 integrin with mucosal addressin cell adhesion molecule-1 (MAdCAM-1) and inhibits the migration of memory T lymphocytes across the endothelium into inflamed gastro-intestinal parenchymal tissue	1. Adult ulcerative colitis (UC) Adult patients with moderately to severely active UC who have had an inadequate response with, lost response to, or were intolerant to a tumor necrosis factor (TNF) blocker or immunomodulator; or had an inadequate response with, were intolerant to, or demonstrated dependence on corticosteroids • inducing and maintaining clinical response • inducing and maintaining clinical remission • improving endoscopic appearance of the mucosa 2. Achieving corticosteroid-free remission adult Crohn's disease (CD) • Adult patients with moderately to severely active CD who have had an inadequate response with, lost response to, or were intolerant to a TNF blocker or immunomodulator; or had an inadequate response with, were intolerant to, or demonstrated dependence on corticosteroids • achieving clinical response • achieving clinical remission • achieving corticosteroid-free remission

[a]Hidradenitis suppuriva is long term skin disease characterized by the occurrence of inflamed and swollen lumps

One other FDA-approved mab, tositumomab (Bexxar) (anti-CD20), was discontinued in 2014 due to lack of demand

[1]Burrill Bernard Crohn (1884 – 1983) was an American gastroenterologist

[2]Friedrich Sigmund Merkel (1845-1919) was a German anatomist and histopathologist

[3]Thomas Hodgkin (1798 – 1866) was a British physician

[4]Albert Sézary (1880 – 1956) was a French dermatologist and syphilogist

[5] Benjamin Castleman (1906 – 1982) was an American physician and pathologist

Small molecule inhibitors FDA-approved for non- disease: examples

- Janus kinase inhibitors – eg, tofacitinib in Crohn's disease, ruxolitinib for steroid-refractory acute graft-versus-host disease
- Bruton's tyrosine kinase inhibitor – eg, ibrutinib for chronic graft-versus-host disease
- Other human tyrosine kinase inhibitors – eg, imatinib for systemic mastocytosis
- Herpes simplex and herpes zoster virus nucleoside analog DNA polymerase inhibitor – eg, acyclovir
- Inhibition of cytomegalovirus DNA polymerases, eg ganciclovir
- Angiogenesis inhibitors – eg, aflibercept for diabetic retinopathy
- Small interfering RNA-based drugs- eg, onasemnogene abeparvovec-xioi (Zolgensma) for familial amyloid polyneuropathy

Enzyme replacement treatments – eg, cerliponase alfa (Brineura) for Batten disease

Enzyme inhibitors – eg, lanadelumab-flyo (Takhzyro) for hereditary angioedema

Anti-sense drugs - eg, fomivirsen for cytomegalovirus retinitis, mipomersen for homozygous familial hypercholesterolemia, eteplirsen for Duchenne muscular dystrophy, nusinersen for spinal muscular atrophy

Cell therapies – eg, allogeneic expanded adipose tissue-derived cells

Alofisel (darvadstrocel, Cx601) has been approved by the European Medicines Agency (EMA) for treating complex perianal fistulas in people with Crohn's disease who have failed standard therapy. It is currently under review by the FDA

Gene-modified cell therapies – eg, Zynteglo (autologous CD34+ cells encoding βA-T87Q-globin gene) to treat transfusion-dependent β-thalassemia has been approved by the EMA for use in Europe. Its manufacturer, Bluebird Bio, has yet to seek FDA approval for the treatment.

Gene therapies – eg, onasemnogene abeparvovec-xioi (Zolgensma) to treat spinal muscular atrophy type 1 has been approved for therapeutic use by the FDA. Voretigene neparvovec-rzyl (Luxturna) to treat congenital retinal dystrophy has also been approved by the FDA

A list of small molecule protein kinase inhibitors approved by the USA FDA for therapeutic use (as of December 2020) are shown in Table 2.

Table 2

Generic name/ trade name	**Target and mechanism of action**	**FDA-approved indication/s**
Abemaciclib/ Verzenio	Cyclin-dependent kinases 4 and 6 (CDK4 and CDK6). CDK4/6 inhibitor activity enforces G1 cell cycle arrest, and thus inhibits cellular proliferation	1. In combination with an aromatase inhibitor as initial endocrine-based therapy for the treatment of postmenopausal women with hormone receptor (HR)-positive, human epidermal growth factor receptor 2 (HER2)-negative advanced or metastatic breast cancer 2. In combination with fulvestrant for the treatment of women with hormone receptor (HR)-positive, human epidermal growth factor receptor 2 (HER2)-negative advanced or metastatic breast cancer with disease progression following endocrine therapy 3. As monotherapy for the treatment of adult patients with HR-positive, HER2-negative advanced or metastatic breast

		cancer with disease progression following endocrine therapy and prior chemotherapy in the metastatic setting
Acalabrutinib/ Calquence	Bruton's tyrosine kinase[1]. (BTK). BTK is a signalling molecule of the B cell antigen receptor (BCR) and cytokine receptor pathways	1. Mantle cell lymphoma (MCL) who have received at least one prior therapy. This indication is approved under accelerated approval based on overall response rate. Continued approval for this indication may be contingent upon verification and description of clinical benefit in confirmatory trials 2. Chronic lymphocytic leukemia (CLL) or small lymphocytic lymphoma (SLL)
Afatinib/ Golotrif	ErbB (derived avian erythroblastosis oncogeneB). Signalling through the ErbB1/2/4 family of receptors promotes cell proliferation and opposes apoptosis. (ErbB is also known as, HER-2, HER-2/neu, HER2, NEU, CD340). Afatinib covalently binds to the kinase domains of EGFR (ErbB1), HER2 (ErbB2), and HER4 (ErbB4) and irreversibly inhibits tyrosine kinase autophosphorylation, resulting in downregulation of ErbB signalling.	1. First-line treatment of patients with metastatic non-small cell lung cancer (NSCLC) whose tumors have non-resistant epidermal growth factor receptor (EGFR) mutations 2. Treatment of patients with metastatic, squamous NSCLC progressing after platinum-based chemotherapy
Alectinib/ Alecensa	ALK, RET. Alectinib is a tyrosine kinase inhibitor that targets ALK and RET. In non-clinical studies, alectinib inhibited ALK phosphorylation and ALK-mediated activation of the downstream signalling proteins STAT3 and AKT, and decreased tumor cell viability in multiple cell lines harboring ALK fusions, amplifications, or activating mutations.	Anaplastic lymphoma kinase (ALK)-positive metastatic non-small cell lung cancer (NSCLC)
Avatpritinib/ AYVAKIT	Kinase inhibitor	Adults with unresectable or metastatic gastrointestinal stromal tumor (GIST) harboring a platelet-derived growth factor receptor alpha (PDGFRA) exon 18 mutation, including PDGFRA D842V mutations
Axitinib/Inlyta	Vascular endothelial growth factor receptors (VEGFR) 1/2/3. Axitinib has been shown to inhibit receptor tyrosine kinases including vascular endothelial growth factor receptors VEGFR-1, VEGFR-2, and VEGFR-3	Advanced renal cell carcinoma after failure of one prior systemic therapy
Baricitinib/ Olumiant	JAK1/2. Janus kinases phosphorylate activated	Adult patients with moderately to severely active rheumatoid arthritis who have had an

	cytokine receptors. These phosphorylated receptors in turn recruit STAT transcrip-tion factors which modulate gene transcription	inadequate response to one or more TNF antagonist therapies
Binimetinib/ Mektovi	MEK1/2. MEK inhibitors inhibit the mitogen-activated protein kinase kinase enzymes MEK1and/or MEK2. They can be used to affect the MAPK/ERK pathway which is often overactive in some cancers	In combination with encorafenib, for the treatment of patients with unresectable or metastatic breast cancer with a BRAF V600E/K mutation
Bosutinib/ Bosulif	BCR-ABL Bosutinib inhibits the BCR-ABL kinase that promotes CML	Treatment of adult patients with chronic, accelerated, or blast phase Ph+ chronic myelogenous leukemia (CML) with resistance or intolerance to prior therapy
Brigatinib/ Alunbrig	ALK. Brigatinib is a tyrosine kinase inhibitor with in vitro activity at clinically achievable concentrations against multiple kinases including ALK, ROS1, insulin-like growth factor-1 receptor (IGF-1R), and FLT-3 as well as EGFR deletion and point mutations. Brigatinib inhibited autophosphorylation of ALK and ALK-mediated phosphorylation of the downstream signalling proteins STAT3, AKT, ERK1/2, and S6 in in vitro and in vivo assays.	Patients with anaplastic lymphoma kinase (ALK)-positive metastatic non-small cell lung cancer (NSCLC) who have progressed on or are intolerant to crizotinib. This indication is approved under accelerated approval based on tumor response rate and duration of response. Continued approval for this indication may be contingent upon verification and description of clinical benefit in a confirmatory trial
Cabozantinib/ Cabometyx	RET, VEGFR2. Cabozantinib inhibits the tyrosine kinase activity of RET, MET, VEGFR-1, -2 and -3, KIT, TRKB, FLT-3, AXL, ROS1, TYRO3, MER, and TIE-2. These receptor tyrosine kinases are involved in both normal cellular function and pathologic processes such as oncogenesis, metastasis, tumor angiogenesis, drug resistance, and maintenance of the tumor microenvironment.	1.Patients with advanced renal cell carcinoma (RCC) 2. Patients with hepatocellular carcinoma (HCC) who have been previously treated with sorafenib
Cabozantinib/ Cometriq	RET, VEGFR2	Patients with progressive, metastatic medullary thyroid cancer (MTC)
Capmatinib/ TABRECTA	Kinase inhibitor that targets MET	Treatment of adult patients with metastatic non-small cell lung cancer (NSCLC) whose tumors have a mutation that leads to mesenchymal-epithelial transition (MET) exon 14 skipping as detected by an FDA-approved test.
Ceritinib/ Zykadia	ALK. Targets of ceritinib inhibition identified in either biochemical or cellular assays at clinically relevant	Patients with metastatic non-small cell lung cancer (NSCLC) whose tumors are anaplastic lymphoma kinase (ALK)-positive

	concentrations include ALK, insulin-like growth factor 1 receptor (IGF-1R), insulin receptor (InsR), and ROS1. Among these, ceritinib is most active against ALK. Ceritinib inhibited autophosphorylation of ALK, ALK-mediated phosphorylation of the downstream signalling protein STAT3, and proliferation of ALK-dependent cancer cells in in vitro and in vivo assays.	
Cobimetinib/ Cotellic	MEK1/2. Cobimetinib is a reversible inhibitor of mitogen-activated protein kinase (MAPK)/extracellular signal regulated kinase 1 (MEK1) and MEK2. MEK proteins are upstream regulators of the extracellular signalrelated kinase (ERK) pathway, which promotes cellular proliferation. BRAF V600E and K mutations result in constitutive activation of the BRAF pathway which includes MEK1 and MEK2.	Patients with unresectable or metastatic breast cancer with a BRAF V600E or V600K mutation, in combination with vemurafenib
Crizotinib/ Xalkori	ALK, ROS1. Crizotinib is an inhibitor of receptor tyrosine kinases including ALK, Hepatocyte growth factor receptor (HGFR, c-Met), ROS1 (c-ros), and Recepteur d'Origine Nantais (RON). Translocations can affect the ALK gene resulting in the expression of oncogenic fusion proteins. The formation of ALK fusion proteins results in activation and dysregulation of the gene's expression and signalling which can contribute to increased cell proliferation and survival in tumors expressing these proteins.	Patients with metastatic non-small cell lung cancer (NSCLC) whose tumors are anaplastic lymphoma kinase (ALK) or ROS1-positive
Dabrafenib/ Tafinlar	B-RAF. Dabrafenib is an inhibitor of some mutated forms of BRAF kinases with in vitro IC50 values of 0.65, 0.5, and 1.84 nM for BRAF V600E, BRAF V600K, and BRAF V600D enzymes, respectively. Dabrafenib also inhibits wild-type BRAF and CRAF kinases with IC50 values of 3.2 and 5.0 nM, respectively, and other kinases such as SIK1, NEK11, and LIMK1 at higher concentrations. Some mutations in the BRAF gene, including those that result in BRAF V600E, can result in constitutively activated BRAF kinases that may stimulate tumor cell growth.	1. Treatment of patients with unresectable or metastatic breast cancer with BRAF V600E or V600K mutations 2. Adjuvant treatment of patients with breast cancer with BRAF V600E or V600K mutations and involvement of lymph node(s), following complete resection. 3. Treatment of patients with metastatic non-small cell lung cancer (NSCLC) with BRAF V600E mutation.
Dacomitinib/ Vizimpro	EGFR. Dacomitinib is an irreversible inhibitor of the kinase activity of the human	First-line treatment of patients with metastatic non-small cell lung cancer (NSCLC) with epidermal

	epidermal growth factor receptor (EGFR) family (EGFR/HER1, HER2, and HER4) and certain EGFR activating mutations (exon 19 deletion or the exon 21 L858R substitution mutation).	growth factor receptor (EGFR) exon 19 deletion or exon 21 L858R substitution mutations
Dasatinib/ Sprycell	BCR-ABL. Dasatinib, at nanomolar concentrations, inhibits the following kinases: BCR-ABL, SRC family (SRC, LCK, YES, FYN), c-KIT, EPHA2, and PDGFR-β. Based on modeling studies, dasatinib is predicted to bind to multiple conformations of the ABL kinase.	1. Newly diagnosed adults with Philadelphia chromosome-positive (Ph+) chronic myeloid leukemia (CML) in chronic phase. The trial is ongoing and further data will be required to determine long-term outcome. 2. Adults with chronic, accelerated, or myeloid or lymphoid blast phase Ph+ CML with resistance or intolerance to prior therapy including imatinib. 3. Adults with Philadelphia chromosome-positive acute lymphoblastic leukemia (Ph+ ALL) with resistance or intolerance to prior therapy
Encorafenib/Braftovi	B-RAF. Encorafenib is a kinase inhibitor that targets BRAF V600E, as well as wild-type BRAF and CRAF in in vitro cell-free assays with IC50 values of 0.35, 0.47, and 0.3 nM, respectively. Mutations in the BRAF gene, such as BRAF V600E, can result in constitutively activated BRAF kinases that may stimulate tumor cell growth. Encorafenib was also able to bind to other kinases in vitro including JNK1, JNK2, JNK3, LIMK1, LIMK2, MEK4, and STK36 and substantially reduce ligand binding to these kinases at clinically achievable concentrations ($\leq$ 0.9 μM).	In combination with binimetinib, for the treatment of patients with unresectable or metastatic breast cancer with a BRAF V600E or V600K mutation
Entrectinib/ Rozlytrek	TRKA/B/C, ROS1, ALK. Entrectinib is an inhibitor of the tropomyosin receptor tyrosine kinases (TRK) TRKA, TRKB, and TRKC (encoded by the neurotrophic tyrosine receptor kinase [NTRK] genes NTRK1, NTRK2, and NTRK3, respectively), proto-oncogene tyrosine-protein kinase ROS1 (ROS1), and anaplastic lymphoma kinase (ALK). Fusion proteins that include TRK, ROS1, or ALK kinase domains can drive tumorigenic potential through hyperactivation of downstream signalling pathways leading to unconstrained cell proliferation.	• Adult patients with metastatic non-small cell lung cancer (NSCLC) whose tumors are ROS1-positive • Adult and pediatric patients 12 years of age and older with solid tumors that: o have a neurotrophic tyrosine receptor kinase (NTRK) gene fusion without a known acquired resistance mutation o are metastatic or where surgical resection is likely to result in severe morbidity o have progressed following treatment or have no satisfactory alternative therapy. This indication is approved under accelerated approval based on tumor response rate and durability

		of response. Continued approval for this indication may be contingent upon verification and description of clinical benefit in the confirmatory trials.
Erdafitinib/ Balversa	FGFR1/2/3/4. Erdafitinib is a kinase inhibitor that binds to and inhibits enzymatic activity of FGFR1, FGFR2, FGFR3 and FGFR4 based on in vitro data. Erdafitinib also binds to RET, CSF1R, PDGFRA, PDGFRB, FLT4, KIT, and VEGFR2. Erdafitinib inhibited FGFR phosphorylation and signalling and decreased cell viability in cell lines expressing FGFR genetic alterations, including point mutations, amplifications, and fusions. Erdafitinib demonstrated antitumor activity in FGFR-expressing cell lines and xenograft models derived from tumor types, including bladder cancer.	Treatment of adult patients with locally advanced or metastatic urothelial carcinoma that has • susceptible FGFR3 or FGFR2 genetic alterations and • progressed during or following at least one line of prior platinum-containing chemotherapy including within 12 months of neoadjuvant or adjuvant platinum-containing chemotherapy. This indication is approved under accelerated approval based on tumor response rate. Continued approval for this indication may be contingent upon verification and description of clinical benefit in confirmatory trials
Erlotinib/ Tarceva	EGFR. The mechanism of the clinical antitumor action of erlotinib is not fully characterized. Erlotinib inhibits the intracellular phosphorylation of tyrosine kinase associated with the epidermal growth factor receptor (EGFR). Specificity of inhibition with regard to other tyrosine kinase receptors has not been fully characterized. EGFR is expressed on the cell surface of normal cells and cancer cells.	1. Maintenance treatment of patients with locally advanced or metastatic non-small cell lung cancer (NSCLC) whose disease has not progressed after four cycles of platinum-based first-line chemotherapy. 2.Treatment of locally advanced or metastatic non-small cell lung cancer after failure of at least one prior chemotherapy regimen. 3.First-line treatment of patients with locally advanced, unresectable or metastatic pancreatic cancer, in combination with gemcitabine
Everolimus/ Afinitor	FKBP12/ mTOR. Everolimus is an inhibitor of mammalian target of rapamycin (mTOR), a serine-threonine kinase, downstream of the PI3K/AKT pathway. The mTOR pathway is dysregulated in several human cancers. Everolimus binds to an intracellular protein, FKBP-12, resulting in an inhibitory complex formation (mTORC1) and thus inhibition of mTOR kinase activity. Everolimus reduced the activity of S6 ribosomal protein kinase (S6K1) and eukaryotic elongation factor 4E-binding protein (4E-BP1), downstream effectors of mTOR, involved in protein synthesis.	Treatment of patients with 1. Advanced renal cell carcinoma (RCC) after failure of treatment with sunitinib or sorafenib. 2. Subependymal giant cell astrocytoma (SEGA) associated with tuberous sclerosis (TS) who require therapeutic intervention but are not candidates for curative surgical resection. The effectiveness of AFINITOR is based on an analysis of change in SEGA volume. Clinical benefit such as improvement in disease-related symptoms or increase in overall survival has not been demonstrated
Fedratinib/ Inrebic	JAK2, FLT3.	Treatment of adult patients with

	Fedratinib is an oral kinase inhibitor with activity against wild type and mutationally activated Janus Associated Kinase 2 (JAK2) and FMS-like tyrosine kinase 3 (FLT3). Fedratinib is a JAK2-selective inhibitor with higher inhibitory activity for JAK2 over family members JAK1, JAK3 and TYK2. Abnormal activation of JAK2 is associated with myeloproliferative neoplasms (MPNs), including myelofibrosis and polycythemia vera	intermediate-2 or high-risk primary or secondary (post-polycythemia vera or post-essential thrombocythemia) myelofibrosis (MF)
Fostamatinib/ Tavalisse	SYK. Fostamatinib is a tyrosine kinase inhibitor with demonstrated activity against spleen tyrosine kinase (SYK). The major metabolite of fostamatinib, R406, inhibits signal transduction of Fc-activating receptors and B cell receptor. The fostamatinib metabolite R406 reduces antibody-mediated destruction of platelets.	Treatment of thrombocytopenia in adult patients with chronic immune thrombocytopenia (ITP) who have had an insufficient response to a previous treatment.
Gefitinib/ Iressa	EGFR. The epidermal growth factor receptor (EGFR) is expressed on the cell surface of both normal and cancer cells and plays a role in the processes of cell growth and proliferation. Some EGFR activating mutations (exon 19 deletion or exon 21 point mutation L858R) within NSCLC cells have been identified as contributing to the promotion of tumor cell growth, blocking of apoptosis, increasing the production of angiogenic factors and facilitating the processes of metastasis. Gefitinib reversibly inhibits the kinase activity of wild-type and certain activating mutations of EGFR, preventing autophosphorylation of tyrosine residues associated with the receptor, thereby inhibiting further downstream signalling and blocking EGFR-dependent proliferation. Gefitinib binding affinity for EGFR exon 19 deletion or exon 21 point mutation L858R mutations is higher than its affinity for the wild-type EGFR. Gefitinib also inhibits IGF and PDGF-mediated signalling at clinically relevant concentrations; inhibition of other tyrosine kinase receptors has not been fully characterized.	First-line treatment of patients with metastatic non-small cell lung cancer (NSCLC) whose tumors have epidermal growth factor receptor (EGFR) exon 19 deletions or exon 21 (L858R) substitution mutations. Limitation of use: the safety and efficacy of IRESSA have not been established in patients whose tumors have EGFR mutations other than exon 19 deletions or exon 21 (L858R) substitution mutations
Gilteritinib/ Xospata	Flt3. Gilteritinib is a small molecule that inhibits multiple receptor tyrosine kinases, including FMS-like tyrosine	Treatment of adult patients who have relapsed or refractory acute myeloid leukemia (AML) with a FLT3 mutation

	kinase 3 (FLT3). Gilteritinib demonstrated the ability to inhibit FLT3 receptor signalling and proliferation in cells exogenously expressing FLT3 including FLT3-ITD, tyrosine kinase domain mutations (TKD) FLT3-D835Y and FLT3-ITD-D835, and it induced apoptosis in leukemic cells expressing FLT3-ITD.	
Ibrutinib/ Imbruvica	BTK. Ibrutinib is a small-molecule inhibitor of BTK. Ibrutinib forms a covalent bond with a cysteine residue in the BTK active site, leading to inhibition of BTK enzymatic activity. BTK is a signalling molecule of the B cell antigen receptor (BCR) and cytokine receptor pathways. BTK's role in signalling through the B cell surface receptors results in activation of pathways necessary for B cell trafficking, chemotaxis, and adhesion. Non-clinical studies show that ibrutinib inhibits B cell proliferation and survival in vivo as well as cell migration and substrate adhesion in vitro.	Treatment of adult patients with: 1. Mantle cell lymphoma (MCL) who have received at least one prior therapy. Accelerated approval was granted for this indication based on overall response rate. Continued approval for this indication may be contingent upon verification and description of clinical benefit in a confirmatory trial. 2. Chronic lymphocytic leukemia (CLL)/Small lymphocytic lymphoma (SLL) Chronic lymphocytic leukemia (CLL)/Small lymphocytic lymphoma (SLL) with 17p deletion 3. Waldenström's macroglobulinemia (WM) 4. Marginal zone lymphoma (MZL) who require systemic therapy and have received at least one prior anti-CD20-based therapy. Accelerated approval was granted for this indication based on overall response rate. Continued approval for this indication may be contingent upon verification and description of clinical benefit in a confirmatory trial. 5. Chronic graft-versus-host disease (cGVHD) after failure of one or more lines of systemic therapy
Imatinib/ Gleevec	BCR-ABL	1. Newly diagnosed adult and pediatric patients with Philadelphia chromosome positive chronic myeloid leukemia (Ph+ CML) in chronic phase 2. Patients with Philadelphia chromosome positive chronic myeloid leukemia (Ph+ CML) in blast crisis (BC), accelerated phase (AP), or in chronic phase (CP) after failure of interferon-alpha therapy 3. Adult patients with relapsed or refractory Philadelphia chromosome positive acute lymphoblastic leukemia (Ph+ ALL)

		4. Pediatric patients with newly diagnosed Philadelphia chromosome positive acute lymphoblastic leukemia (Ph+ ALL) in combination with chemotherapy 5. Adult patients with myelodysplastic/myeloproliferative diseases (MDS/MPD) associated with platelet-derived growth factor receptor (PDGFR) gene re-arrangements 6. Adult patients with aggressive systemic mastocytosis (ASM) without the D816V c-Kit mutation or with c-Kit mutational status unknown 7. Adult patients with hypereosinophilic syndrome (HES) and/or chronic eosinophilic leukemia (CEL) who have the FIP1L1-PDGFR-α fusion kinase and for patients with HES and/or CEL who are FIP1L1 PDGFR-α fusion kinase negative or unknown 8. Adult patients with unresectable, recurrent and/or metastatic dermatofibrosarcoma protuberans (DFSP) 9. Patients with kit (CD117) positive unresectable and/or metastatic gastrointestinal stromal tumors (GIST) 10. Adjuvant treatment of adult patients following resection of kit (CD117) positive GIST
Lapatinib/ Tykerb	EGFR, ErbB2/HER2. Lapatinib is a 4-anilinoquinazoline kinase inhibitor of the intracellular tyrosine kinase domains of both Epidermal Growth Factor Receptor (EGFR [ErbB1]) and of Human Epidermal Receptor Type 2 (HER2 [ErbB2]). Lapatinib inhibits ErbB-driven tumor cell growth in vitro and in various animal models.	1. In combination with capecitabine for the treatment of patients with advanced or metastatic breast cancer whose tumors overexpress human epidermal growth factor receptor 2 (HER2) and who have received prior therapy including an anthracycline, a taxane, and trastuzumab. Limitations of use: patients should have disease progression on trastuzumab prior to initiation of treatment with TYKERB in combination with capecitabine. 2. In combination with letrozole for the treatment of postmenopausal women with hormone receptor-positive metastatic breast cancer that overexpresses the HER2 receptor for whom hormonal therapy is indicated.
Larotrectinib/ Vitrakvi	TRKA/B/C. Larotrectinib is an inhibitor of the	Treatment of adult and pediatric patients with solid tumors that

	tropomyosin receptor kinases (TRK), TRKA, TRKB, and TRKC. In a broad panel of purified enzyme assays, larotrectinib inhibited TRKA, TRKB, and TRKC. TRKA, B, and C are encoded by the genes NTRK1, NTRK2, and NTRK3. Chromosomal rearrangements involving in-frame fusions of these genes with various partners can result in constitutively-activated chimeric TRK fusion proteins that can act as an oncogenic driver, promoting cell proliferation and survival in tumor cell lines.	• have a neurotrophic receptor tyrosine kinase (NTRK) gene fusion without a known acquired resistance mutation • are metastatic or where surgical resection is likely to result in severe morbidity, and • have no satisfactory alternative treatments or that have progressed following treatment. This indication is approved under accelerated approval based on overall response rate and duration of response. Continued approval for this indication may be contingent upon verification and description of clinical benefit in confirmatory trials.
Lenvatinib/ Lenvima	VEGFR, FGFR, RET, PDGFR, KIT. Lenvatinib is a kinase inhibitor that inhibits the kinase activities of vascular endothelial growth factor (VEGF) receptors VEGFR1 (FLT1), VEGFR2 (KDR), and VEGFR3 (FLT4). Lenvatinib inhibits other kinases that have been implicated in pathogenic angiogenesis, tumor growth, and cancer progression in addition to their normal cellular functions, including fibroblast growth factor (FGF) receptors FGFR1, 2, 3, and 4; platelet derived growth factor receptor alpha (PDGFRα), KIT, and RET. Lenvatinib also exhibited antiproliferative activity in hepatocellular carcinoma cell lines dependent on activated FGFR signalling with a concurrent inhibition of FGF-receptor substrate 2α (FRS2α) phosphorylation. The combination of lenvatinib and everolimus showed increased antiangiogenic and antitumor activity as demonstrated by decreases in human endothelial cell proliferation, tube formation, and VEGF signalling in vitro, and by decreases in tumor volume in mouse xenograft models of human renal cell cancer that were greater than those with either drug alone.	Treatment of patients with 1. Locally recurrent or metastatic, progressive, radioactive iodine-refractory differentiated thyroid cancer (DTC). 2. In combination with everolimus, for the treatment of patients with advanced renal cell carcinoma (RCC) following one prior antiangiogenic therapy. 3. For the first-line treatment of patients with unresectable hepatocellular carcinoma (HCC)
Lorlatinib/ Lorbrena	ALK, ROS1 and others. Lorlatinib is a kinase inhibitor with in vitro activity against ALK and ROS1 as well as TYK1, FER, FPS, TRKA, TRKB, TRKC, FAK, FAK2, and ACK. Lorlatinib demonstrated in vitro activity against multiple mutant forms of the ALK enzyme, including some mutations detected in tumors at the	Treatment of patients with anaplastic lymphoma kinase (ALK)-positive metastatic non-small cell lung cancer (NSCLC) whose disease has progressed on • crizotinib and at least one other ALK inhibitor for metastatic disease • or on alectinib as the first ALK

	time of disease progression on crizotinib and other ALK inhibitors.	inhibitor therapy for metastatic disease • or on ceritinib as the first ALK inhibitor therapy for metastatic disease. This indication is approved under accelerated approval based on tumor response rate and duration of response. Continued approval for this indication may be contingent upon verification and description of clinical benefit in a confirmatory trial.
Midostaurin/ Rydapt	Flt3. Midostaurin is a small molecule that inhibits multiple receptor tyrosine kinases. In vitro biochemical or cellular assays have shown that midostaurin or its major human active metabolites CGP62221 and CGP52421 inhibit the activity of wild type FLT3, FLT3 mutant kinases (ITD and TKD), KIT (wild type and D816V mutant), PDGFRα/β, VEGFR2, as well as members of the serine/threonine kinase PKC (protein kinase C) family.	Treatment of adult patients with: newly diagnosed acute myeloid leukemia (AML) that is FLT3 mutation-positive in combination with standard cytarabine and daunorubicin induction and cytarabine consolidation. Limitations of use: RYDAPT is not indicated as a single-agent induction therapy for the treatment of patients with AML, aggressive systemic mastocytosis (ASM), systemic mastocytosis with associated hematological neoplasm (SM-AHN), or mast cell leukemia (MCL).
Neratinib/ Nerlynx	ErbB2/HER2. A kinase inhibitor that irreversibly binds to Epidermal Growth Factor Receptor (EGFR), Human Epidermal Growth Factor Receptor 2 (HER2), and HER4. In vitro, neratinib reduces EGFR and HER2 autophosphorylation, downstream MAPK and AKT signalling pathways, and showed antitumor activity in EGFR and/or HER2 expressing carcinoma cell lines. Neratinib human metabolites M3, M6, M7 and M11 inhibited the activity of EGFR, HER2 and HER4 in vitro. In vivo, oral administration of neratinib inhibited tumor growth in mouse xenograft models with tumor cell lines expressing HER2 and EGFR.	The extended adjuvant treatment of adult patients with early stage HER2-overexpressed/amplified breast cancer, to follow adjuvant trastuzumab-based therapy
Netarsudil/ Rhopressa	ROCK1/2 (Rho associated coiled-coil containing protein kinase 1) Netarsudil is a rho kinase inhibitor, which is believed to reduce intra-ocular pressure (IOP) by increasing the outflow of aqueous humor through the trabecular meshwork route. The exact mechanism is unknown.	RHOPRESSA® (netarsudil ophthalmic solution) 0.02% is a Rho kinase inhibitor indicated for the reduction of elevated intraocular pressure in patients with open-angle glaucoma or ocular hypertension
Nilotinib/ Tasigna	BCR-ABL. Nilotinib is an inhibitor of the BCR-ABL kinase.	1. Treatment of newly diagnosed adult patients with Philadelphia chromosome positive chronic

		myeloid leukemia (Ph+ CML) in chronic phase. 2. Treatment of chronic phase (CP) and accelerated phase (AP) Ph+ CML in adult patients resistant to or intolerant to prior therapy that included imatinib.
Nintedanib/ Vargatef	Multiple kinases. Nintedanib is a small molecule that inhibits multiple receptor tyrosine kinases (RTKs) and non-receptor tyrosine kinases (nRTKs). Nintedanib inhibits the following RTKs: platelet-derived growth factor receptor (PDGFR) α and β, fibroblast growth factor receptor (FGFR) 1-3, vascular endothelial growth factor receptor (VEGFR) 1-3, and Fms-like tyrosine kinase-3 (FLT3). Among them, FGFR, PDGFR, and VEGFR have been implicated in IPF pathogenesis. Nintedanib binds competitively to the adenosine triphosphate (ATP) binding pocket of these receptors and blocks the intracellular signalling which is crucial for the proliferation, migration, and transformation of fibroblasts representing essential mechanisms of the IPF pathology.	The treatment of idiopathic pulmonary fibrosis (IPF).
Osimertinib/ Tagrisso	EGFR Osimertinib is a kinase inhibitor of the epidermal growth factor receptor (EGFR), which binds irreversibly to certain mutant forms of EGFR (T790M, L858R, and exon 19 deletion) at approximately 9- fold lower concentrations than wild-type. In vitro, osimertinib also inhibited the activity of HER2, HER3, HER4, ACK1, and BLK at clinically relevant concentrations. In cultured cells and animal tumor implantation models, osimertinib exhibited anti-tumor activity against NSCLC lines harboring EGFR-mutations (T790M/L858R, L858R, T790M/exon 19 deletion, and exon 19 deletion) and, to a lesser extent, wild-type EGFR amplifications	1. The first-line treatment of patients with metastatic NSCLC whose tumors have epidermal growth factor receptor (EGFR) exon 19 deletions or exon 21 L858R mutations 2. The treatment of patients with metastatic EGFR T790M mutation-positive NSCLC whose disease has progressed on or after EGFR TKI therapy
Palbociclib/ Ibrance	CDK4/6	The treatment of adult patients with hormone receptor (HR)-positive, human epidermal growth factor receptor 2 (HER2)-negative advanced or metastatic breast cancer in combination with: 1. An aromatase inhibitor as initial endocrine-based therapy in postmenopausal women or in men, or 2. Fulvestrant in patients with

		disease progression following endocrine therapy.
Pazopanib/ Votrient	VEGFR1/2/3 Pazopanib is a multi-tyrosine kinase inhibitor of vascular endothelial growth factor receptor (VEGFR)-1, VEGFR-2, VEGFR-3, platelet-derived growth factor receptor (PDGFR)-α and -ß, fibroblast growth factor receptor (FGFR) -1 and -3, cytokine receptor (Kit), interleukin-2, receptor inducible T cell kinase (Itk), leukocyte-specific protein tyrosine kinase (Lck), and transmembrane glycoprotein receptor tyrosine kinase (c-fms). In vitro, pazopanib inhibited ligand-induced autophosphorylation of VEGFR-2, Kit and PDGFR-β receptors. In vivo, pazopanib inhibited VEGF-induced VEGFR-2 phosphorylation in mouse lungs, angiogenesis in a mouse model, and the growth of some human tumor xenografts in mice.	The treatment of patients with: 1. Advanced renal cell carcinoma 2. Advanced soft tissue sarcoma who have received prior chemotherapy. Limitations of use: the efficacy of VOTRIENT for the treatment of patients with adipocytic soft tissue sarcoma or gastrointestinal stromal tumors has not been demonstrated.
Pemigatinib/ PEMAZYRE	Kinase inhibitor targets FGFR1, 2 and 3	Treatment of adults with previously treated, unresectable locally advanced or metastatic cholangiocarcinoma with a fibroblast growth factor receptor 2 (FGFR2) fusion or other rearrangement as detected by an FDA-approved test.
Pexidartinib/ Turalio	Multiple kinases. Pexidartinib is a small molecule tyrosine kinase inhibitor that targets colony stimulating factor 1 receptor (CSF1R), KIT proto-oncogene receptor tyrosine kinase (KIT), and FMS-like tyrosine kinase 3 (FLT3) harboring an internal tandem duplication (ITD) mutation. Overexpression of the CSF1R ligand promotes cell proliferation and accumulation in the synovium. In vitro, pexidartinib inhibited proliferation of cell lines dependent on CSF1R and ligand-induced autophosphorylation of CSF1R. Pexidartinib also inhibited the proliferation of a CSF1R dependent cell line in vivo.	The treatment of adult patients with symptomatic tenosynovial giant cell tumor (TGCT) associated with severe morbidity or functional limitations and not amenable to improvement with surgery.
Pralsetinib/ GAVRETO™	Kinase inhibitor of wild-type RET and oncogenic RET fusions (CCDC6-RET) and mutations (RET V804L, RET V804M and RET M918T)	Treatment of adult patients with metastatic rearranged during transfection (RET) fusion- positive nonsmall cell lung cancer (NSCLC) as detected by an FDA approved test. This indication is approved

		under accelerated approval based on overall response rate and duration of response. Continued approval for this indication may be contingent upon verification and description of clinical benefit in confirmatory trials
Ponatinib/ Iclusig	ABL Ponatinib inhibited the in vitro tyrosine kinase activity of ABL and T315I mutant ABL with IC50 concentrations of 0.4 and 2.0 nM, respectively. Ponatinib inhibited the in vitro activity of additional kinases with IC50 concentrations between 0.1 and 20 nM, including members of the VEGFR, PDGFR, FGFR, EPH receptors and SRC families of kinases, and KIT, RET, TIE2, and FLT3. Ponatinib inhibited the in vitro viability of cells expressing native or mutant BCR-ABL, including T315I. In mice, treatment with ponatinib reduced the size of tumors expressing native or T315I mutant BCR-ABL when compared to controls.	Iclusig is a kinase inhibitor indicated for the: 1. Treatment of adult patients with chronic phase, accelerated phase, or blast phase chronic myeloid leukemia (CML) or Ph+ ALL for whom no other tyrosine kinase inhibitor (TKI) therapy is indicated. 2. Treatment of adult patients with T315I-positive CML (chronic phase, accelerated phase, or blast phase) or T315I-positive Philadelphia chromosome positive acute lymphoblastic leukemia (Ph+ ALL)
Regorafenib/ Tafinlar	VEGFR1/2/3 Regorafenib is a small molecule inhibitor of multiple membrane-bound and intracellular kinases involved in normal cellular functions and in pathologic processes such as oncogenesis, tumor angiogenesis, and maintenance of the tumor microenvironment. In in vitro biochemical or cellular assays, regorafenib or its major human active metabolites M-2 and M-5 inhibited the activity of RET, VEGFR1, VEGFR2, VEGFR3, KIT, PDGFR-alpha, PDGFR-beta, FGFR1, FGFR2, TIE2, DDR2, Trk2A, Eph2A, RAF-1, BRAF, BRAFV600E , SAPK2, PTK5, and Abl at concentrations of regorafenib that have been achieved clinically. In in vivo models, regorafenib demonstrated anti-angiogenic activity in a rat tumor model, and inhibition of tumor growth as well as anti-metastatic activity in several mouse xenograft models including some for human colorectal carcinoma.	Metastatic colorectal cancer (CRC) who have been previously treated with fluoropyrimidine-, oxaliplatin- and irinotecan-based chemotherapy, an anti-VEGF therapy, and, if KRAS wild type, an anti-EGFR therapy
Ribociclib/ Kisqali	CDK4/6 Ribociclib is an inhibitor of cyclin-dependent kinase (CDK) 4 and 6. These kinases are activated upon	KISQALI is a kinase inhibitor indicated in combination with: 1. an aromatase inhibitor for the treatment of pre/perimenopausal

	binding to Dcyclins and play a crucial role in signalling pathways which lead to cell cycle progression and cellular proliferation. The cyclin D-CDK4/6 complex regulates cell cycle progression through phosphorylation of the retinoblastoma protein (pRb). In vitro, ribociclib decreased pRb phosphorylation leading to arrest in the G1 phase of the cell cycle and reduced cell proliferation in breast cancer cell lines. In vivo, treatment with single agent ribociclib in a rat xenograft model with human tumor cells led to decreased tumor volumes, which correlated with inhibition of pRb phosphorylation.	or postmenopausal women with hormone receptor (HR)-positive, human epidermal growth factor receptor 2 (HER2)-negative advanced or metastatic breast cancer, as initial endocrine-based therapy, or 2. fulvestrant for the treatment of postmenopausal women with HR-positive, HER2-negative advanced or metastatic breast cancer, as initial endocrine-based therapy or following disease progression on endocrine therapy
Repritinib/ QINLOCK	Kinase inhibitor	Treatment of adult patients with advanced gastrointestinal stromal tumor (GIST) who have received 3 or more kinase inhibitors, including imatinib
Ruxolitinib/ Jakafi	JAK1/2/3,Tyk Ruxolitinib, a kinase inhibitor, inhibits Janus Associated Kinases (JAKs) JAK1 and JAK2 which mediate the signalling of a number of cytokines and growth factors that are important for hematopoiesis and immune function. JAK signalling involves recruitment of STATs (signal transducers and activators of transcription) to cytokine receptors, activation and subsequent localization of STATs to the nucleus leading to modulation of gene expression. Myelofibrosis (MF) is a myeloproliferative neoplasm (MPN) known to be associated with dysregulated JAK1 and JAK2 signalling. In a mouse model of JAK2V617F-positive MPN, oral administration of ruxolitinib prevented splenomegaly, preferentially decreased JAK2V617F mutant cells in the spleen and decreased circulating inflammatory cytokines (eg, TNF-α, IL-6).	Jakafi is a kinase inhibitor indicated for treatment of patients with intermediate or high-risk myelofibrosis, including primary myelofibrosis, post-polycythemia vera myelofibrosis and post-essential thrombocythemia myelofibrosis
Selpercatinib/ RETEVMOTM	Kinase inhibitor of wild-type RET and multiple mutated RET isoforms as well as VEGFR1 and VEGFR3	Treatment of: • Adult patients with metastatic RET fusion-positive non-small cell lung cancer (NSCLC)1 • Adult and pediatric patients 12 years of age and older with advanced or metastatic RET-mutant medullary thyroid cancer (MTC) who require systemic

		therapy1 • Adult and pediatric patients 12 years of age and older with advanced or metastatic RET fusion-positive thyroid cancer who require systemic therapy and who are radioactive iodine-refractory (if radioactive iodine is appropriate). This indication is approved under accelerated approval based on overall response rate and duration of response. Continued approval for this indication may be contingent upon verification and description of clinical benefit in confirmatory trial(s)
Selumetinib/ KOSELUGO	Inhibitor of mitogen-activated protein kinases 1 and 2 (MEK1/2). MEK1/2 proteins are upstream regulators of the extracellular signal-related kinase (ERK) pathway. Both MEK and ERK are critical components of the RAS-regulated RAF-MEK-ERK pathway, which is often activated in different types of cancers	Treatment of pediatric patients 2 years of age and older with neurofibromatosis type 1 (NF1) who have symptomatic, inoperable plexiform neurofibromas (PN)
Sirolimus/ Rapamycin	FKBP12/mTOR Sirolimus inhibits T-lymphocyte activation and proliferation that occurs in response to antigenic and cytokine (interleukin [IL]-2, IL-4, and IL-15) stimulation by a mechanism that is distinct from that of other immunosuppressants. Sirolimus also inhibits antibody production. In cells, sirolimus binds to the immunophilin, FK Binding Protein-12 (FKBP-12), to generate an immunosuppressive complex. The sirolimus-FKBP-12 complex has no effect on calcineurin activity. This complex binds to and inhibits the activation of the mammalian Target Of Rapamycin (mTOR), a key regulatory kinase. This inhibition suppresses cytokine-driven T cell proliferation, inhibiting the progression from the G1 to the S phase of the cell cycle. Studies in experimental models show that sirolimus prolongs allograft (kidney, heart, skin, islet, small bowel, pancreatico-duodenal, and bone marrow) survival in mice, rats, pigs, and/or primates. Sirolimus reverses	Rapamune is an mTOR inhibitor immunosuppressant indicated for 1.The prophylaxis of organ rejection in patients aged ≥13 years receiving renal transplants: (a) Patients at low- to moderate-immunologic risk - use initially with cyclosporine (CsA) and corticosteroids. CsA withdrawal is recommended 2-4 months after transplantation. (b) Patients at high-immunologic risk - use in combination with CsA and corticosteroids for the first 12 months following transplantation. Safety and efficacy of CsA withdrawal has not been established in high risk patients. 2.Rapamune is an mTOR inhibitor indicated for the treatment of patients with lymphangioleiomyomatosis

	acute rejection of heart and kidney allografts in rats and prolongs the graft survival in presensitized rats. In some studies, the immunosuppressive effect of sirolimus lasts up to 6 months after discontinuation of therapy. This tolerization effect is alloantigen-specific. Lymphangioleiomyom-atosis involves lung tissue infiltration with smooth muscle-like cells that harbor inactivating mutations of the tuberous sclerosis complex (TSC) gene (LAM cells). Loss of TSC gene function activates the mTOR signalling pathway, resulting in cellular proliferation and release of lymphangiogenic growth factors. Sirolimus inhibits the activated mTOR pathway and thus the proliferation of LAM cells.	
Sorafenib/ Nexavar	VEGFR1/2/3 Sorafenib has been shown to inhibit multiple intracellular (c-CRAF, BRAF and mutant BRAF) and cell surface kinases (KIT, FLT- 3, RET, RET/PTC, VEGFR-1, VEGFR- 2, VEGFR- 3, and PDGFR-ß). Several of these kinases are thought to be involved in tumor cell signalling, angiogenesis and apoptosis. Sorafenib inhibited tumor growth of HCC, RCC, and DTC human tumor xenografts in immunocompromised mice. Reductions in tumor angiogenesis were seen in models of HCC and RCC upon sorafenib treatment, and increases in tumor apoptosis were observed in models of HCC, RCC, and DTC.	Treatment of 1.Unresectable hepatocellular carcinoma (HCC) 2. Advanced renal cell carcinoma (RCC) 3. Locally recurrent or metastatic, progressive, differentiated thyroid carcinoma (DTC) refractory to radioactive iodine treatment
Sunitinib/ Sutent	Multiple kinases. Sunitinib is a small molecule that inhibits multiple receptor tyrosine kinases (RTKs), some of which are implicated in tumor growth, pathologic angiogenesis, and metastatic progression of cancer. Sunitinib was evaluated for its inhibitory activity against a variety of kinases (>80 kinases) and was identified as an inhibitor of platelet-derived growth factor receptors (PDGFRα and PDGFRβ), vascular endothelial growth factor receptors (VEGFR1, VEGFR2 and VEGFR3), stem cell factor receptor (KIT), Fms-like tyrosine kinase-3 (FLT3), colony stimulating factor receptor Type 1 (CSF-1R), and the glial cell-line derived neurotrophic factor receptor	The treatment of: 1. Gastrointestinal stromal tumor (GIST) after disease progression on or intolerance to imatinib mesylate. 2. Advanced renal cell carcinoma (RCC). 3. Progressive, well-differentiated pancreatic neuroendocrine tumors (pNET) in patients with unresectable locally advanced or metastatic disease

	(RET). Sunitinib inhibited the phosphorylation of multiple RTKs (PDGFRβ, VEGFR2, KIT) in tumor xenografts expressing RTK targets in vivo and demonstrated inhibition of tumor growth or tumor regression and/or inhibited metastases in some experimental models of cancer. Sunitinib demonstrated the ability to inhibit growth of tumor cells expressing dysregulated target RTKs (PDGFR, RET, or KIT) in vitro and to inhibit PDGFRβ- and VEGFR2-dependent tumor angiogenesis in vivo.	
Temsirolimus/ Torisel	FKBP12/mTOR. Temsirolimus is an inhibitor of mTOR (mammalian target of rapamycin). Temsirolimus binds to an intracellular protein (FKBP-12), and the protein-drug complex inhibits the activity of mTOR that controls cell division. Inhibition of mTOR activity resulted in a G1 growth arrest in treated tumor cells. When mTOR was inhibited, its ability to phosphorylate p70S6k and S6 ribosomal protein, which are downstream of mTOR in the PI3 kinase/AKT pathway was blocked. In in vitro studies using renal cell carcinoma cell lines, temsirolimus inhibited the activity of mTOR and resulted in reduced levels of the hypoxia-inducible factors HIF-1 and HIF-2 alpha, and the vascular endothelial growth factor.	Treatment of advanced renal cell carcinoma (RCC)
Tofacitinib/ Xeljanz/ Xeljanz XR	JAK Tofacitinib is a Janus kinase (JAK) inhibitor. JAKs are intracellular enzymes which transmit signals arising from cytokine or growth factor-receptor interactions on the cellular membrane to influence cellular processes of hematopoiesis and immune cell function. Within the signalling pathway, JAKs phosphorylate and activate Signal Transducers and Activators of Transcription (STATs) which modulate intracellular activity including gene expression. Tofacitinib modulates the signalling pathway at the point of JAKs, preventing the phosphorylation and activation of 26 Reference ID: 4467787 STATs. JAK enzymes transmit cytokine signalling through pairing of JAKs (e.g., JAK1/JAK3, JAK1/JAK2, JAK1/TyK2, JAK2 /JAK2). Tofacitinib inhibited the in	1. Rheumatoid arthritis: XELJANZ/XELJANZ XR is indicated for the treatment of adult patients with moderately to severely active rheumatoid arthritis who have had an inadequate response or intolerance to methotrexate. It may be used as monotherapy or in combination with methotrexate or other nonbiologic disease-modifying antrheumatic drugs (DMARDs). ○ Limitations of use: use of XELJANZ/XELJANZ XR in combination with biologic DMARDs or potent immunosuppressants such as azathioprine and cyclosporine is not recommended. 2. Psoriatic arthritis: XELJANZ/XELJANZ XR is indicated for the treatment of adult patients with active psoriatic

	vitro activities of JAK1/JAK2, JAK1/JAK3, and JAK2/JAK2 combinations with IC50 of 406, 56, and 1377 nM, respectively. However, the relevance of specific JAK combinations to therapeutic effectiveness is not known.	arthritis who have had an inadequate response or intolerance to methotrexate or other disease-modifying anti-rheumatic drugs (DMARDs). ○ Limitations of use: use of XELJANZ/XELJANZ XR in combination with biologic DMARDs or potent immunosuppressants such as azathioprine and cyclosporine is not recommended. 3. Ulcerative colitis: XELJANZ is indicated for the treatment of adult patients with moderately to severely active ulcerative colitis (UC), who have had an inadequate response or who are intolerant to TNF blockers. ○ Limitations of use: use of XELJANZ in combination with biological therapies for UC or with potent immunosuppressants such as azathioprine and cyclosporine is not recommended.
Trametinib/ Mekinist	MEK1/2 Trametinib is a reversible inhibitor of mitogen-activated extracellular signal-regulated kinase 1 (MEK1) and MEK2 activation and of MEK1 and MEK2 kinase activity. MEK proteins are upstream regulators of the extracellular signal-related kinase (ERK) pathway, which promotes cellular proliferation. BRAF V600E mutations result in constitutive activation of the BRAF pathway which includes MEK1 and MEK2. Trametinib inhibits cell growth of various BRAF V600 mutation-positive tumors in vitro and in vivo. Trametinib and dabrafenib target two different kinases in the RAS/RAF/MEK/ERK pathway. Use of trametinib and dabrafenib in combination resulted in greater growth inhibition of BRAF V600 mutation-positive tumor cell lines in vitro and prolonged inhibition of tumor growth in BRAF V600 mutation positive tumor xenografts compared with either drug alone.	MEKINIST is a kinase inhibitor indicated as a single agent 1. For the treatment of patients with unresectable or metastatic breast cancer with BRAF V600E or V600K mutations. 2. MEKINIST is indicated, in combination with dabrafenib, for • The treatment of patients with unresectable or metastatic breast cancer with BRAF V600E or V600K mutations. • The adjuvant treatment of patients with breast cancer with BRAF V600E or V600K mutations and involvement of lymph node(s), following complete resection. 3. The treatment of patients with metastatic non-small cell lung cancer (NSCLC) with BRAF V600E mutation.
Tucatinib/ TUKYSATM	Tyrosine kinase inhibitor of HER2. In vitro, tucatinib inhibits phosphorylation of HER2 and HER3, resulting in inhibition of downstream MAPK and AKT signaling and cell proliferation, and showed antitumor activity in HER2 expressing tumor cells	In combination with trastuzumab and capecitabine for treatment of adult patients with advanced unresectable or metastatic HER2-positive breast cancer, including patients with brain metastases, who have received one or more prior anti-HER2-based regimens

		in the metastatic setting
Vemurafenib/ Zelboraf	B-Raf Vemurafenib is a low molecular weight, orally available inhibitor of some mutated forms of BRAF serine-threonine kinase, including BRAF V600E. Vemurafenib also inhibits other kinases in vitro such as CRAF, ARAF, wild-type BRAF, SRMS, ACK1, MAP4K5, and FGR at similar concentrations. Some mutations in the BRAF gene including V600E result in constitutively activated BRAF proteins, which can cause cell proliferation in the absence of growth factors that would normally be required for proliferation. Vemurafenib has anti-tumor effects in cellular and animal models of breast cancers with mutated BRAF V600E.	The treatment of patients with unresectable or metastatic breast cancer with BRAF V600E mutation as detected. Limitation of use: ZELBORAF is not indicated for treatment of patients with wild-type BRAF breast cancer.
Upadacitinib/Rinvaq	Janus kinase inhibitor	The treatment of adults with moderately to severely active rheumatoid arthritis who have had an inadequate response or intolerance to methotrexate. Limitation of use: use of RINVOQ in combination with other JAK inhibitors, biologic DMARDs, or with potent immunosuppressants such as azathioprine and cyclosporine is not recommended

[1]Ogden Carr Bruton (1908 - 2003) was an American pediatrician

Summary of treatments derived from of the biological discoveries in the 20th Century

82 monoclonal antibodies (including biosimilars) and 55 small molecule protein kinase inhibitors are now FDA-approved for therapeutic purposes. Additional classes of therapeutics include new cellular therapies including gene-modified cellular therapies and gene therapies that have also been FDA-approved for therapeutic use All these agents will be described in detail in each book on diseases for which they have been approved.

This book deals with their use in **breast cancer.** It is one in a series of books on the impact of targeted biological treatments across the whole field of medicine as a series called Medicine 2020.

3. The biology of non-malignant human cells

Information in this section was adapted in part from Wikipedia Cell Biology (https://en.wikipedia.org/wiki/Cell_biology) and Wikipedia DNA replication (https://en.wikipedia.org/wiki/DNA_replication).

To fully understand how these new therapeutic agents work it is useful to understand how cells work – in particular what signalling pathways they use. Normal cells and cells in tissues affected by non- diseases use signalling pathways often different from those used by cells.

All human cells are derived from a single totipotent stem cell which is produced by the fusion of a single sperm with a single ovum. This totipotent stem cell has all the genes on its chromosomes responsible for the future growth and development of the fetus, including reproductive capacity. Cell biology is concerned with the physiological properties, metabolic processes, signalling pathways, life cycle, chemical composition and interactions of cells with their environment. Cell biology involves genetics, biochemistry, molecular biology, immunology and cytochemistry. Human cells are eukaryotes - they contain organelles. The generalized structure of a eukaryotic cell is shown in Figure 2.

Figure 2. A diagram of a mammalian cell.

This image, reproduced here from Wikimedia Commons, has been released into the public domain by its author, LadyofHats (Mariana Ruiz). Source: own work using Adobe Illustrator. Image renamed from Image:Animal cell structure.svg. https://commons.wikimedia.org/wiki/File:Animal_cell_structure_en.svg.

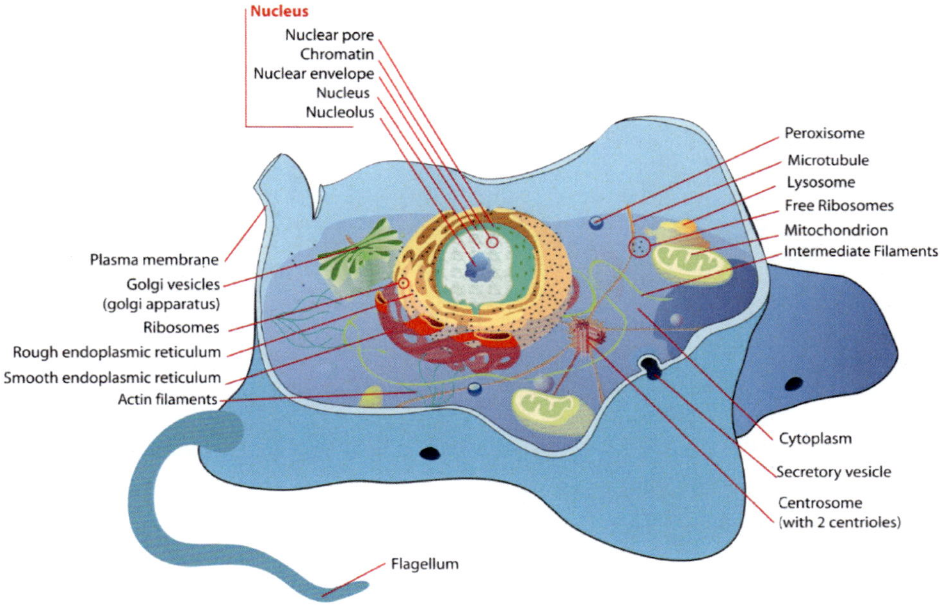

Most of the processes of eukaryotic cells are performed by a mixture of small organic molecules, inorganic ions, hormones and water. Approximately 75-85% of the cell's volume is due to water making it an indispensable solvent as a result of its polarity and structure. The shape of cells are generally round and spherical or oval.

The main constituents of the cell include proteins and lipids which are either free-flowing or membrane-bound, along with different internal compartments known as organelles. The cytoplasm is all of the material within a cell, enclosed by the cell membrane, except for the cell nucleus. The material inside the nucleus and contained within the nuclear membrane is termed the nucleoplasm. A cell's DNA, contained on the cell's chromosomes, is located within the cell's nucleus. The main components of the cytoplasm are cytosol – a gel-like substance, the organelles – the cell's internal sub-structures - and various cytoplasmic inclusions. Cell are composed of hydrophilic and hydrophobic regions. The hydrophilic regions of the cell are on both the inside and outside of the cell, while the hydrophobic regions are within the phospholipid bilayer of the cell membrane. A diagram of a mammalian cell membrane is shown in Figure 3

Figure 3. A diagram of a mammalian cell membrane.

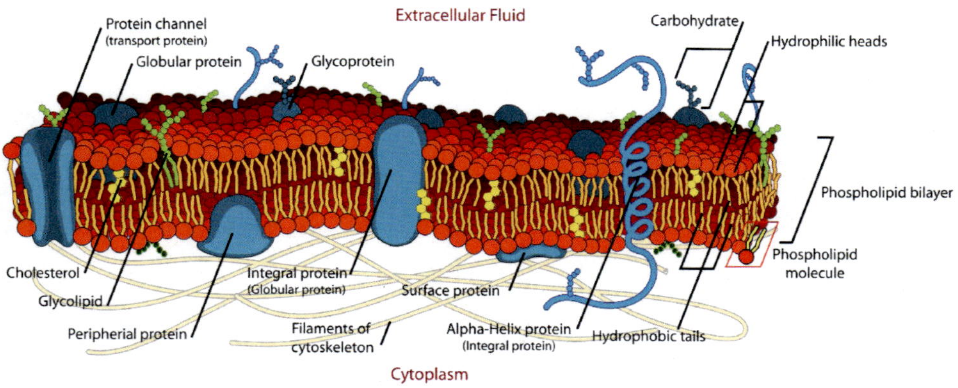

The figure shows the detailed diagram of the lipid bilayer of the cell membrane. The cell membrane, also called the plasma membrane or plasmalemma, is a semipermeable lipid bilayer common to all living cells. It contains a variety of biological molecules, primarily proteins and lipids, which are involved in a vast array of cellular processes. It also serves as the attachment point for both the intracellular cytoskeleton and, if present, the cell wall. This image, reproduced here from Wikimedia Commons, has been released into the public domain by its author, LadyofHats (Mariana Ruiz). Source: Own work. Image renamed from File:Cell membrane detailed diagram.svg.
https://commons.wikimedia.org/wiki/File:Cell_membrane_detailed_diagram_en.svg

In order for molecules to participate in reactions within the cell, they need to be able to cross this membrane layer to get into the cell. They accomplish this process of gaining access to the cell via osmotic pressure, diffusion, concentration gradients, and membrane channels. Inside the cell are extensive internal subcellular membrane-bounded compartments called organelles as well as a complex signalling network.

Figure 4. Some of the cell surface structures and internal signalling pathways of a normal human cell.

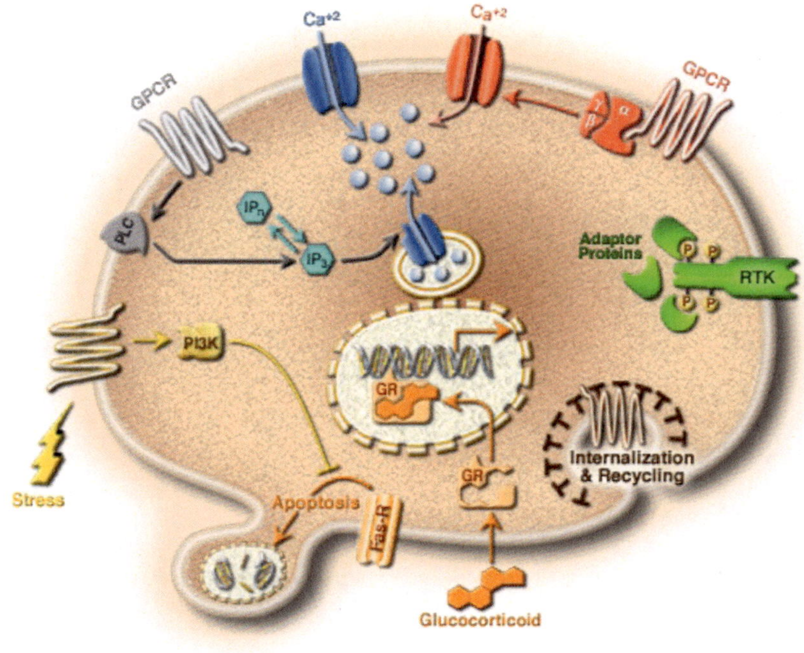

This image, reproduced here from Wikimedia Commons is in the public domain in the United States because it is a work prepared by an officer or employee of the United States Government as part of that person's official duties under the terms of Title 17, Chapter 1, Section 105 of the US Code. Source: http://dir.niehs.nih.gov/dirlst/imagemap/cell.jpg.

https://commons.wikimedia.org/wiki/File:NIEHScell.jpg

Cell growth pertains to the increase in the number of cells present in an organism as it grows and develops; in order for the organism to grow the number of cells present must increase. To enable cell growth and development the cell goes through the steps of the cell cycle: DNA replication, cell division, regeneration, specialization, and cell death. The cell cycle is divided into four distinct phases, G1, S, G2, and M. The G phases (cell growth) make up approximately 95% of the cycle. After proliferation cells then differentiate to become specialized in order to form specialized tissues, then organs and ultimately systems. The G phases along with the S phase – DNA replication, damage and repair - are considered to be the interphase portion of the cycle. While the M phase (mitosis and cytokinesis) is the cell division portion of the cycle. The cell cycle is regulated by a series of signalling factors and complexes such as cyclin-dependent kinases and p53. When the cell has completed its growth process, and if it is found to be damaged or altered, it undergoes cell death, either by apoptosis or necrosis, in order to eliminate the threat it can cause to the organism's survival. Some of the main cell surface structures and internal signalling processes are shown in Figure 4.

Essential cell processes include

- Active transport and passive transport – the movement of molecules into and out of cells
- Adhesion - holding cells and tissues together
- Cell movement - chemotaxis, contraction and cilia
- Cell signalling - regulation of cell behaviour by signals from outside and inside the cell
- Division – the process by which cells reproduce either by mitosis (to produce clones of the parent cell) or meiosis (to produce haploid gametes either male [sperm)] or female [ova]) dependent on the gender of the organism
- DNA repair - cell death and cell senescence
- Metabolism - glycolysis, respiration, photosynthesis, and chemosynthesis
- Signal transduction - the process by which the activities in the cell are regulated
- Transcription and mRNA splicing - gene expression

Three of the most important processes – signal transduction, gene expression and apoptosis (also known as programmed cell death) - are described further below. Some of the most important pathways for understanding the basis of targeted therapies, such as the pathways for angiogenesis, interkeukin (IL) 4, IL-12 and IL-23 and the TNF pathways are described in chapters dealing with the therapeutic use of molecules involved in these pathways.

Signal transduction and cell signalling pathways

Signal transduction is the process by which a chemical or physical signal is transmitted through a cell as a series of molecular events, most commonly protein phosphorylation catalyzed by protein kinases, which ultimately results in a cellular response. Proteins responsible for detecting stimuli such as ligands are termed receptors The changes elicited by ligand binding to a receptor give rise to a biochemical cascade otherwise known as a signalling path. A simplified representation of major signal transduction pathways in mammals

Figure 5. A simplified representation of major signal transduction pathways in mammals.

This image is reproduced here from Wikimedia Commons since permission has been granted by its creator, Cybertory, to copy, distribute and/or modify this document under the terms of the GNU Free Documentation License, Version 1.2 or any later version published by the Free Software Foundation;

Author: By Cybertory - This file was derived from: Signal transduction v1.png, CC BY-SA 3.0, https://commons.wikimedia.org/w/index.php?curid=12081090

https://en.wikipedia.org/wiki/Creative_Commons_license. No change has been made to the image.

Figure 5. A simplified representation of major signal transduction pathways in mammals

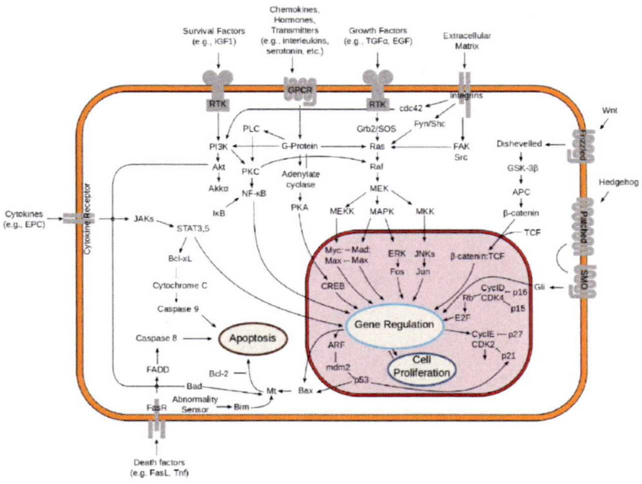

When signalling pathways interact with one another they form networks, which allow cellular responses to be coordinated, often by combinatorial signalling events. At the molecular level, such responses include changes in the transcription or translation of genes, and post-translational and conformational changes in proteins, as well as changes in their location. These molecular events are the basic mechanisms controlling cell growth, proliferation, metabolism and many other processes. In multicellular organisms, signal transduction pathways have evolved to regulate cell communication in a wide variety of ways.

Each component (or node) of a signalling pathway is classified according to the role it plays with respect to the initial stimulus. Ligands are termed first messengers, while receptors are the signal transducers, which then activate primary effectors. Such effectors are often linked to second messengers, which can activate secondary effectors, and so on. Depending on the efficiency of the nodes, a signal can be amplified (a concept known as signal gain), so that one signalling molecule can generate a response involving hundreds to millions of molecules With the advent of computational biology, the analysis of signalling pathways and networks has become an essential tool to understand cellular functions and disease, including signalling rewiring mechanisms underlying responses to acquired drug resistance.

Ligands

The majority of signal transduction pathways involve the binding of signalling molecules, known as ligands, to receptors that trigger events inside the cell. The binding of a signalling molecule with a receptor causes a change in the conformation of the receptor, known as receptor activation. Most ligands are soluble molecules from the extracellular medium which bind to cell surface receptors. These include growth factors, cytokines and neurotransmitters. Components of the extracellular matrix such as fibronectin and hyaluronan can also bind to such receptors (integrins and CD44, respectively). In addition, some molecules such as steroid hormones are lipid-soluble and thus cross the plasma membrane to reach nuclear receptors.

Some receptors such as HER2/neu are capable of ligand-independent activation when overexpressed or mutated. This leads to constitutive activation of the pathway, which may or may not be overturned by compensation mechanisms. In the case of HER2, which acts as a dimerization partner of other EGFRs, constitutive activation leads to hyperproliferation and cancer – primarily some cases of breast cancer and gastric cancer (HER2/neu is also known as receptor tyrosine-protein kinase erbB-2, CD340, proto-oncogene Neu and ERBB2).

Figure 6. A ribbon diagram of the Fab fragment of trastuzumab, a monoclonal antibody, bound to the extracellular domain of HER2.

This image, reproduced here from Wikimedia Commons, is in the public domain because its creator, Fvasconcellos, has placed it there. https://commons.wikimedia.org/wiki/File:Trastuzumab_Fab-HER2_complex_1N8Z.png#/media/File:Trastuzumab_Fab-HER2_complex_1N8Z.png; https://commons.wikimedia.org/wiki/User:Fvasconcellos. Created using Accelrys DS Visualizer Pro 1.6 and GIMP. More information: Cho HS, Mason K, Ramyar KX, et al. (2003). "Structure of the extracellular region of HER2 alone and in complex with the Herceptin Fab". Nature 421 (6924): 756–60. PMID 12610629. doi:10.1038/nature01392.

Figure 6. A ribbon diagram of the Fab fragment of trastuzumab, a monoclonal antibody, bound to the extracellular domain of HER2.

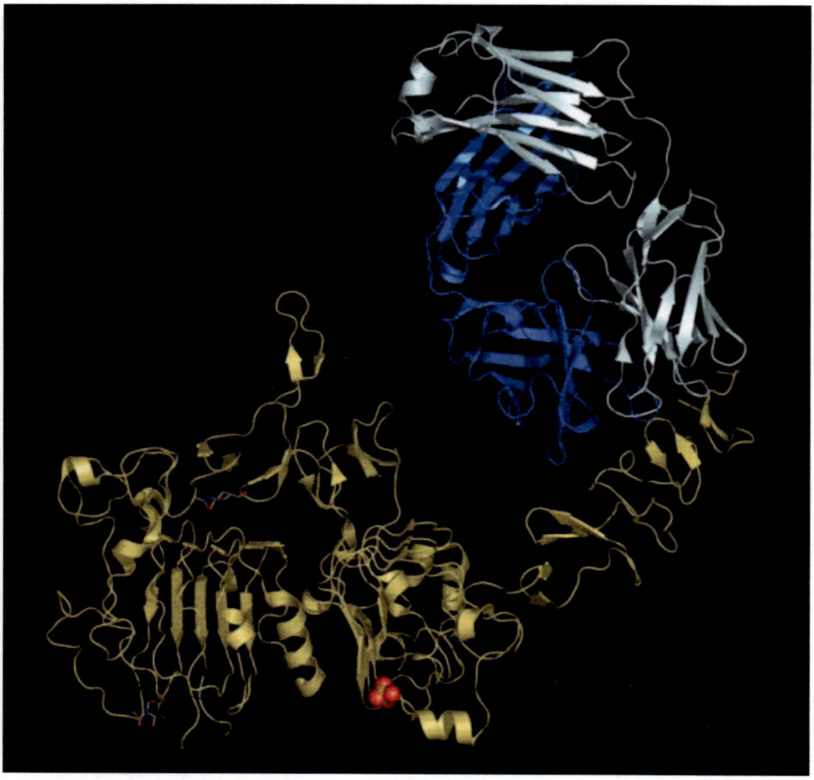

Legend: ▌ Trastuzumab Fab fragment, heavy chain ▯ ; Trastuzumab Fab fragment, light chain ▯ ; HER2, extracellular domain

Extracellular receptors, ligand binding, messengers and adaptor proteins

Extracellular receptors are integral transmembrane proteins that span the plasma membrane (Figure 2) of the cell, with one part of the receptor on the outside of the cell and the other on the inside. Signal transduction occurs as a result of a ligand binding to the outside region of the receptor (the ligand does not pass through the membrane). Ligand-receptor binding induces a change in the conformation of the inside part of the receptor, a process sometimes called "receptor activation". This results in either the activation of an enzyme domain of the receptor or the exposure of a binding site for other intracellular signalling proteins within the cell, eventually propagating the signal through the cytoplasm (Figure 5).

In mammalian cells most intracellular proteins activated by a ligand/receptor interaction possess an enzymatic activity; examples include tyrosine kinases and phosphatases. Often such enzymes are covalently linked to the receptor. Some of them create second messengers such as cyclic AMP and IP3, the latter controlling the release of intracellular calcium stores into the cytoplasm. Other activated proteins interact with adaptor proteins (an example is shown Figure 4) that facilitate signalling protein interactions and coordination of signalling complexes necessary to respond to a particular stimulus. Enzymes and adaptor proteins are both responsive to various second messenger molecules.

Many adaptor proteins and enzymes activated as part of signal transduction possess specialized protein domains that bind to specific secondary messenger molecules. For example, calcium ions bind to the EF hand domains of calmodulin, allowing it to bind and activate calmodulin-dependent kinase.

The following major extracellular receptor/ligand binding pathways will be discussed in more detail below:

- Tyrosine, seronine/threonine- and histidine-specific protein kinases
- Integrins
- Toll-like receptors
- Ligand-gated ion binding channels
- G protein-coupled receptors

G protein–coupled receptors (GPCRs) are a family of integral transmembrane proteins that possess seven transmembrane domains and are linked to a heterotrimeric G protein. G proteins, also known as guanine nucleotide-binding proteins, are a family of proteins that act as molecular switches inside cells, and are involved in transmitting signals from a variety of stimuli outside a cell to its interior. Their activity is regulated by factors that control their ability to bind to and hydrolyze guanosine triphosphate (GTP) to guanosine diphosphate (GDP). When they are bound to GTP, they are 'on', and, when they are bound to GDP, they are 'off'. A ribbon diagram of a G protein is shown in Figure 7 below.

Figure 7. Beta and gamma subunits of G-protein are shown by blue and red, respectively, in the phosducin-transducin beta-gamma complex. (Phosducin binds tightly to the beta gamma subunits (Gt beta gamma) of the heterotrimeric G protein transducin, preventing Gt beta gamma reassociation with Gt alpha-GDP and thereby inhibiting the G-protein cycle).

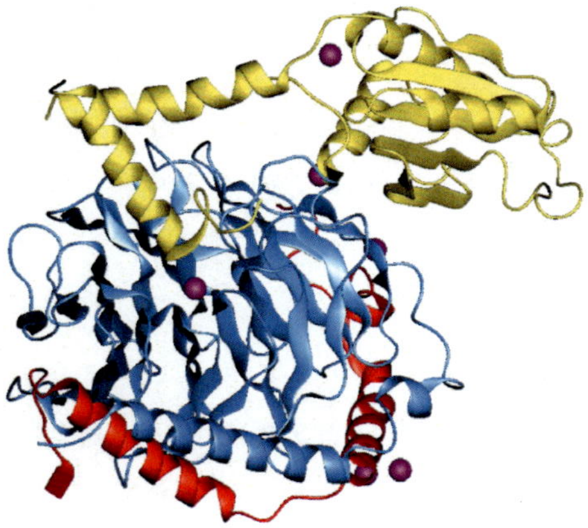

This image, reproduced here from Wikimedia Commons, has been released into the public domain by its creator, Andrei Lomize, has placed it there. By Andrei Lomize - Own work, Public Domain, https://commons.wikimedia.org/w/index.php?curid=34114642

https://commons.wikimedia.org/wiki/File:1b9x_opm.png#/media/File:1b9x_opm.png

Tyrosine and seronine/threonine-specific protein kinases

Receptor tyrosine kinases (RTKs) are transmembrane proteins with an intracellular kinase domain and an extracellular domain that binds ligands (Figure 4); examples include growth factor receptors such as the insulin receptor. To perform signal transduction, RTKs need to form dimers in the plasma membrane. The dimer is stabilized by ligands binding to the receptor. The interaction between the cytoplasmic domains stimulates the autophosphorylation of tyrosine residues within the intracellular kinase domains of the RTKs, causing conformational changes. Subsequent to this, the receptors' kinase domains are activated, initiating phosphorylation signalling cascades of downstream cytoplasmic molecules that facilitate various cellular processes such as cell differentiation and metabolism. Many serine/threonine and dual-specificity protein kinases are important for signal transduction, either acting downstream of receptor tyrosine kinases, or as membrane-embedded or cell-soluble versions in their own right. The process of signal transduction involves around 560 known protein kinases and pseudokinanases, encoded by the human kinome.

The kinome of an organism is the complete set of protein kinases encoded in its genome

As is the case with GPCRs, proteins that bind GTP play a major role in signal transduction from the activated RTK into the cell. In this case, the G proteins are members of the Ras, Rho (see Figure 4 above), and Raf families, referred to collectively as small G proteins. They act as molecular switches usually tethered to membranes by isoprenyl groups linked to their carboxyl ends. Upon activation, they assign proteins to specific membrane subdomains where they participate in signalling. Activated RTKs in turn activate small G proteins that activate guanine nucleotide exchange factors such as SOS1. Once activated, these exchange factors can activate more small G proteins, thus amplifying the receptor's initial signal. The mutation of certain RTK genes, as with that of GPCRs, can result in the expression of receptors that exist in a constitutively activated state. Such mutated genes may act as oncogenes. An example is the BCR-ABL gene, which is translated to the BCR-ABL protein, a growth factor responsible for the development of chronic myeloid leukemia (CML). The first tyrosine kinase inhibitor developed that was therapeutically successful is imatinib, now routinely used as first-line treatment of CML, obviating the need in many cases of the only curative treatment for CML – allogeneic hematopoietic stem cell transplantaion, a procedure that had a treatment-related mortality of 20-30%.

Integrins

Integrins are produced by a wide variety of cells. They play a role in cell attachment to other cells and the extracellular matrix and in the transduction of signals from extracellular matrix components such as fibronectin and collagen (Figure 8).

Figure 8. An overview of integrin-mediated signal transduction, adapted from Hehlgens et al. (2007).

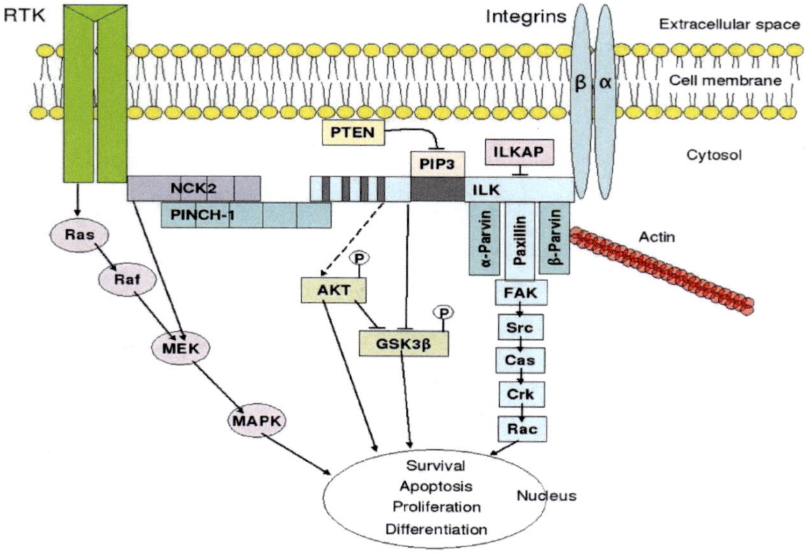

This image, reproduced here from Wikimedia Commons, has been released into the public domain by its author, K.murphy at English Wikipedia. https://commons.wikimedia.org/wiki/File:Integrin_sig_trans_overview.jpeg

Original source: Hehlgans S, Haase M, Cordes N (Jan 2007). "Signalling via integrins: implications for cell survival and anticancer strategies". Biochimica et Biophysica Acta. 1775 (1): 163–80. doi:10.1016/j.bbcan.2006.09.001. PMID 17084981.

Ligand binding to the extracellular domain of integrins changes the protein's conformation, clustering it at the cell membrane to initiate signal transduction. Integrins lack kinase activity; hence, integrin-mediated signal transduction is achieved through a variety of intracellular protein kinases and adaptor molecules, the main coordinator being integrin-linked kinase. As shown in Figure 8, cooperative integrin-RTK signalling determines the timing of cellular survival, apoptosis, proliferation and differentiation.

Toll-like receptors

When activated, toll-like receptors (TLRs) take adapter molecules within the cytoplasm of cells in order to propagate a signal.

Figure 9. Cellular signalling pathways activated by Toll-like receptors. Dashed lines represent unknown associations.

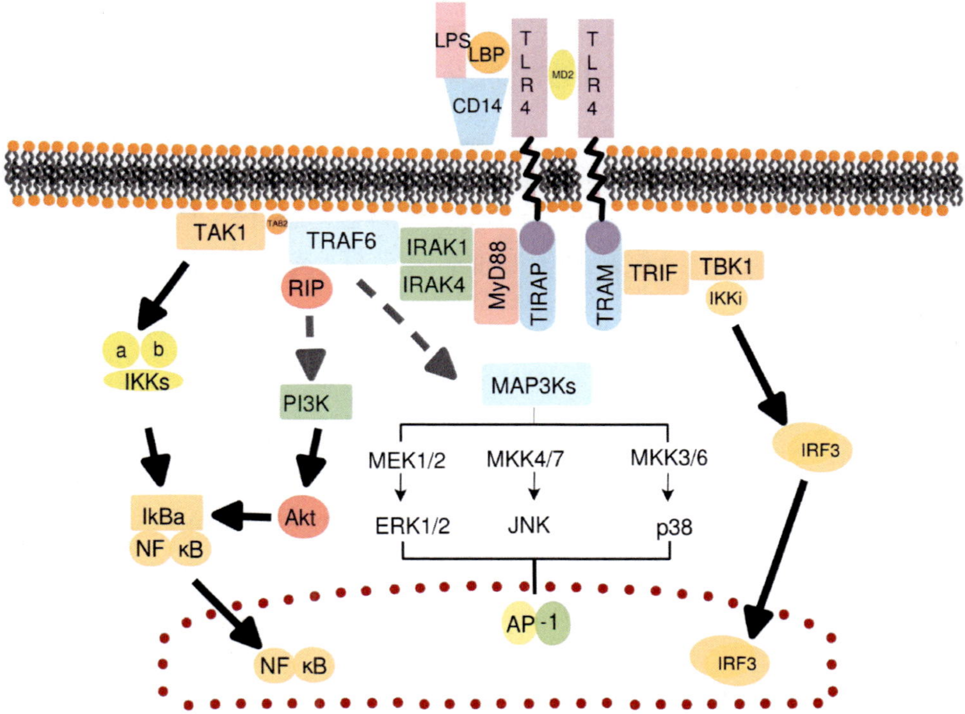

Four adaptor molecules are known to be involved in signalling. These are Myd88, TIRAP, TRIF, and TRAM. These adapter molecules activate other intracellular molecules such as IRAK1, IRAK4, TBK1, and IKKi that amplify the signal, eventually leading to the induction or suppression of genes that cause certain responses. Thousands of genes are activated by TLR signalling, implying that this method constitutes an important gateway for gene modulation. The signalling pathways of toll-like receptors are shown in Figure 9 above.

Messenger systems

First messengers are the signalling molecules (hormones, neurotransmitters and paracrine/autocrine agents) that reach the cell from the extracellular fluid and bind to thier specific receptors.

Second messengers are the substances that enter the cytoplasm and act within the cell to trigger a response. Second messengers serve as chemical relays from the plasma membrane to the cytoplasm, thus carrying out intracellular signal transduction.

Calcium

The release of calcium ions from the endoplasmic reticulum into the cytosol results in its binding to signalling proteins that are then activated. It is then sequestered in the smooth endoplasmic reticulum and the mitochondria (Figure 1). Calcium is used in many processes including muscle contraction, neurotransmitter release from nerve endings, and cell migration. The three main pathways that lead to its activation are GPCR pathways, RTK pathways, and gated ion channels. It regulates proteins either directly or by binding to an enzyme.

Cellular responses

Gene activations and metabolism alterations are examples of cellular responses to extracellular stimulation that require signal transduction. Gene activation leads to further cellular effects, since the products of responding genes include instigators of activation. Transcription factors produced as a result of a signal transduction cascade can activate even more genes. Hence, an initial stimulus can trigger the expression of a large number of genes, leading to physiological events. Examples are the increased uptake of glucose from the blood stream and the migration of neutrophils to sites of infection.

Mammalian cells require stimulation for cell division and survival. In the absence of growth factor, apoptosis (programmed cell death – see below) ensues. Such requirements for extracellular stimulation are necessary for controlling cell behavior. Signal transduction pathways are perceived to be so central to biological processes that a large number of diseases are attributed to their dysregulation. Three basic types of signals determine cellular growth:

1. Stimulatory signals (growth factors)

Transcription-dependent response
Steroids are an example of this. They bind DNA, which needs to be transcribed. The produced mRNA needs to be translated, and the produced protein/peptide can undergo posttranslational modification (PMT).

Transcription-independent response
Epidermal growth factor (EGF) is an example. It binds to the epidermal growth factor receptor (EGFR), which causes dimerization and autophosphorylation of the EGFR, which in turn activates the intracellular signalling pathway.

2. Inhibitory signals (cell-cell contact)

3. Permissive signals (cell-matrix interactions)

The combination of these signals are integrated in an altered cytoplasmic machinery which leads to altered cell behaviour.

Major cell signalling pathways

The following are some of the major cell signalling pathways, demonstrating how ligands binding to their receptors can affect second messengers and eventually result in altered cellular responses.

- MAPK/ERK pathway: a pathway that couples intracellular responses to the binding of growth factors to cell surface receptors. This pathway is very complex and includes many protein components. In many cell types, activation of this pathway promotes cell division, and many forms of cancer are associated with aberrations in it.

- cAMP-dependent pathway: cAMP works by activating protein kinase A (PKA, cAMP-dependent protein kinase. Further effects depend mainly on cAMP-dependent protein kinase, which vary based on the type of cell involved.

- IP3/DAG pathway: PLC cleaves the phospholipid phosphatidylinositol 4,5-bisphosphate (PIP2), yielding diacyl glycerol (DAG) and inositol 1,4,5-triphosphate (IP3). DAG remains bound to the membrane, and IP3 is released as a soluble structure into the cytosol. IP3 then diffuses through the cytosol to bind to IP3 receptors, particular calcium channels in the endoplasmic reticulum (ER). These channels are specific to calcium and allow the passage of only calcium to move through. This causes the cytosolic concentration of calcium to increase, in turn precipitating a cascade of intracellular changes and activity. In addition, calcium and DAG together work to activate PKC, which then phosphorylates other molecules, leading to altered cellular activity.

DNA, RNA and genes

DNA is a molecule composed of two chains that coil around each other to form a double helix carrying the genetic instructions used in the growth, development, functioning, and reproduction of all known organisms and many viruses. DNA and ribonucleic acid (RNA) are nucleic acids. Nucleic acids, together with proteins, lipids and complex carbohydrates (polysaccharides), are one of the four major types of macromolecules that are essential for all known forms of life.

The two DNA strands are also known as polynucleotides as they are composed of simpler monomeric units called nucleotides. Each nucleotide is composed of one of four nitrogen-containing nucleobases (cytosine [C], guanine [G], adenine [A] or thymine [T]), a sugar called deoxyribose, and a phosphate group. The nucleotides are joined to one another in a chain by covalent bonds between the sugar of one nucleotide and the phosphate of the next, resulting in an alternating sugar-phosphate

Figure 10 is a graphic of DNA replication

By LadyofHats - Own work, CC0,

https://commons.wikimedia.org/w/index.php?curid=8011953

Figure 10. A graphic of DNA replication.

.

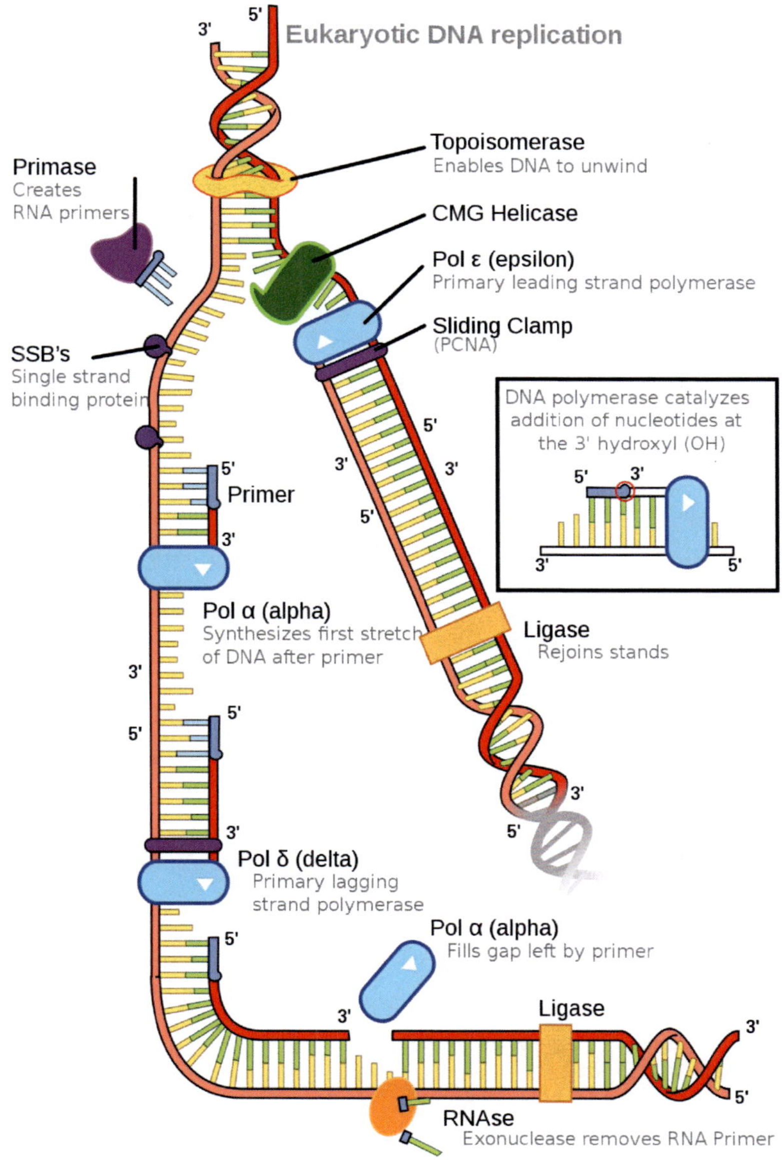

The nitrogenous bases of the two separate polynucleotide strands are bound together, according to base pairing rules (A with T and C with G), with hydrogen bonds to make double-stranded DNA in a helical form.

As seen in Figure 10, many enzymes are involved in DNA replication.

Genes

A gene is a sequence of nucleotides in DNA or RNA that codes for a molecule that has a function, although it is important to realize that not all genes do this.

Genes are contained on the chromosomes in the cell nucleus. During gene expression, the DNA is first copied into RNA. The RNA can be directly functional or be the intermediate template for a protein that performs a function.
A chromosome consists of a long strand of DNA containing many genes. A human chromosome can have up to 500 million base pairs of DNA with thousands of genes. Gene expression is the process by which information from a gene is used in the synthesis of a functional gene product. These products are often proteins. When the end-product is a protein, genes are first transcribed into RNA, and this transcript is then translated into protein. Several steps in the gene expression process may be modulated, including transcription, RNA splicing, translation and post-translational modification of the protein. Gene regulation gives the cell control over structure and function, and is the basis for cellular differentiation, morphogenesis and the versatility and adaptability of any organism.

Genes are expressed by being transcribed into RNA, and this transcript may then be translated into protein. Figure 11 shows how translation of messenger RNA and protein synthesis takes place in ribosomes.

Figure 11. Diagram showing how translation of messenger RNA and protein synthesis takes place in ribosomes. This work has been released into the public domain by its author, LadyofHats. By LadyofHats - Own work based on:[1], [2], [3], [4], [5], [6], [7], and [8]., Public Domain,
https://commons.wikimedia.org/w/index.php?curid=4889777;
https://en.wikipedia.org/wiki/Translation_(biology)#/media/File:Ribosome_mRNA_translation_en.svg

Figure 11. Diagram showing how translation of messenger RNA and protein synthesis takes place in ribosomes.

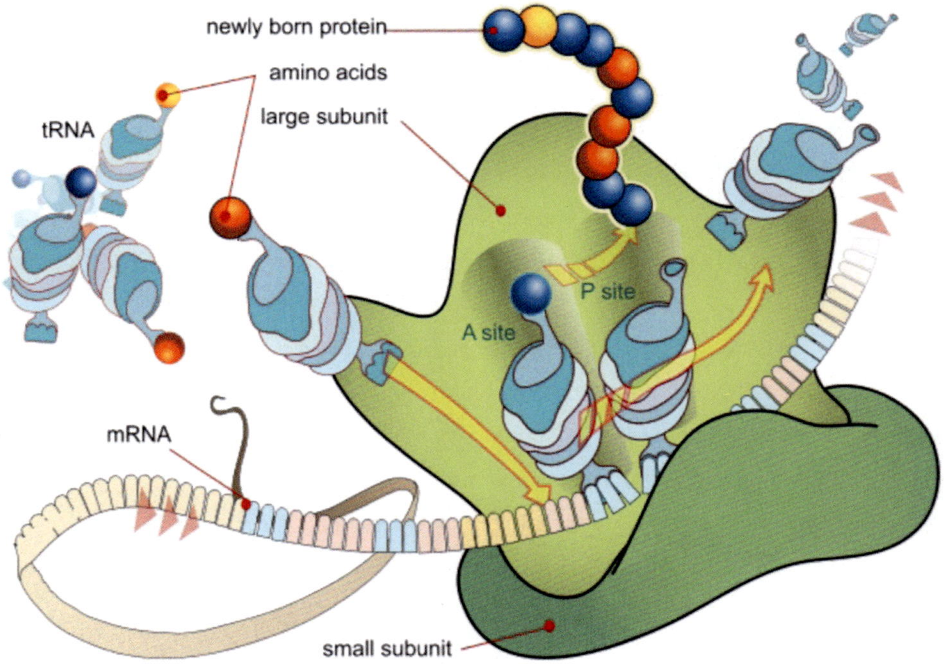

Protein folding

A polypeptide (protein) folds into its characteristic and functional three-dimensional structure from a random coil. Each protein exists as an unfolded polypeptide or random coil when translated from a sequence of messenger (m) RNA into a linear chain of amino acids (Figure 12, left hand image). Amino acids interact with each other to produce a well-defined three-dimensional structure.

Figure 12 shows a protein before (left) and after (right) folding.

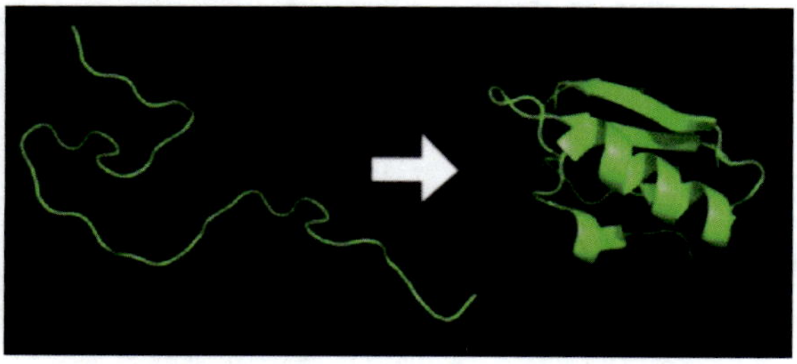

This image, reproduced here from Wikimedia Commons, is in the public domain because

its creator has placed it there. By No machine-readable author provided. DrKjaergaard assumed (based on copyright claims). - No machine-readable source provided. Own work assumed (based on copyright claims). Public Domain, https://commons.wikimedia.org/w/index.php?curid=1967109. https://en.wikipedia.org/wiki/Protein_folding#/media/File:Protein_folding.png

4. The biology ofmalignant human cells

Some of the material in this chapter was derived from https://en.wikipedia.org/wiki/Carcinogenesis#Cause

and

https://en.wikipedia.org/wiki/Cancer#Pathophysiology.

Malignant human cells

Defects in genes (DNA), epigenetic factors and mismatch repair systems can all cause human cells to become malignant.

Genes

With the exception of congenital disorders, all human malignant cells have an abnormality of their genetic systems, and differ in this regard to abnormal, but non-malignant, human cells. Carcinogenesis is the formation of a cancer, whereby normal cells are transformed into cancer cells. The process is characterized by changes at the cellular, genetic, and epigenetic levels and abnormal cell division. Cell division is a physiological process that occurs in almost all tissues and under a variety of circumstances. Normally the balance between proliferation and programmed cell death, in the form of apoptosis, is maintained to ensure the integrity of tissues and organs. According to the prevailing accepted theory of carcinogenesis, the somatic mutation theory, mutations in DNA and epimutations that lead to cancer disrupt these orderly processes by disrupting the programming regulating the processes, upsetting the normal balance between proliferation and cell death. This results in uncontrolled cell division and the evolution of those cells by natural selection in the body. Only certain mutations lead to cancer whereas the majority of mutations do not.

A series of several mutations to certain classes of genes is usually required before a normal cell will transform into a malignant cell.

In order for a normal cell to transform into a malignant cell, the genes that regulate cell growth and differentiation must be altered.

The affected genes are divided into two broad categories. Oncogenes are genes that promote cell growth and reproduction. Tumor suppressor genes are genes that inhibit cell division and survival. Transformation can occur through the formation of novel oncogenes, the inappropriate over-expression of normal oncogenes, or by the under-expression or disabling of tumor suppressor genes. Typically, changes in multiple genes are required to transform a normal cell into a cancer cell (Figure 13).

This image, reproduced here from Wikimedia Commons, is in the public domain because it is a work prepared by an officer or employee of the United States Government as part of that person's official duties under the terms of Title 17, Chapter 1, Section 105 of the US Code. By National Cancer Institute, Public Domain, https://commons.wikimedia.org/w/index.php?curid=1972023. (Figure 13).

Figure 13 illustrates that cancers are caused by a series of mutations. Each mutation alters the behavior of the cell somewhat.

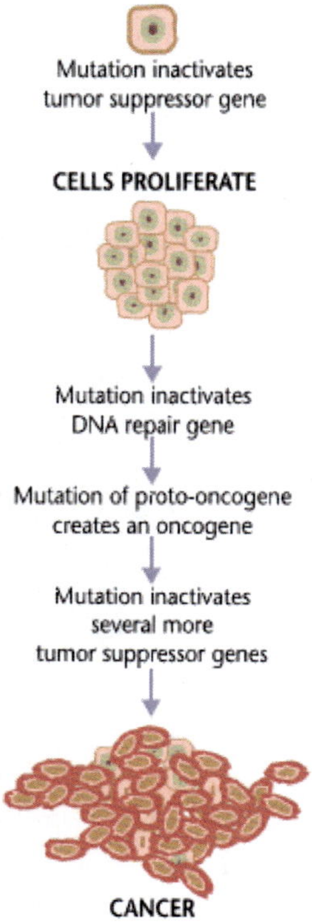

The abnormal biological properties of human malignant cells can be summarized as follows:

- Acquisition of self-sufficiency in growth signals, leading to unchecked growth.
- Loss of sensitivity to anti-growth signals, also leading to unchecked growth.
- Loss of capacity for apoptosis, allowing growth despite genetic errors and external anti-growth signals.
- Loss of capacity for senescence, leading to limitless replicative potential (immortality).
- Acquisition of sustained angiogenesis, allowing the tumor to grow beyond the limitations of passive nutrient diffusion.
- Acquisition of ability to invade neighbouring tissues, the defining property of invasive carcinoma.

- Acquisition of ability to seed metastases at distant sites, a late-appearing property of some tumors (carcinomas or others).

Involved in these steps is

- Loss of capacity to repair genetic errors, leading to an increased mutation rate (genomic instability), thus accelerating all the above changes.

Often, the multiple genetic changes that result in cancer may take many years to accumulate. During this time, the biological behavior of the pre- cells slowly changes from the properties of normal cells to those with cancer-like properties (Figure 14).

Figure 14

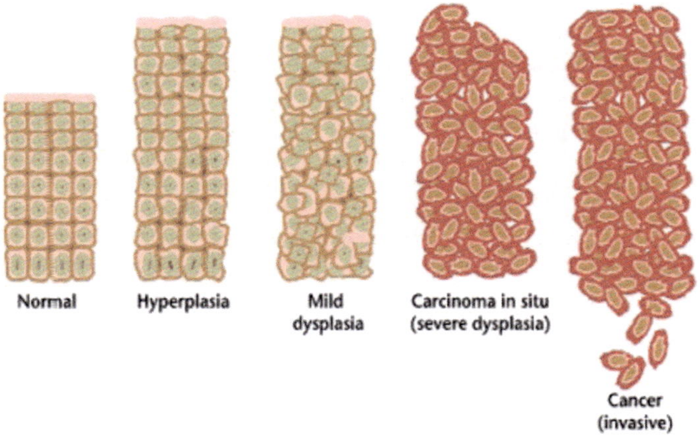

Figure 14 shows that tissue can be organized in a continuous spectrum from normal to malignant. This image, reproduced here from Wikimedia Commons, is in the public domain because it is a work prepared by an officer or employee of the United States Government as part of that person's official duties under the terms of Title 17, Chapter 1, Section 105 of the US Code. By Unknown author - National Cancer Institute (archived), Public Domain, https://commons.wikimedia.org/w/index.php?curid=658483

Epigenetic factors also plays a major role in the development of human cancers.

Epigenetic modifications to the DNA of cancer cells do not involve a change in the nucleotide sequence, but instead involve a change in the way the genetic code is expressed. Epigenetic alterations may be just as important, or even more important, than genetic mutations in a cell's transformation to malignancy. In malignant cells loss of expression of genes occurs about 10 times more frequently by transcription silencing (caused by epigenetic promoter hypermethylation of CpG islands) than by mutations. In different types of cancer, a variety of epigenetic mechanisms can be perturbed, such as silencing of tumor suppressor genes and activation of oncogenes by altered CpG island methylation patterns, histone modifications, and dysregulation of DNA-binding proteins (Figure 15)

Figure 15 shows epigenetics patterns in a normal and cancer cells.

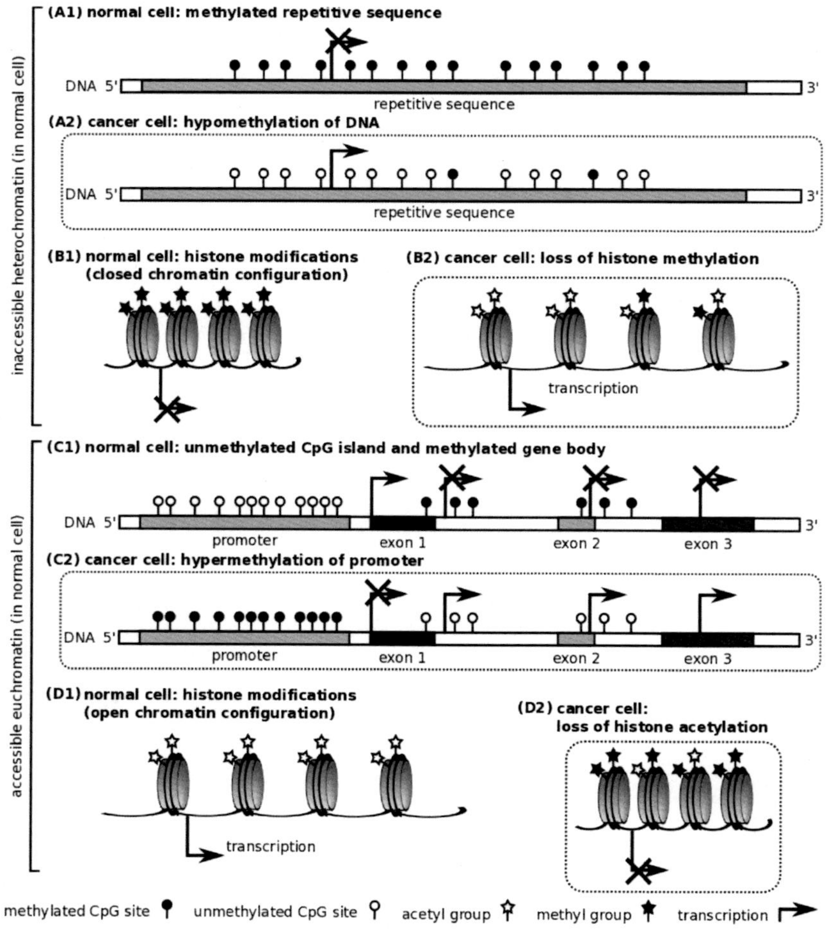

This image, reproduced here from Wikimedia Commons, was made by By Philippe Hupé - Emmanuel Barillot, Laurence Calzone, Philippe Hupé, Jean-Philippe Vert, Andrei Zinovyev, Computational Systems Biology of Cancer Chapman & Hall/CRC who have licensed the file under the Creative Commons Attribution-Share Alike 3.0 Unported license. https://creativecommons.org/licenses/by-sa/3.0/deed.en; https://commons.wikimedia.org/w/index.php?curid=18769951. No change has been made to this image.

Figure 16 shows a DNA molecule that is methylated on both strands on the center cytosine. DNA methylation plays an important role for epigenetic gene regulation in development and cancer. [Details: The picture shows the crystal structure of a short DNA helix with sequence "accgcCGgcgcc", which is methylated on both strands at the center cytosine. The structure was taken from the Protein Data Bank (accession number 329D), rendering was performed with VMD (Visual Molecular Dynamics rendering program) and post-processing was done in Photoshop]. This image, reproduced here from Wikimedia Commons, is by Christoph Bock, Max Planck Institute for Informatics - Own work, licensed under the Creative Commons Attribution-Share Alike 3.0 Unported license. https://creativecommons.org/licenses/by-sa/3.0/deed.en; https://commons.wikimedia.org/w/index.php?curid=17066877. No change has been made to this image.

Figure 16. A DNA molecule that is methylated on both strands on the center cytosine

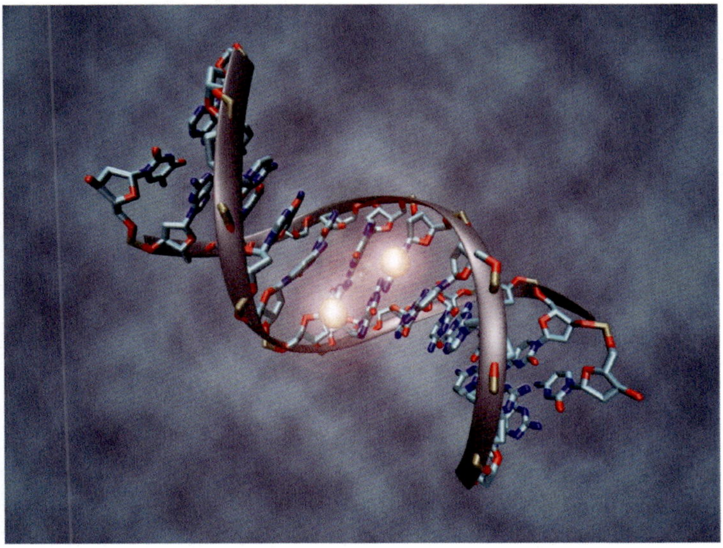

DNA mismatch repair systems

If DNA repair is deficient, DNA damage tends to accumulate. Such excess DNA damage can increase mutational errors during DNA replication due to error-prone translesion synthesis. Excess DNA damage can also increase epigenetic alterations due to errors during DNA repair. Such mutations and epigenetic alterations can give rise to malignancy. Germ line mutations in DNA repair genes cause only 2–5% of colon cancer cases. However, altered expression of microRNAs, causing DNA repair deficiencies, are frequently associated with cancers and may be an important causal factor for such cancers.

In non-hereditary cancers, a deficiency in DNA repair is occasionally found to be due to a mutation in a DNA repair gene, but reduced or absent expression of DNA repair genes is much more frequently due to epigenetic alterations that reduce or silence gene expression.

Cancer therapy procedures such as chemotherapy and radiotherapy work by overwhelming the capacity of the cells to repair DNA damage, resulting in their death. Cells that are most rapidly dividing – most typically cancer cells – are preferentially affected. An important side-effect is that other non-cancerous but rapidly dividing cells such as progenitor cells in the gut, skin, and hematopoietic system are also affected. Modern cancer treatments attempt to localize the DNA damage to cells and tissues only associated with cancer, either by physical means (concentrating the therapeutic agent in the region of the tumor) or by biochemical means (exploiting a feature unique to cancer cells in the body).

This book describes FDA-approved targeted biologic therapeutic agents for breast cancer.

5. Clinical and pathological features of breast cancer

Some information in this section was taken from Wikipedia Breast Cancer: https://en.wikipedia.org/wiki/Breast_cancer

Breast cancer is cancer that develops in breast tissue. Signs of breast cancer may include a lump in the breast, a change in breast shape, dimpling of the skin, fluid coming from the nipple, a newly inverted nipple, or a red or scaly patch of skin. In those with distant spread of the disease, there may be bone pain, swollen lymph nodes, shortness of breath, or jaundice.

Risk factors for developing breast cancer include being female, obesity, a lack of physical exercise, alcoholism, hormone replacement therapy during menopause, ionizing radiation, an early age at first menstruation, having children late in life or not at all, older age, having a prior history of breast cancer, and a family history of breast cancer.

Breast cancer most commonly develops in epithelial cells that form the lining of milk ducts and the lobules that supply these ducts with milk. Cancers developing from the ducts are known as ductal carcinomas, while those developing from lobules are known as lobular carcinomas. There are more than 18 other sub-types of breast cancer. Some, such as ductal carcinoma in situ, develop from pre-invasive lesions. The diagnosis of breast cancer is confirmed by taking a biopsy of the concerning tissue. Once the diagnosis is made, further tests are done to determine if the cancer has spread beyond the breast and which treatments are most likely to be effective.

A 2009 review for the US Preventive Services Task Force found evidence of benefit for mammographic screening in women 40 to 70 years of age, and the organization recommends screening every two years in women 50 to 74 years of age.

Outcomes for breast cancer vary depending on the cancer type, the extent of disease, and the person's age. The five-year survival rates in England and the United States are between 80 and 90%. Worldwide, breast cancer is the leading type of cancer in women, accounting for 25% of all cases. In 2018 it resulted in 2 million new cases and 627,000 deaths. It is more than 100 times more common in women than in men.

Signs and symptoms

Figure 17. Breast cancer showing an inverted nipple, lump, and skin dimpling.

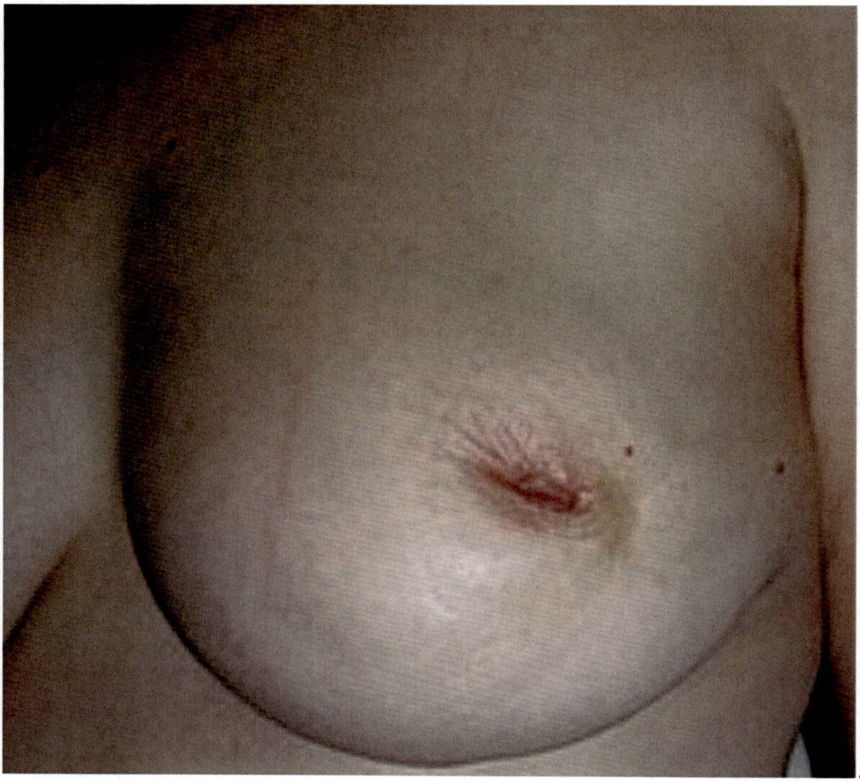

This image is by Hic et nunc - Own work, CC BY-SA 3.0, https://commons.wikimedia.org/w/index.php?curid=9722580. https://en.wikipedia.org/wiki/Breast_cancer#/media/File:Breast_cancer.jpg. This file is licensed under the Creative Commons Attribution-Share Alike 3.0 Unported license. No changes have been made to this imageb

Breast cancer most commonly presents as a lump that feels different from the rest of the breast tissue. More than 80% of cases are discovered when a person detects such a lump with the fingertips. The earliest breast cancers, however, are detected by a mammography. Lumps found in lymph nodes located in the armpits may also indicate breast cancer.

Inflammatory breast cancer accounts for less than 5% of breast cancer but it is an aggressive form of breast cancer characterized by the swollen, red areas formed on the top of the reast. As inflammatory breast cancer does not present as a lump there can sometimes be a delay in diagnosis. It is referred to as "inflammatory" due to its frequent presentation with symptoms resembling a skin inflammation, such as the streptococcal infection erysipelas (Figure 18).

Figure 18. Erysipelas involving the skin of the right lower leg.

Figure 18. Erysipelas involving the skin of the right lower leg.

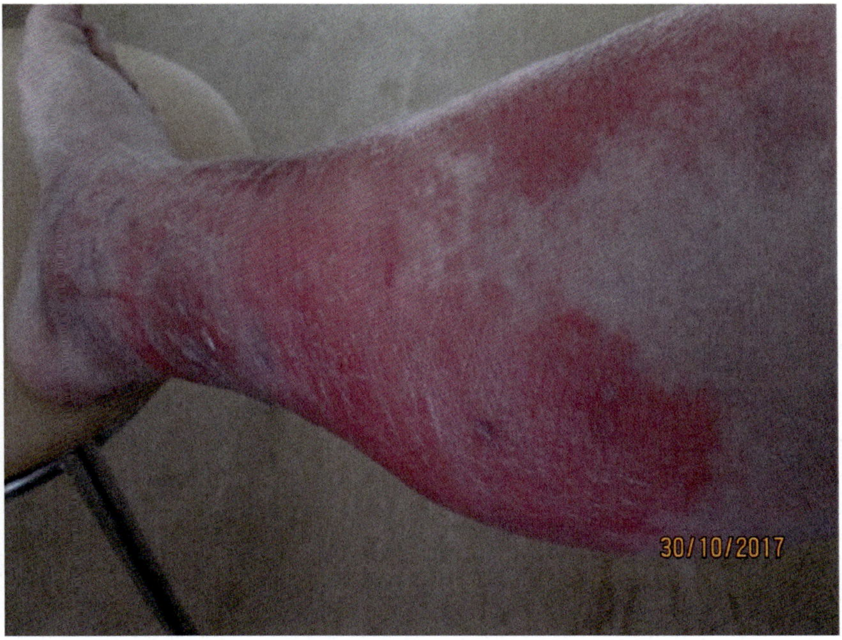

The symptoms caused by metastatic breast cancer will depend on the location of metastasis. Common sites of metastasis include bone, liver, lung, and brain.

Types of breast cancer

Figure 19. Pie chart of the incidence and prognosis of histopathologic breast cancer types.

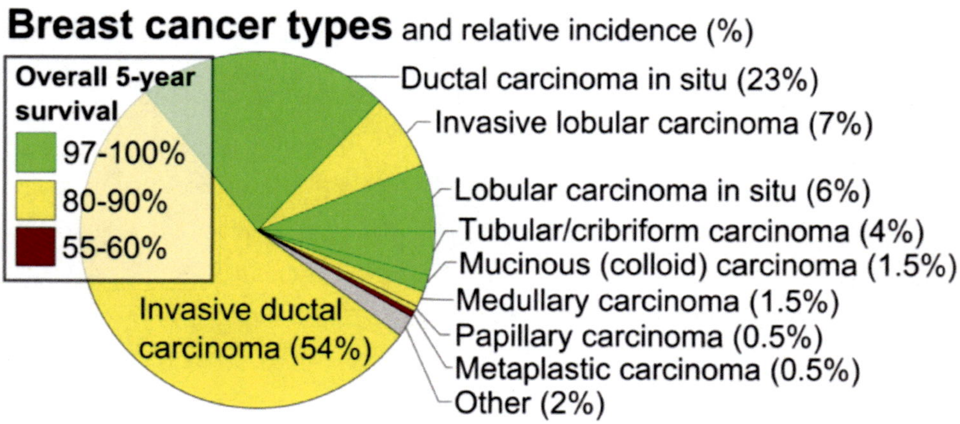

This image is by Mikael Häggström, M.D.- Author info- Reusing imagesMikael Häggström - Own work. https://commons.wikimedia.org/wiki/File:Pie_chart_of_incidence_and_prognosis_of_histopathologic_breast_cancer_types.png. Its author has placed it in the public domain. No changes were made to this image.

Staging of breast cancer (Figure 20 and 21)

Breast cancer staging using the TNM system is based on the size of the tumor (T), whether or not the tumor has spread to the lymph nodes (N) in the armpits, and whether the tumor has metastasized (M) (i.e. spread to a more distant part of the body). Larger size, nodal spread, and metastasis have a larger stage number and a worse prognosis.

Figure 20. The five stages of breast cancer.

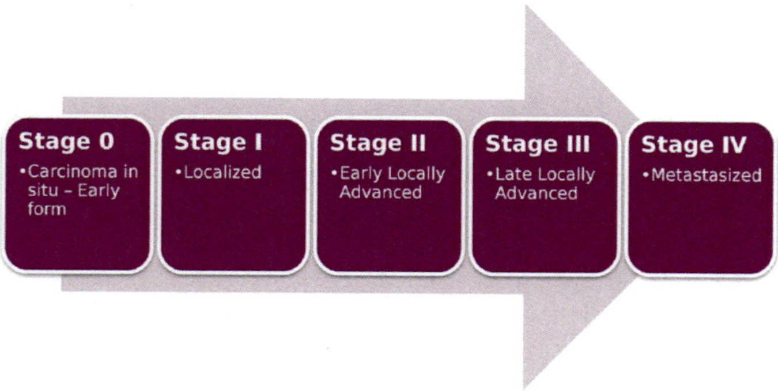

This image is by By Original drawing created by User:Simplyanon. Vectorized by User:忍者猫 - Vectorized version of File:Cancer stages.png, CC BY-SA 3.0, https://commons.wikimedia.org/w/index.php?curid=101222874https://en.wikipedia.org/wiki/Cancer_staging#/media/File:Cancer_stages.svg. This file is licensed under the Creative Commons Attribution-Share Alike 3.0 Unported license. No changes were made to this image.

Figure 21. 3D Medical illustration showing the TNM (tumor, node, metastasis) stages in breast cancer.

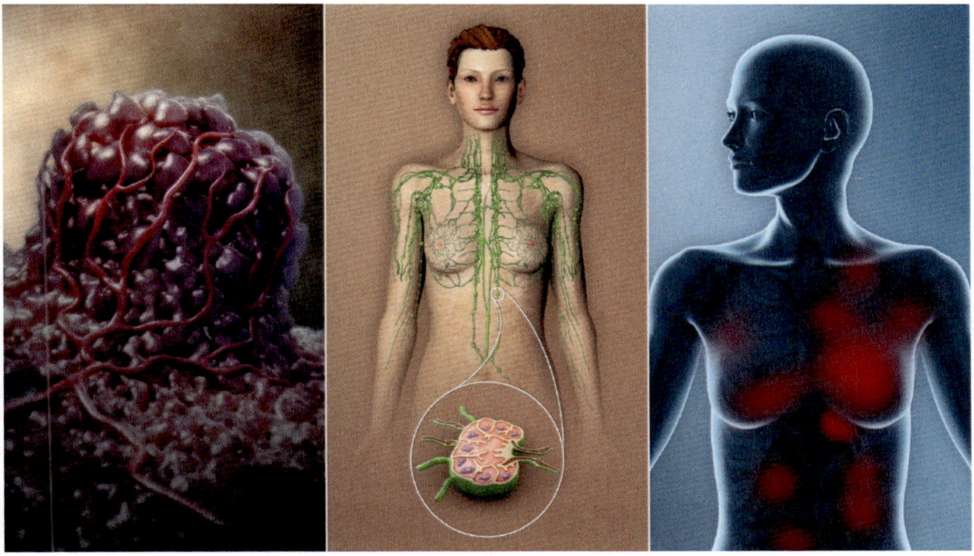

This image is by https://www.scientificanimations.com - https://www.scientificanimations.com/wiki-images/, CC BY-SA 4.0, https://commons.wikimedia.org/w/index.php?curid=85862273. https://en.wikipedia.org/wiki/Cancer_staging#/media/File:3D_medical_animation_TNM_Staging_System.jpg. This file is licensed under the Creative Commons Attribution-Share Alike 4.0 International license. No changes were made to this image.

Receptor status

Breast cancer cells have receptors on their surface and in their cytoplasm and nucleus. Chemical messengers such as hormones bind to receptors, and this causes changes in the cell. Breast cancer cells may or may not have three important receptors: estrogen receptor (ER), progesterone receptor (PR), and human epidermal growth factor receptor 2 (HER2). Receptor status of an individual breast cancer determines the suitability or otherwise for receiving additional treatment in addition to surgery, chest wall irradiation and chemotherapy. Such treatment is often called endocrine treatment (ET).

7. Overview of breast cancer treatment

Treatment for breast cancer depends on many factors especially the stage of the disease at diagnosis (Figures 20 and 21). A major key factor is whether the ipsilateral axillary lymph glands are involved by the tumour. A second key factor is whether metastatic disease is present at diagnosis. Breast cancer should be treated in a major hospital and, before any elective treatment is given, each new case should be reviewed by a **multi-disciplinary team** compising breast cancer surgeons, readiation oncologists, medical oncologists, the pathologist who examined the tissue biopsy, nursing and other allied staff. This ensures that the most appropriate treatment plan for an individual patient is devised and it serves an important role as a quality assurance tool.

Breast cancer is usually treated initially with surgery, which may be followed by chemotherapy or radiation therapy, or both. A multidisciplinary approach is preferable. Additionally, **hormone receptor-positive** cancers are usually treated with hormone-blocking therapy over courses of several years. Breast cancers that overexpress **HER2** are usualy given the monoclonal antibody trastuzumab, or a trastuzumab-based medication, in addition to all their other treatments.

Other immune-modulating treatments, may be administered in certain cases of metastatic and other advanced stages of breast cancer.

Non-metastatic breast cancer

Stage 1 cancers (and DCIS, lobular carcinoma in situ [LCIS]) are generally treated with lumpectomy and are sometimes with radiation to the ipsilateral chst wall.

Stage 2 and 3 cancers have a poorer prognosisand are generally treated with surgery followed by chemotherapy (plus trastuzumab for HER2+ cancers) and sometimes radiation to the chest wall.

Patients with hormone receptor-positive breast cancer should receive adjuvant endocrine therapy.

Most patients with locally advanced breast cancer are treated with neoadjuvant systemic therapy prior to proceeding with primary surgery.

Following surgery (with or without neoadjuvant systemic therapy), all patients who undergo breast-conserving surgery should undergo adjuvant RT to maximize locoregional control.

Patients with HER2-positive breast cancer and a complete response to neoadjuvant treatment should receive one year of trastuzumab, with or without pertuzumab, following completion of surgery. If residual disease is present, ado-trastuzumab emtansine should be administered, rather than trastuzumab.

For some patients with ER-positive breast cancer, in whom surgery is not an option or life expectancy is limited, primary hormonal treatment with either tamoxifen or an aromatase inhibitor without surgery can be used.

Metastatic breast cancer (MBC)

Stage 4 metastatic cancer has a poor prognosis and is managed by various combination of treatments including surgery, radiation, chemotherapy and targeted therapies.

For most patients with hormone-positive MBC, endocrine therapy with or without targeted treatments is preferred to chemotherapy

In general, single-agent chemotherapy, used in sequence, is preferable to combination chemotherapy, since the single-agent chemotherapy is reasonably likely to induce palliation with fewer side effects.

Women who progress ≥12 months from the end of adjuvant ET and patients who present with de novo metastatic breast cancer can be offered first-line ET or ET in combination with a cyclin-dependent kinase (CDK) 4/6 inhibitor. Other acceptable options include single-agent fulvestrant or anastrozole, or fulvestrant in combination with an AI or ribociclib.

For patients who have previously experienced progression on an AI and CDK 4/6 inhibitor, the approach should consider the patient's tumor phosphatidylinositol-4,5-

bisphosphate 3-kinase catalytic subunit alpha (PIK3CA) status: for those with PIK3CA-mutant cancers progressive on the combination of AIs and CDK 4/6 inhibitors, the combination of fulvestrant with the alpha isoform-specific phosphoinositide 3-kinase (PI3K) inhibitor alpelisib can be used.

For those with PIK3CA-mutant cancers progressive on the combination of AIs and CDK 4/6 inhibitors, options include fulvestrant monotherapy or everolimus-based combinations, with a choice between them driven by side-effect profiles.

For patients with HER2-positive breast cancer, HER2-directed therapy should be incorporated in their first-line treatment.

For patients with metastatic, HER2-negative breast cancer with germline BRCA mutations who have previously been treated with chemotherapy an oral inhibitor of poly (ADP-ribose) polymerase (PARP) is recommended.

Surgery

Surgery involves the physical removal of the tumor, typically along with some of the surrounding tissue. One or more lymph nodes may be biopsied during the surgery; increasingly, lymph node sampling is performed by a sentinel lymph node biopsy.

Standard surgical procedures include either:

Mastectomy – removal of the whole breast or lumpectomy - removal of a small part of the breast. Figure 22). Appearance of the chest wall after a right mastectomy.

This image is by Acrocynus - Acrocynus, CC BY-SA 3.0, https://commons.wikimedia.org/w/index.php?curid=3616194. https://en.wikipedia.org/wiki/Breast_cancer#/media/File:Mastectomie_02.jpg. This file is licensed under the Creative Commons Attribution-Share Alike 3.0 Unported, 2.5 Generic, 2.0 Generic and 1.0 Generic license. No changes have been made to this image.

Figure 22 shows the appearance of the chest wall after a right mastectomy.

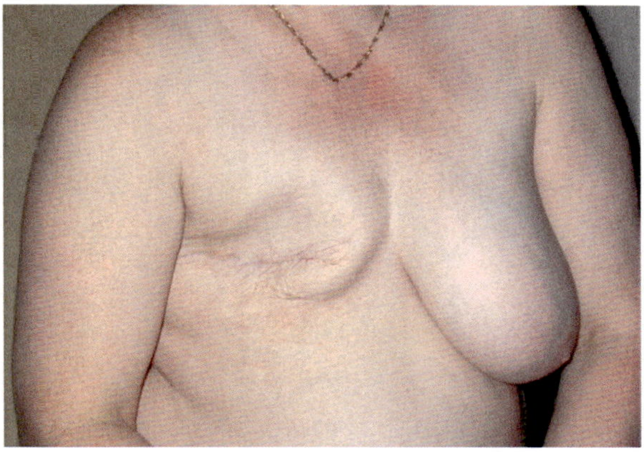

The decision regarding mastectomy or lumpectomy depends on the stage and grade of the breast cancer, as well as the patient's wishes and the surgeon's advice.

Once the tumor has been removed, if the person desires, breast reconstruction surgery, a type of plastic surgery, may then be performed to improve the aesthetic appearance of the treated site.

Figure 23. The appearance of the breast after bilateral nipple-sparing lumpectomy and implant reconstruction for bilateral breast cancer in a 57-year-old woman.

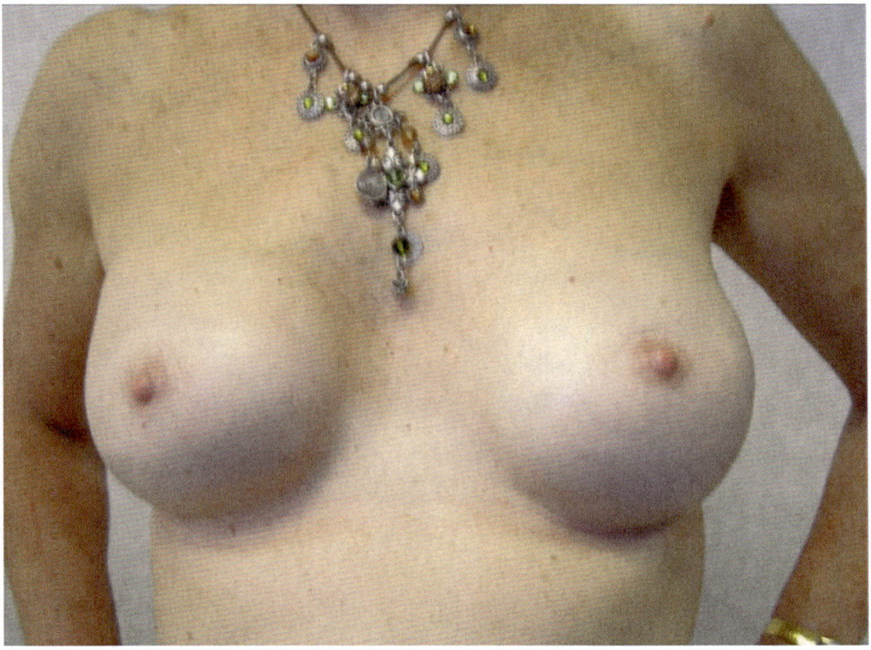

This image is by Sara Reefy, Neill Patani, Anne Anderson, Gwyne Burgoyne, Hisham Osman, KefahMokbel. - Sara Reefy, Neill Patani, Anne Anderson, Gwyne Burgoyne, Hisham Osman, KefahMokbel: Oncological outcome and patient satisfaction with skin-sparing Lumpectomy andimmediate breast reconstruction: a prospective observational study. In: BMC Cancer 2010, 10:171 doi:10.1186/1471-2407-10-171 [1] [2] Open Access, CC BY-SA 2.0, https://commons.wikimedia.org/w/index.php?curid=10254346. https://en.wikipedia.org/wiki/Breast_cancer#/media/File:Breast_reconstruction_15.jpg. This file is licensed under the Creative Commons Attribution-Share Alike 2.0 Generic license. No changes were made to this image

Medications

Medications used after and in addition to surgery are called adjuvant therapy. Chemotherapy or other types of therapy prior to surgery are called neoadjuvant therapy.

There are currently three main groups of medications used for adjuvant breast cancer treatment: hormone-blocking agents, chemotherapy, and monoclonal antibodies.

Hormonal therapy (sometimes called endocrine therapy or ET)

Some breast cancers require the female hormone estrogen to continue growing. They can be identified by the presence of estrogen receptors (ER+) and progesterone receptors (PR+) on their surface. These ER+ cancers can be treated with drugs that either block the receptors, e.g. tamoxifen, or alternatively that block the production of estrogen with an aromatase inhibitor, e.g. anastrozole or letrozole. The use of tamoxifen is recommended for 10 years. Tamoxifen can be used in either pre- or post- menopausal women. Tamoxifen increases the risk of postmenopausal bleeding, endometrial polyps, hyperplasia, and endometrial cancer. Letrozole is recommended for 5 years.

Aromatase inhibitors are only suitable for women after the menopause; however, in this group, they appear better than tamoxifen. This is because the active aromatase in postmenopausal women is different from the prevalent form in premenopausal women, and therefore these agents are ineffective in inhibiting the predominant aromatase of premenopausal women. Aromatase inhibitors should not be given to premenopausal women with intact ovarian function (unless they are also on treatment to stop their ovaries from working. Cyclin-dependent kinase (CDK) inhibitors can be used in combination with endocrine or aromatase therapy. A CDK inhibitor is any chemical that inhibits the function of CDKs. They are used to treat cancers by preventing overproliferation of cancer cells. The US FDA approved the first drug of this type, palbociclib (Ibrance), a CDK4/6 inhibitor, in February 2015, for use in postmenopausal women with breast cancer that is estrogen receptor positive and HER2 negative.

Chemotherapy

Chemotherapy is predominantly used for cases of breast cancer in stages 2–4 and is particularly beneficial in estrogen receptor-negative (ER-) disease. The chemotherapy medications are administered in combinations, usually for periods of 3–6 months. One of the most common regimens, known as "AC", combines cyclophosphamide with adriamycin (aka doxorubicin). Sometimes a taxane drug, such as docetaxel, is added, and the regime is then known as "CAT". Most chemotherapy medications work by destroying fast-growing and/or fast-replicating cancer cells, either by causing DNA damage upon replication or by other mechanisms. However, the medications also damage fast-growing normal cells, which may cause serious side effects. Damage to the heart muscle is the most dangerous complication of doxorubicin.

Monoclonal antibodies

Trastuzumab, a monoclonal antibody to HER2, has improved the 5-year disease free survival of stage 1–3 HER2-positive breast cancers to about 87% (overall survival 95%). Between 25% and 30% of breast cancers overexpress the HER2 gene or its protein product. Overexpression of HER2 in breast cancer is associated with increased disease recurrence and a worse prognosis. Trastuzumab, however, may cause serious side effects (approximately 2% of people who receive it develop significant heart damage). Another antibody pertuzumab prevents HER2 dimerization and is recommended together with trastuzumab and chemotherapy in severe disease.

Radiation

Radiotherapy is given after surgery to the region of the tumor bed and regional lymph nodes, to destroy microscopic tumor cells that may have escaped surgery. Radiation therapy is usually delivered as external beam radiotherapy. Conventionally radiotherapy is given after the operation for breast cancer. Radiation can reduce the risk of recurrence by 50–66% (1/2 – 2/3 reduction of risk) and is considered essential when breast cancer is treated by removing only the lump (lumpectomy or wide local excision).

Sometimes, women, especially if old and frail, do not seek medical help for their breast tumor until late in its course (Figure 22)

Figure 24. An extreme example of an advanced recurrent breast cancer with an ulcerating axillary mass.

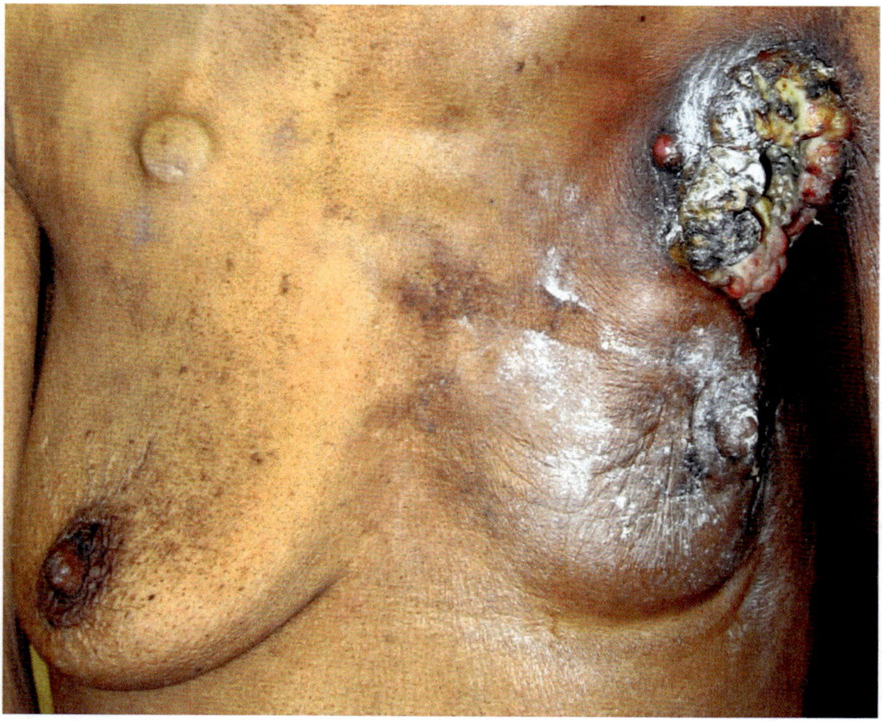

By James Heilman, MD - Own work, CC BY-SA 3.0, https://commons.wikimedia.org/w/index.php?curid=8824650. https://en.wikipedia.org/wiki/Breast cancer#/media/File:RecurrentbreastCA1.gif This file is licensed under the Creative Commons Attribution-Share Alike 3.0 Unported license. No changes have been made to this image.

Advanced cases like this, particularly in elderly women, can be treated by tamoxifen alone, sometimes with a surprisingly good outcome.

Prognostic factors

The stage of the breast cancer is the most important component of traditional classification methods of breast cancer, because it has a greater effect on the prognosis than the other considerations. Staging takes into consideration size, local involvement, lymph node status and whether metastatic disease is present. The higher the stage at diagnosis, the poorer the prognosis. The stage is raised by the invasiveness of disease to lymph nodes, chest wall, skin or beyond, and the aggressiveness of the cancer cells. The stage is lowered by the presence of cancer-free zones and close-to-normal cell behaviour (grading). Size is not a factor in staging unless the cancer is invasive. For example, ductal carcinoma in situ (DCIS) involving the entire breast will still be stage zero and consequently have an excellent outcome

6. The pathogenesis of breast cancer and the development of targeted agents based on understanding its pathogenesis

Normal cells divide as many times as needed and stop. They attach to other cells and stay in place in tissues. Cells become cancerous when they lose their ability to stop dividing, to attach to other cells, to stay where they belong, and to die at the proper time. Normal cells will self-destruct, a process known programmed cell death or apoptosis, when they are no longer needed. Until then, cells are protected from programmed death by several protein clusters and pathways. One of the protective pathways is the PI3K/AKT pathway; another is the RAS/MEK/ERK pathway. Sometimes the genes along these protective pathways are mutated in a way that turns them permanently "on", rendering the cell incapable of self-destructing when it is no longer needed. This is one of the steps that causes cancer in combination with other mutations. Normally, the PTEN protein turns off the PI3K/AKT pathway when the cell is ready for programmed cell death. In some breast cancers, the gene for the PTEN protein is mutated, so the PI3K/AKT pathway is stuck in the "on" position, and the cancer cell does not self-destruct. An overview of signal transduction pathways involved in programmed cell death is shown in Figure 25. Mutations leading to loss of this ability can lead to cancer formation.

Figure 25. A diagram of some of the key cellular signalling pathways controlling gene regulation, cell proliferation, and apoptosis (also shown earlier in this book as Figure 5).

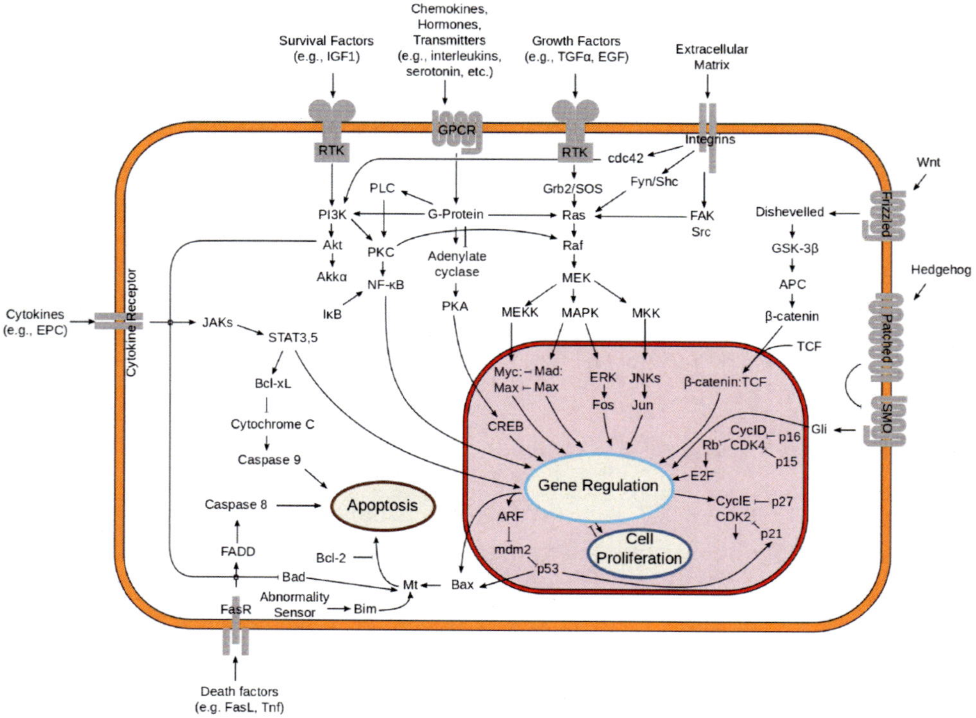

This image is by cybertory - This file was derived from: Signal transduction v1.png, CC BY-SA 3.0, https://commons.wikimedia.org/w/index.php?curid=12081090. https://en.wikipedia.org/wiki/Breast_cancer#/media/File:Signal_transduction_pathways.svg. This file is licensed under the Creative Commons Attribution-Share Alike 3.0 Unported license. No changes were made to this image.

About 5–10% of breast cancer cases are the result of a genetic predisposition inherited from a person's parents, including the BRCA1 and BRCA2 genes. Other significant mutations predisposing to breast cancer include include p53, PTEN, STK11, CHEK2, ATM, BRIP1, CDH1 and PALB2.

Abnormalities such as overexpression of cell surface molecules (eg, HER2), the inheritance of BRCA1 and BRCA2 as well as mutations in p53, PTEN, STK11, CHEK2, ATM, BRIP1, CDH1 and PALB2 predispose to breast cancer and provide drug targets for the development of therapeutic agents.

7. Overview of treatment of breast cancer with drugs

Treatment of breast cancer is tailored to the individual patient but can include surgery, radiation therapy, chemotherapy, hormone therapy and the use of targeted biological drugs such as monoclonal antibodies and small molecule inhibitors.

This book deals only with targeted biological agents for breast cancer – monoclonal antibodies and small molecule inhibitors. It does not deal with hormone inhibitors or chemotherapeutic agents

As of January 22nd, 2021 the USA National Cancer Institute issued the following list of FDA-approved drugs for breast cancer. Some on this list are duplicated since they are listed separately by their generic and brand names

Abemaciclib

Abraxane (Paclitaxel Albumin-stabilized Nanoparticle Formulation)

Ado-Trastuzumab Emtansine

Afinitor (Everolimus)
Afinitor Disperz (Everolimus)

Alpelisib

Anastrozole

Aredia (Pamidronate Disodium)

Arimidex (Anastrozole)

Aromasin (Exemestane)

Atezolizumab

Capecitabine

Cyclophosphamide

Docetaxel

Doxorubicin Hydrochloride

Ellence (Epirubicin Hydrochloride)

Enhertu (Fam-Trastuzumab Deruxtecan-nxki)

Epirubicin Hydrochloride

Eribulin Mesylate

Everolimus

Exemestane

5-FU (Fluorouracil Injection)

Fam-Trastuzumab Deruxtecan-nxki

Fareston (Toremifene)

Faslodex (Fulvestrant)

Femara (Letrozole)

Fluorouracil Injection

Fulvestrant

Gemcitabine Hydrochloride

Gemzar (Gemcitabine Hydrochloride)

Goserelin Acetate

Halaven (Eribulin Mesylate)

Herceptin Hylecta (Trastuzumab and Hyaluronidase-oysk)

Herceptin (Trastuzumab)

Ibrance (Palbociclib)

Infugem (Gemcitabine Hydrochloride)

Ixabepilone

Ixempra (Ixabepilone)

Kadcyla (Ado-Trastuzumab Emtansine)

Keytruda (Pembrolizumab)

Kisqali (Ribociclib)

Lapatinib Ditosylate

Letrozole

Lynparza (Olaparib)

Margenza (Margetuximab-cmkb)

Margetuximab-cmkb

Megestrol Acetate

Methotrexate Sodium

Neratinib Maleate

Nerlynx (Neratinib Maleate)

Olaparib

Paclitaxel

Paclitaxel Albumin-stabilized Nanoparticle Formulation

Palbociclib

Pamidronate Disodium

Pembrolizumab

Perjeta (Pertuzumab)

Pertuzumab

Pertuzumab, Trastuzumab, and Hyaluronidase-zzxf

Phesgo (Pertuzumab, Trastuzumab, and Hyaluronidase-zzxf)

Piqray (Alpelisib)

Ribociclib

Sacituzumab Govitecan-hziy

Soltamox (Tamoxifen Citrate)

Talazoparib Tosylate

Talzenna (Talazoparib Tosylate)

Tamoxifen Citrate

Taxotere (Docetaxel)

Tecentriq (Atezolizumab)

Tepadina (Thiotepa)

Thiotepa

Toremifene

Trastuzumab

Trastuzumab and Hyaluronidase-oysk

Trexall (Methotrexate Sodium)

Trodelvy (Sacituzumab Govitecan-hziy)

Tucatinib

Tukysa (Tucatinib)

Tykerb (Lapatinib Ditosylate)

Verzenio (Abemaciclib)

Vinblastine Sulfate

Xeloda (Capecitabine)

Zoladex (Goserelin Acetate)

This list includes chemotherapy agents, drugs that interfere with the estrogen receptor on breast cancer cells, drugs used to prevent or treat osteoporosis which is common in postmenopausal women, especially after chemotherapy, and drugs that are targeted to a specific protein on the cell surface and small molecules that are designed to specifically target cell processes within breast cancer cells.

Many of these drugs are also used to treat other cancers. There are 82 drugs on this list but many are listed twice – once by their generic name and again by the brand name. The total individual drugs that are currently FDA-approved for the treatment of breast cancer is 57. Of these, 20 are chemotherapeutic agents, 16 are small inhibitory molecules, 7 are monoclonal antibodies, 5 are monoclonal antibody-drug conjugates, 6 are hormone therapies, 2 are for the treatment of osteoporosis/slowing down the rate of growth of bone metastases and 1 is a gonadotropin-releasing hormone agonist.

This book deals only with monoclonal antibodies and small molecule inhibitors (sometimes known as the "mabs, nibs and ribs": together they make up the targeted biological therapeutic armamentarium. (Receptor blockers – the 'cepts' are another type of targeted biological treatment, but none are yet FDA-approved for the treatment of breast cancer: etanercept is an example of a "cept").

8. Introduction to FDA-approved targeted biologic agents for breast cancer

8.1. Important notes

In this section it is important to state clearly that all the information from the FDA's approved label for each biologic (which is the public domain) is taken verbatim from the label. However, I have made some minor changes to the format of each label:

i. I have brought the **"MECHANISM OF ACTION"** and "**DESCRIPTION**" sections forward to be placed immediately after the biologic's name, since how the drug works and what it is composed of, is key to understanding it.

ii. I have **not** generally included data from clinical trials, nor dosage, nor recommended administration schedules. This book is not a clinical manual but rather aims to give an overview of the astonishing development of targeted biological agents in breast cancer

iii. I have put a few other salient facts in **bold type** to emphasize them.

iv. I have **also added some material** in this section that is **not** in the FDA approval label to illustrate certain points and to break up the many pages of words. Please note that in these cases, ***I have put all such added text in italics.***

v. The FDA approval labels do **not** generally contain illustrations. The exceptions in their Approval Label for drugs licensed to be used for brest cancer are Figure 131 and Figure 142 – the chemical structures for taxane and talazoparib respectively. All figures or images added to this section are **not** from the FDA label and the legends to these figures are also ***in italics***. They are, however, are attributed in the normal way as requested by their creator.

As of January 2021, the following biological targeted agents were FDA-approved for the treatment of breast cancer.

9. FDA-approved targeted biologic treatments for breast cancer

9.1. ABEMACICLIB (VERZENIO™)

VERZENIO™ (abemaciclib) tablets, for oral use. Initial U.S. Approval: 2017.

MECHANISM OF ACTION

Cyclin-dependent kinase (CDK) inhibitors, the newest class of interest for advanced breast cancer, work by specifically inhibiting CDK4/6 proteins and blocking the transition from the G1 to the S phase of the cell cycle. This drug class inhibits kinase activity, which phosphorylates the retinoblastoma protein pathway. Figure 26 shows an example selective cyclin-dependent kinase 2 inhibitor from the library of pyrrolone-fused benzosuberene compounds.

Figure 26. Selective cyclin-dependent kinase 2 inhibitor from the library of pyrrolone-fused benzosuberene compounds.

This image is by Rahulbioinfowiki - Own work, CC BY-SA 4.0, https://commons.wikimedia.org/w/index.php?curid=105296406. https://en.wikipedia.org/wiki/CDK_inhibitor#/media/File:CDK2-Selective_inhibitor.png. This file is licensed under the Creative Commons Attribution-Share Alike 4.0 International license. No changes have been made to this image.

Figure 26. Selective cyclin-dependent kinase 2 inhibitor from the library of pyrrolone-fused benzosuberene compounds.

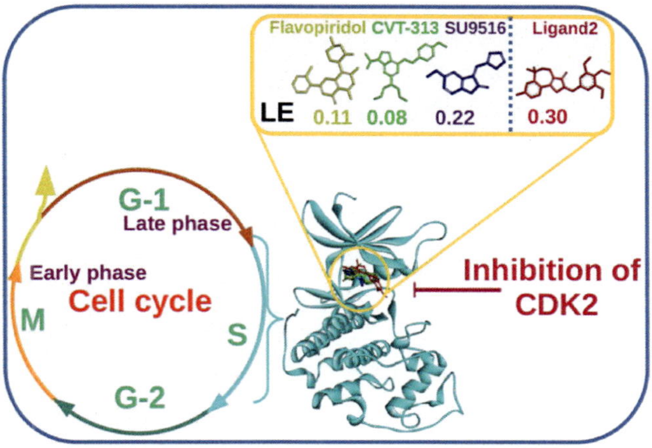

To place this figure in the context of signal transduction pathways that lead to a cellular response, Figure 27 is shown.

Figures 27. (Also previously shown as Figures 5 and 25). Signal transduction pathways that lead to a cellular response.

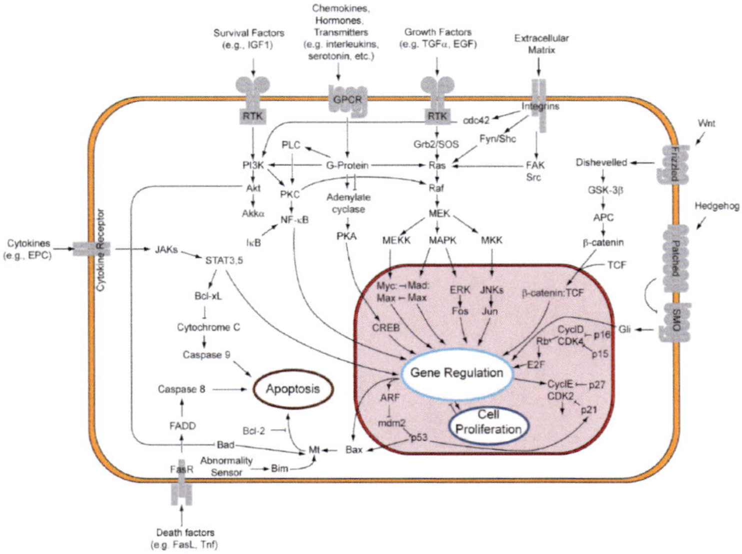

This image is By Boghog2 at English Wikipedia - Transferred from en.wikipedia to Commons. Public Domain, https://commons.wikimedia.org/w/index.php?curid=4851717. https://en.wikipedia.org/wiki/Cell_signalling#/media/File:Signal_transduction_pathwa

ys.png. This work has been released into the public domain by its author, Boghog2 at English Wikipedia. No changes have been made to this image.

RECENT MAJOR CHANGES

INDICATIONS AND USAGE

VERZENIO™ is a kinase inhibitor indicated:

• in combination with an aromatase inhibitor as initial endocrine-based therapy for the treatment of postmenopausal women with hormone receptor (HR)-positive, human epidermal growth factor receptor 2 (HER2)-negative advanced or metastatic breast cancer.

• in combination with fulvestrant for the treatment of women with hormone receptor (HR)-positive, human epidermal growth factor receptor 2 (HER2)-negative advanced or metastatic breast cancer with disease progression following endocrine therapy. *(Fulvestrant is a selective estrogen receptor degrader (SERD) and was first-in-class to be approved. It works by binding to the estrogen receptor and destabilizing it, causing the cell's normal protein degradation processes to destroy it).*

• as monotherapy for the treatment of adult patients with HR positive, HER2-negative advanced or metastatic breast cancer with disease progression following endocrine therapy and prior chemotherapy in the metastatic setting.

CONTRAINDICATIONS: None.

WARNINGS AND PRECAUTIONS

• Diarrhea: instruct patients at the first sign of loose stools to initiate antidiarrheal therapy, increase oral fluids, and notify their healthcare provider.

• Neutropenia: monitor complete blood counts prior to the start of VERZENIO therapy, every 2 weeks for the first 2 months, monthly for the next 2 months, and as clinically indicated.

• Hepatotoxicity: increases in serum transaminase levels have been observed. Perform liver function tests (LFTs) before initiating treatment with VERZENIO. Monitor LFTs every two weeks for the first two months, monthly for the next 2 months, and as clinically indicated.

• Venous Thromboembolism: monitor patients for signs and symptoms of thrombosis and pulmonary embolism and treat as medically appropriate.

• Embryo-fetal toxicity: can cause fetal harm. Advise patients of potential risk to a fetus and to use effective contraception.

ADVERSE REACTIONS

The most common adverse reactions (incidence ≥20%) were diarrhea, neutropenia, nausea, abdominal pain, infections, fatigue, anemia, leukopenia, decreased appetite, vomiting, headache, alopecia, and thrombocytopenia.

Abemaciclib is an inhibitor of cyclin-dependent kinases 4 and 6 (CDK4 and CDK6). These kinases are activated upon binding to D-cyclins. In estrogen receptor-positive (ER+) breast cancer cell lines, cyclin D1 and CDK4/6 promote phosphorylation of the retinoblastoma protein (Rb), cell cycle progression, and cell proliferation. In vitro, continuous exposure to abemaciclib inhibited Rb phosphorylation and blocked progression from G1 into S phase of the cell cycle, resulting in senescence and apoptosis. In breast cancer xenograft models, abemaciclib dosed daily without interruption as a single agent or in combination with antiestrogens resulted in reduction of tumor size.

INDICATIONS AND USAGE

VERZENIO™ (abemaciclib) is indicated:

• in combination with an aromatase inhibitor as initial endocrine-based therapy for the treatment of postmenopausal women with hormone receptor (HR)-positive, human epidermal growth factor receptor 2 (HER2)-negative advanced or metastatic breast By Rahulbioinfowiki - Own work, CC BY-SA 4.0, https://commons.wikimedia.org/w/index.php?curid=105296406 cancer.

• in combination with fulvestrant for the treatment of women with hormone receptor (HR)-positive, human epidermal growth factor receptor 2 (HER2)-negative advanced or metastatic breast cancer with disease progression following endocrine therapy.

• as monotherapy for the treatment of adult patients with HR-positive, HER2-negative advanced or metastatic breast cancer with disease progression following endocrine therapy and prior chemotherapy in the metastatic setting.

Dose modification for use with strong CYP3A inhibitors

Avoid concomitant use of the strong CYP3A inhibitor ketoconazole. With concomitant use of other strong CYP3A inhibitors, in patients with recommended starting doses of 200 mg twice daily or 150 mg twice daily, reduce the VERZENIO dose to 100 mg twice daily. In patients who have had a dose reduction to 100 mg twice daily due to adverse reactions, further reduce the VERZENIO dose to 50 mg twice daily. If a patient taking VERZENIO discontinues a strong CYP3A inhibitor, increase the VERZENIO dose (after 3-5 half-lives of the inhibitor) to the dose that was used before starting the strong inhibitor.

Dose modification for patients with severe hepatic impairment

For patients with severe hepatic impairment (Child Pugh-C *score*), reduce the VERZENIO dosing frequency to once daily. Refer to the Full Prescribing Information for coadministered aromatase inhibitor or fulvestrant for dose modification requirements for severe hepatic impairment.

CONTRAINDICATIONS: None.

More detail on **WARNINGS AND PRECAUTIONS**

Diarrhea

Diarrhea occurred in 81% of patients receiving VERZENIO plus an aromatase inhibitor in *(the trial)* MONARCH 3, 86% of patients receiving VERZENIO plus fulvestrant in MONARCH 2, and 90% of patients receiving VERZENIO alone in MONARCH 1. Grade 3 diarrhea occurred in 9% of patients receiving VERZENIO plus an aromatase inhibitor in MONARCH 3, 13% of patients receiving VERZENIO plus fulvestrant in MONARCH 2, and in 20% of patients receiving VERZENIO alone in MONARCH 1.

Episodes of diarrhea have been associated with dehydration and infection.

Diarrhea incidence was greatest during the first month of VERZENIO dosing. In MONARCH 3, the median time to onset of the first diarrhea event was 8 days, and the median duration of diarrhea for Grades 2 and 3 were 11 and 8 days, respectively. In MONARCH 2, the median time to onset of the first diarrhea event was 6 days, and the median duration of diarrhea for Grades 2 and 3 were 9 days and 6 days, respectively [see Dosage and Administration (2.2) and Patient Counseling Information (17)]. In MONARCH 3, 19% of patients with diarrhea required a dose omission and 13% required a dose reduction.

In MONARCH 2, 22% of patients with diarrhea required a dose omission and 22% required a dose reduction. The time to onset and resolution for diarrhea were similar across MONARCH 3, MONARCH 2, and MONARCH 1.

Instruct patients that at the first sign of loose stools, they should start antidiarrheal therapy such as loperamide, increase oral fluids, and notify their healthcare provider for further instructions and appropriate follow up. For Grade 3 or 4 diarrhea, or diarrhea that requires hospitalization, discontinue VERZENIO until toxicity resolves to ≤Grade 1, and then resume VERZENIO at the next lower dose.

Neutropenia

Neutropenia occurred in 41% of patients receiving VERZENIO plus an aromatase inhibitor in MONARCH 3, 46% of patients receiving VERZENIO plus fulvestrant in MONARCH 2, and 37% of patients receiving VERZENIO alone in MONARCH 1.

A Grade ≥3 decrease in neutrophil count (based on laboratory findings) occurred in 22% of patients receiving VERZENIO plus an aromatase inhibitor in MONARCH 3, 32% of patients receiving VERZENIO plus fulvestrant in MONARCH 2, and in 27% of patients receiving VERZENIO in MONARCH 1.

In MONARCH 3, the median time to first episode of Grade ≥3 neutropenia was 33 days, and in MONARCH 2 and MONARCH 1 was 29 days. In MONARCH 3, median duration of Grade ≥3 neutropenia was 11 days, and for MONARCH 2 and MONARCH 1 was 15 days. Monitor complete blood counts prior to the start of VERZENIO therapy, every 2 weeks for the first 2 months, monthly for the next 2 months, and as clinically indicated. Dose interruption, dose reduction, or delay in starting treatment cycles is recommended for patients who develop Grade 3 or 4 neutropenia.

Febrile neutropenia has been reported in <1% of patients exposed to VERZENIO in the MONARCH studies. Two deaths due to neutropenic sepsis were observed in MONARCH 2. Inform patients to promptly report any episodes of fever to their healthcare provider.

DRUG INTERACTIONS

Effect of other drugs on VERZENIO

Strong CYP3A inhibitors

Strong CYP3A4 inhibitors increased the exposure of abemaciclib plus its active metabolites to a clinically meaningful extent and may lead to increased toxicity.
Ketoconazole

Avoid concomitant use of ketoconazole. Ketoconazole is predicted to increase the AUC of abemaciclib by up to 16-fold.

Other strong CYP3A inhibitors

In patients with recommended starting doses of 200 mg twice daily or 150 mg twice daily, reduce the VERZENIO dose to 100 mg twice daily with concomitant use of other strong CYP3A inhibitors. In patients who have had a dose reduction to 100 mg twice daily due to adverse reactions, further reduce the VERZENIO dose to 50 mg twice daily with concomitant use of other strong CYP3A inhibitors. If a patient taking VERZENIO discontinues a strong CYP3A inhibitor, increase the VERZENIO dose (after 3-5 half-lives of the inhibitor) to the dose that was used before starting the strong inhibitor.

Patients should avoid grapefruit products.

Strong CYP3A inducers

Coadministration of VERZENIO with rifampin, a strong CYP3A inducer, decreased the plasma concentrations of abemaciclib plus its active metabolites and may lead to reduced activity. Avoid concomitant use of strong CYP3A inducers and consider alternative agents

USE IN SPECIFIC POPULATIONS

Pregnancy risk summary

Based on findings in animals and its mechanism of action, VERZENIO can cause fetal harm when administered to a pregnant woman. There are no available human data informing the drug-associated risk. Advise pregnant women of the potential risk to a fetus. In animal reproduction studies, administration of abemaciclib during organogenesis was teratogenic and caused decreased fetal weight at maternal exposures that were similar to human clinical exposure based on AUC at the maximum recommended human dose. Advise pregnant women of the potential risk to a fetus. The background risk of major birth defects and miscarriage for the indicated population is unknown. However, the background risk in the U.S. general population of major birth defects is 2 to 4% and of miscarriage is 15 to 20% of clinically recognized pregnancies.

Animal data

In an embryo-fetal development study, pregnant rats received oral doses of abemaciclib up to 15 mg/kg/day during the period of organogenesis. Doses ≥4 mg/kg/day caused decreased fetal body weights and increased incidence of cardiovascular and skeletal malformations and variations. These findings included absent innominate artery and aortic arch, malpositioned subclavian artery, unossified sternebra, bipartite ossification of thoracic centrum, and rudimentary or nodulated ribs. At 4 mg/kg/day in rats, the maternal systemic exposures were approximately equal to the human exposure (AUC) at the recommended dose.

Lactation risk summary

There are no data on the presence of abemaciclib in human milk, or its effects on the breastfed child or on milk production. Because of the potential for serious adverse reactions in breastfed infants from VERZENIO, advise lactating women not to breastfeed during VERZENIO treatment and for at least 3 weeks after the last dose.

Females and males of reproductive potential

Pregnancy testing

Based on animal studies, VERZENIO can cause fetal harm when administered to a pregnant woman. Pregnancy testing is recommended for females of reproductive potential prior to initiating treatment with VERZENIO.

Contraception

Females

VERZENIO can cause fetal harm when administered to a pregnant woman. Advise females of reproductive potential to use effective contraception during VERZENIO treatment and for at least 3 weeks after the last dose.

Infertility

Males

Based on findings in animals, VERZENIO may impair fertility in males of reproductive potential.

Pediatric use

The safety and effectiveness of VERZENIO have not been established in pediatric patients.

Geriatric use

Of the 900 patients who received VERZENIO in MONARCH 1, MONARCH 2, and MONARCH 3, 38% were 65 years of age or older and 10% were 75 years of age or older. The most common adverse reactions (≥5%) Grade 3 or 4 in patients ≥65 years of age across MONARCH 1, 2, and 3 were neutropenia, diarrhea, fatigue, nausea, dehydration, leukopenia, anemia, infections, and ALT increased. No overall differences in safety or effectiveness of VERZENIO were observed between these patients and younger patients.

Renal impairment

No dosage adjustment is required for patients with mild or moderate renal impairment (CLcr ≥30-89 mL/min, estimated by Cockcroft-Gault [C-G]). The pharmacokinetics of abemaciclib in patients with severe renal impairment (CLcr<30mi/min [C-G], end stage renal disease, or in patients on dialysis is unknown.

Patients with hepatic impairment

Following a single 200 mg oral dose of abemaciclib, the relative potency adjusted unbound AUC0-INF of abemaciclib plus its active metabolites (M2, M18, M20) in plasma increased 1.2-fold in subjects with mild hepatic impairment (Child-Pugh *(score)* A, n=9), 1.1-fold in subjects with moderate hepatic impairment (Child-Pugh B, n=10), and 2.4-fold in subjects with severe hepatic impairment (Child-Pugh C, n=6) relative to subjects with normal hepatic function (n=10).

In subjects with severe hepatic impairment, the mean plasma elimination half-life of abemaciclib increased to 55 hours compared to 24 hours in subjects with normal hepatic function.

Drug interaction studies effects of other drugs on abemaciclib

Strong CYP3A Inhibitors

Ketoconazole (a strong CYP3A inhibitor) is predicted to increase the AUC of abemaciclib by up to 16-fold.

Itraconazole (a strong CYP3A inhibitor) is predicted to increase the relative potency adjusted unbound AUC of abemaciclib plus its active metabolites (M2, M18 and M20) by 2.2-fold.

Coadministration of 500 mg twice daily doses of clarithromycin (a strong CYP3A inhibitor) with a single 50 mg dose of VERZENIO (0.3 times the approved recommended 150 mg dosage) increased the relative potency adjusted unbound AUC0-INF of abemaciclib plus its active metabolites (M2, M18, and M20) by 1.7-fold relative to abemaciclib alone in cancer patients.

Moderate CYP3A inhibitors

Diltiazem and verapamil (moderate CYP3A inhibitors) are predicted to increase the relative potency adjusted unbound AUC of abemaciclib plus its active metabolites (M2, M18, and M20) by 1.7-fold and 1.3-fold, respectively.

Strong CYP3A inducers

Coadministration of 600 mg daily doses of rifampin (a strong CYP3A inducer) with a single 200 mg dose of VERZENIO decreased the relative potency adjusted unbound AUC0-INF of abemaciclib plus its active metabolites (M2, M18, and M20) by 67% in healthy subjects.

Moderate CYP3A inducers

The effect of moderate CYP3A inducers on the pharmacokinetics of abemaciclib is unknown.

Endocrine therapies

In clinical studies in patients with breast cancer, there was no clinically relevant effect of fulvestrant, anastrozole, letrozole, or exemestane on abemaciclib pharmacokinetics.

Effects of abemaciclib on other drugs

Loperamide

In a clinical drug interaction study in healthy subjects, coadministration of a single 8 mg dose of loperamide with a single 400 mg abemaciclib (2.7 times the approved recommended 150 mg dosage) increased loperamide AUC0-INF by 9% and Cmax by 35% relative to loperamide alone. These increases in loperamide exposure are not considered clinically relevant.

Metformin

In a clinical drug interaction study in healthy subjects, co-administration of a single 1000 mg dose of metformin, a clinically relevant substrate of renal OCT2, MATE1, and MATE2-K transporters, with a single 400 mg dose of abemaciclib (2.7 times the approved recommended 150 mg dosage) increased metformin AUC0-INF by 37% and Cmax by 22% relative to metformin alone. Abemaciclib reduced the renal clearance and renal secretion of metformin by 45% and 62%, respectively, relative to metformin alone, without any effect on glomerular filtration rate (GFR) as measured by iohexol clearance and serum cystatin C.

Endocrine therapies

In clinical studies in patients with breast cancer, there was no clinically relevant effect of abemaciclib on the pharmacokinetics of fulvestrant, anastrozole, letrozole, or exemestane.

Therapeutic efficacy of abemaciclib in the management of breast cancer

Since September 2017 Abemaciclib is approved in the US for "adult patients who have hormone receptor (HR)-positive, human epidermal growth factor receptor 2 (HER2)-negative advanced or metastatic breast cancer that has progressed after taking therapy that alters a patient's hormones".

9.2. ADO-TRASTUZUMAB EMTANSINE (KADCYLA™)

KADCYLA™ (ado-trastuzumab emtansine) for injection, for intravenous use

Initial U.S. Approval: {YYYY}

MECHANISM OF ACTION

Ado-trastuzumab emtansine is a HER2-targeted antibody-drug conjugate. The antibody is the humanized anti-HER2 IgG1, trastuzumab. The small molecule cytotoxin, DM1, is a microtubule inhibitor. Upon binding to sub-domain IV of the HER2 receptor, ado-trastuzumab emtansine undergoes receptor-mediated internalization and subsequent lysosomal degradation, resulting in intracellular release of DM1-containing cytotoxic catabolites. Binding of DM1 to tubulin disrupts microtubule networks in the cell, which results in cell cycle arrest and apoptotic cell death. In addition, in vitro studies have shown that similar to trastuzumab, ado-trastuzumab emtansine inhibits HER2 receptor signalling, mediates antibody-dependent cell-mediated cytotoxicity and inhibits shedding of the HER2 extracellular domain in human breast cancer cells that overexpress HER2.

DESCRIPTION

KADCYLA (ado-trastuzumab emtansine) is a HER2-targeted antibody-drug conjugate (ADC) which contains the humanized anti-HER2 IgG1, trastuzumab, covalently linked to the microtubule inhibitory drug DM1 (a maytansine derivative) via the stable thioether linker MCC (4-[N-maleimidomethyl] cyclohexane-1-carboxylate). Emtansine refers to the MCC-DM1 complex. The antibody trastuzumab, is a well characterized recombinant monoclonal antibody product produced by mammalian (Chinese hamster ovary) cells, and the small molecule components (DM1 and MCC) are produced by chemical synthesis. Ado-trastuzumab emtansine contains an average of 3.5 DM1 molecules per antibody.

WARNING: HEPATOTOXICITY, CARDIAC TOXICITY, EMBRYO-FETAL TOXICITY. See full prescribing information for complete boxed warning

- Do not substitute KADCYLA for or with trastuzumab.

• Hepatotoxicity, liver failure and death have occurred in KADCYLA-treated patients. Monitor hepatic function prior to initiation and prior to each dose. Institute dose modifications or permanently discontinue as appropriate.

• KADCYLA may lead to reductions in left ventricular ejection fraction (LVEF). Assess LVEF prior to initiation. Monitor and withhold dosing or discontinue as appropriate.

• Can cause fetal harm. Advise women of potential risk to the fetus.

INDICATIONS AND USAGE

KADCYLA is a HER2-targeted antibody and microtubule inhibitor conjugate indicated, as a single agent, for the treatment of patients with HER2-positive, metastatic breast cancer who previously received trastuzumab and a taxane, separately or in combination. Patients should have either:

• Received prior therapy for metastatic disease, or

• Developed disease recurrence during or within six months completing adjuvant therapy.

CONTRAINDICATIONS: None.

Further details on **WARNINGS AND PRECAUTIONS**

• Pulmonary Toxicity: permanently discontinue KADCYLA in patients diagnosed with interstitial lung disease or pneumonitis.

• Infusion-related reactions, hypersensitivity reactions: monitor for signs and symptoms during and after infusion. If significant infusion-related reactions or hypersensitivity reactions occur, slow or interrupt the infusion and administer appropriate medical therapies. Permanently discontinue KADCYLA for life threatening infusion-related reaction.

• Thrombocytopenia: monitor platelet counts prior to each KADCYLA dose. Institute dose modifications as appropriate.

• Neurotoxicity: monitor for signs or symptoms. Withhold dosing temporarily for patients experiencing Grade 3 or 4 peripheral neuropathy.

• HER2 Testing: perform using FDA-approved tests by laboratories with demonstrated proficiency.

ADVERSE REACTIONS

The most common adverse drug reactions (frequency > 25%) with KADCYLA (n=884 treated patients) were fatigue, nausea, musculoskeletal pain, thrombocytopenia, headache, increased transaminases, and constipation.

FULL PRESCRIBING INFORMATION

Do Not Substitute KADCYLA for or with Trastuzumab

Further details on **WARNING: HEPATOTOXICITY, CARDIAC TOXICITY, EMBRYO-FETAL TOXICITY**

Hepatotoxicity: serious hepatotoxicity has been reported, including liver failure and death in patients treated with KADCYLA. Monitor serum transaminases and bilirubin prior to initiation of KADCYLA treatment and prior to each KADCYLA dose. Reduce dose or discontinue KADCYLA as appropriate in cases of increased serum transaminases or total bilirubin.

• Cardiac toxicity: KADCYLA administration may lead to reductions in left ventricular ejection fraction (LVEF) (Figures 28, 29 and 30). Evaluate left ventricular function in all patients prior to and during treatment with KADCYLA. Withhold treatment for clinically significant decrease in left ventricular function.

Figure 28. Model of a normal heart (left); and a weakened heart, with over-stretched muscle and dilation of left ventricle (right); both during diastole. This image is by https://www.scientificanimations.com - http://www.scientificanimations.com/wiki-images/, CC BY-SA 4.0, https://commons.wikimedia.org/w/index.php?curid=63766023. https://en.wikipedia.org/wiki/Heart_failure#/media/File:Right_side_heart_failure.jpg. This file is licensed under the Creative Commons Attribution-Share Alike 4.0 International license. No changes have been made to this image.

Figure 28. Model of a normal heart (left); and a weakened heart, with over-stretched muscle and dilation of left ventricle (right); both during diastole.

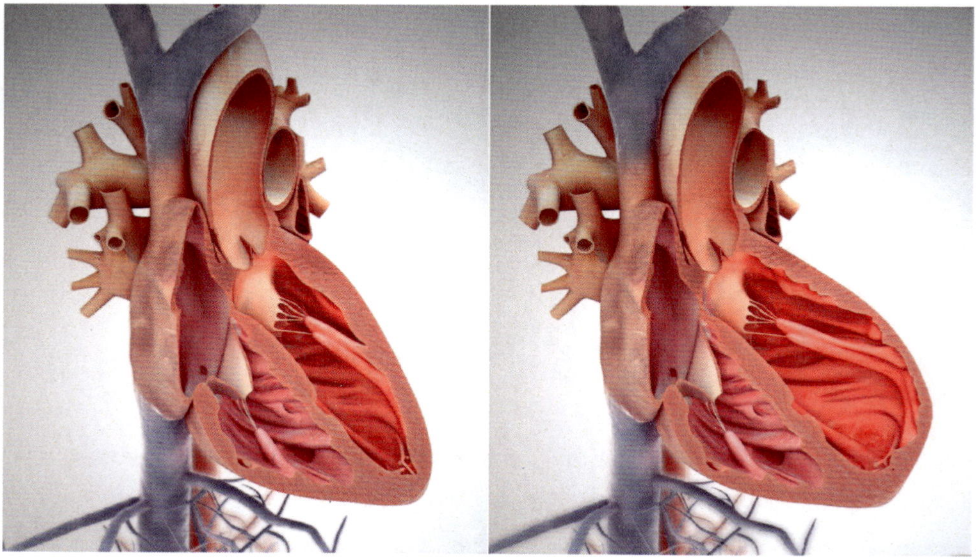

Figure 29. Ultrasound showing severe systolic heart failure.

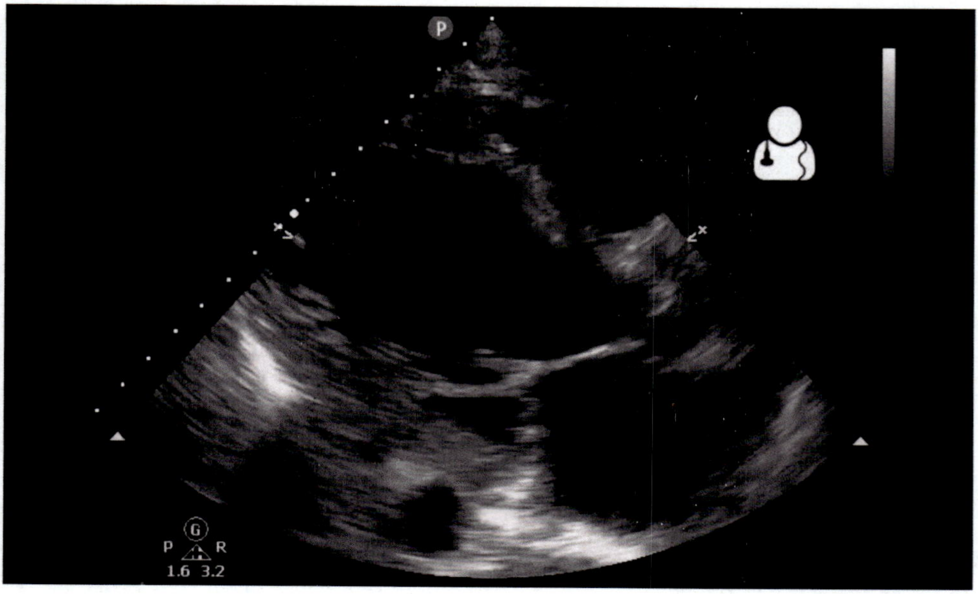

_Ultrasound_of_the_Week_5.jpg. This file is licensed under the Creative Commons Attribution-Share Alike 4.0 International license. Attribution: Ben Smith https://www.ultrasoundoftheweek.com. https://www.coreultrasound.com/category/ultrasound-of-the-week/

Figure 30. Kerley B lines in acute cardiac decompensation. The short, horizontal lines can be found everywhere in the right lung.

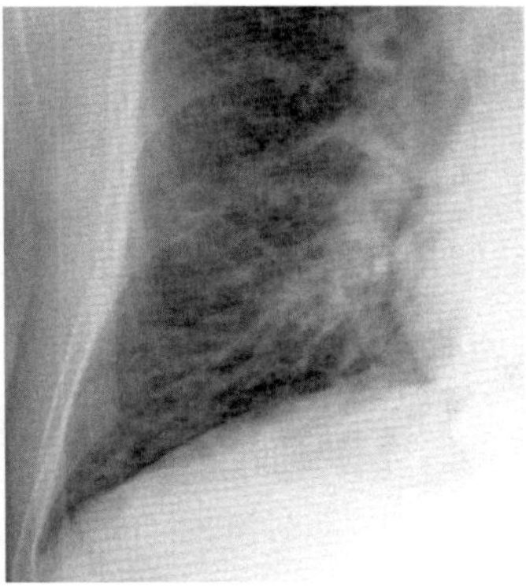

This image is by Hellerhoff - Own work, CC BY-SA 3.0, https://commons.wikimedia.org/w/index.php?curid=37883875. https://en.wikipedia.org/wiki/Heart_failure#/media/File:Kerley-B-Linien.jpg. This file is licensed under the Creative Commons Attribution-Share Alike 3.0 Unported license. No changes have been made to this image.

• Embryo-fetal toxicity: Exposure to KADCYLA can result in embryo-fetal death or birth defects. Advise patients of these risks and the need for effective contraception.

USE IN SPECIFIC POPULATIONS

• Nursing mothers

Discontinue nursing or discontinue KADCYLA taking into consideration the importance of the drug to the mother.

• Females of reproductive potential

Counsel females on pregnancy prevention and planning.

INDICATIONS AND USAGE

KADCYLA™, as a single agent, is indicated for the treatment of patients with HER2-positive, metastatic breast cancer who previously received trastuzumab and a taxane, separately or in combination. Patients should have either:

- Received prior therapy for metastatic disease, or
- Developed disease recurrence during or within six months of completing adjuvant therapy

FULL PRESCRIBING INFORMATION

Do Not Substitute KADCYLA for or with Trastuzumab

Further details on **WARNING: HEPATOTOXICITY, CARDIAC TOXICITY, EMBRYO-FETAL TOXICITY**

- Hepatotoxicity

Serious hepatotoxicity has been reported, including liver failure and death in patients treated with KADCYLA. Monitor serum transaminases and bilirubin prior to initiation of KADCYLA treatment and prior to each KADCYLA dose. Reduce dose or discontinue KADCYLA as appropriate in cases of increased serum transaminases or total bilirubin.

- Cardiac Toxicity

KADCYLA administration may lead to reductions in left ventricular ejection fraction (LVEF). Evaluate left ventricular function in all patients prior to and during treatment with KADCYLA. Withhold treatment for clinically significant decrease in left ventricular function.

- Embryo-fetal toxicity

Exposure to KADCYLA can result in embryo-fetal death or birth defects. Advise patients of these risks and the need for effective contraception.

INDICATIONS AND USAGE

KADCYLA™, as a single agent, is indicated for the treatment of patients with HER2-positive, metastatic breast cancer who previously received trastuzumab and a taxane, separately or in combination. Patients should have either:

• Received prior therapy for metastatic disease, or

• Developed disease recurrence during or within six months of completing adjuvant therapy.

DOSAGE AND ADMINISTRATION

Recommended Doses and Schedules

The recommended dose of KADCYLA is 3.6 mg/kg given as an intravenous infusion every 3 weeks (21-day cycle) until disease progression or unacceptable toxicity. Do not administer KADCYLA at doses greater than 3.6 mg/kg. Do not substitute KADCYLA for or with trastuzumab. Closely monitor the infusion site for possible subcutaneous infiltration during drug administration.

First infusion

Administer infusion over 90 minutes. Patients should be observed during the infusion and for at least 90 minutes following the initial dose for fever, chills, or other infusion related reactions.

Subsequent infusions: administer over 30 minutes if prior infusions were well tolerated. Patients should be observed during the infusion and for at least 30 minutes after infusion.

Dose Modifications

KADCYLA dose should not be re-escalated after a dose reduction is made. If a planned dose is delayed or missed, it should be administered as soon as possible; do not wait until the next planned cycle. The schedule of administration should be adjusted to maintain a 3-week interval between doses. The infusion may be administered at the dose and rate the patient tolerated in the most recent infusion. The infusion rate of KADCYLA should be slowed or interrupted if the patient develops an infusion-related reaction. Permanently discontinue KADCYLA for life-threatening infusion-related reactions.

Management of increased serum transaminases, hyperbilirubinemia, left ventricular dysfunction, thrombocytopenia, pulmonary toxicity, or peripheral neuropathy may require temporary interruption, dose reduction or treatment discontinuation of KADCYLA as per guidelines provided in Tables 1 to 5.

Recommended dose reduction schedule for adverse events

Dose reduction schedule dose level starting dose 3.6 mg/kg:

First dose reduction 3 mg/kg

Second dose reduction 2.4 mg/kg

Requirement for further dose reduction: discontinue treatment

Hepatotoxicity

Hepatotoxicity, predominantly in the form of asymptomatic, transient increases in the concentrations of serum transaminases, has been observed in clinical trials with KADCYLA. Serious hepatobiliary disorders, including at least two fatal cases of severe drug-induced liver injury and associated hepatic encephalopathy, have been reported in 5 of 21 clinical trials with KADCYLA. Some of the observed cases may have been confounded by comorbidities and/or concomitant medications with known hepatotoxic potential. Monitor serum transaminases and bilirubin prior to initiation of KADCYLA treatment and prior to each KADCYLA dose. Patients with known active hepatitis B virus or hepatitis C virus were excluded from Study 1. Reduce the dose or discontinue KADCYLA as appropriate in cases of increased serum transaminases and/or total bilirubin. Permanently discontinue KADCYLA treatment in patients with serum transaminases > 3 x ULN and concomitant total bilirubin > 2 x ULN. KADCYLA has not been studied in patients with serum transaminases > 2.5 x ULN or bilirubin > 1.5 x ULN prior to the initiation of treatment. In clinical trials of KADCYLA, cases of nodular regenerative hyperplasia (NRH) of the liver have been identified from liver biopsies (3 cases out of 884 treated patients). Two of these three cases of NRH were observed in the randomized trial (Study 1). NRH is a rare liver condition characterized by widespread benign transformation of hepatic parenchyma into small regenerative nodules; NRH may lead to non-cirrhotic portal hypertension. The diagnosis of NRH can be confirmed only by histopathology. NRH should be considered in all patients with clinical symptoms of portal hypertension but with normal transaminases and no manifestations of cirrhosis. Upon diagnosis of NRH, KADCYLA treatment must be permanently discontinued.

Left ventricular dysfunction

Patients treated with KADCYLA are at increased risk of developing left ventricular dysfunction (see Figures 45, 46 and 47). A decrease of LVEF to < 40% has been observed in patients treated with KADCYLA. In the randomized trial (Study 1), left ventricular dysfunction occurred in 1.8% of patients in the KADCYLA-treated group and 3.3% of patients in the lapatinib plus capecitabine-treated group. Assess LVEF prior to initiation of KADCYLA and at regular intervals (e.g. every three months) during treatment to ensure the LVEF is within the institution's normal limits. Treatment with KADCYLA has not been studied in patients with LVEF < 50% prior to initiation of treatment. If, at routine monitoring, LVEF is < 40%, or is 40% to 45% with a 10% or greater absolute decrease below the pretreatment value, withhold KADCYLA and repeat LVEF assessment within approximately 3 weeks. Permanently discontinue KADCYLA if the LVEF has not improved or has declined further. Patients with a history of symptomatic congestive heart failure (CHF), serious cardiac arrhythmia, or history of myocardial infarction or unstable angina within 6 months were excluded from Study 1.

Embryo-fetal toxicity

KADCYLA can cause fetal harm when administered to a pregnant woman. There are no adequate and well-controlled studies of KADCYLA in pregnant women and no reproductive and developmental toxicology studies have been conducted with ado-trastuzumab emtansine. Nevertheless, treatment with trastuzumab, the antibody component of KADCYLA, during pregnancy in the postmarketing setting has resulted in oligohydramnios (*Oligohydramnios is a condition in pregnancy characterized by a deficiency of amniotic fluid), some associated with fatal pulmonary hypoplasia (Figures 31 and 32), skeletal abnormalities and neonatal death).* DM1, the cytotoxic component of KADCYLA, can be expected to cause Embryo-fetal toxicity based on its mechanism of action. If KADCYLA is used during pregnancy, or if the patient becomes pregnant while receiving KADCYLA, apprise the patient of the potential hazard to the fetus. Verify pregnancy status prior to the initiation of KADCYLA. Advise patients of the risks of embryo-fetal death and birth defects and the need for contraception during and after treatment. Advise patients to contact their healthcare provider immediately if they suspect they may be pregnant. Encourage women who may be exposed during pregnancy to enroll in the MotHER Pregnancy Registry by contacting 1-800-690-6720.

Pulmonary hypoplasia is incomplete development of the lungs, resulting in an abnormally low number or size of bronchopulmonary segments (Figure 31) or alveoli (Figure 32).

Figure 31. A bronchopulmonary segment is a portion of lung supplied by a specific segmental bronchus and its vessels.

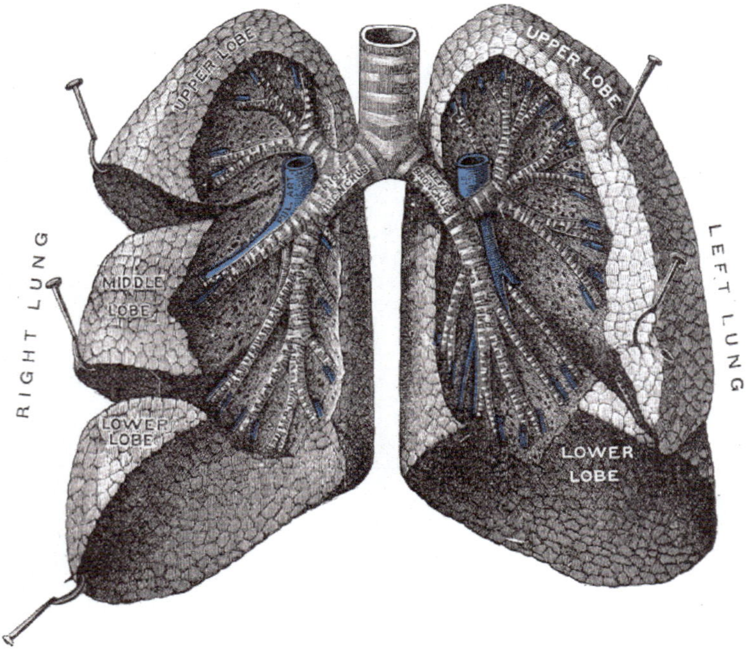

This image is by Henry Vandyke Carter - Henry Gray (1918) Anatomy of the Human Body (See " Book" section below)Bartleby.com: Gray's Anatomy, Plate 962, Public Domain, https://commons.wikimedia.org/w/index.php?curid=566896. https://en.wikipedia.org/wiki/Bronchopulmonary_segment#/media/File:Gray962.png. This work is in the public domain in its country of origin and other countries and areas where the copyright term is the author's life plus 100 years or fewer.This work is in the public domain in the United States because it was published (or registered

with the registered with the U.S. Copyright Office) before January 1, 1926 (PD1925). No changes have been made to this image.

Figure 32. An alveolus (plural: alveoli, from Latin alveus, "little cavity"), is an anatomical structure that has the form of a hollow cavity. Mainly found in the lung, the pulmonary alveoli are spherical outcroppings of the respiratory bronchioles and are the primary sites of gas exchange with the blood.

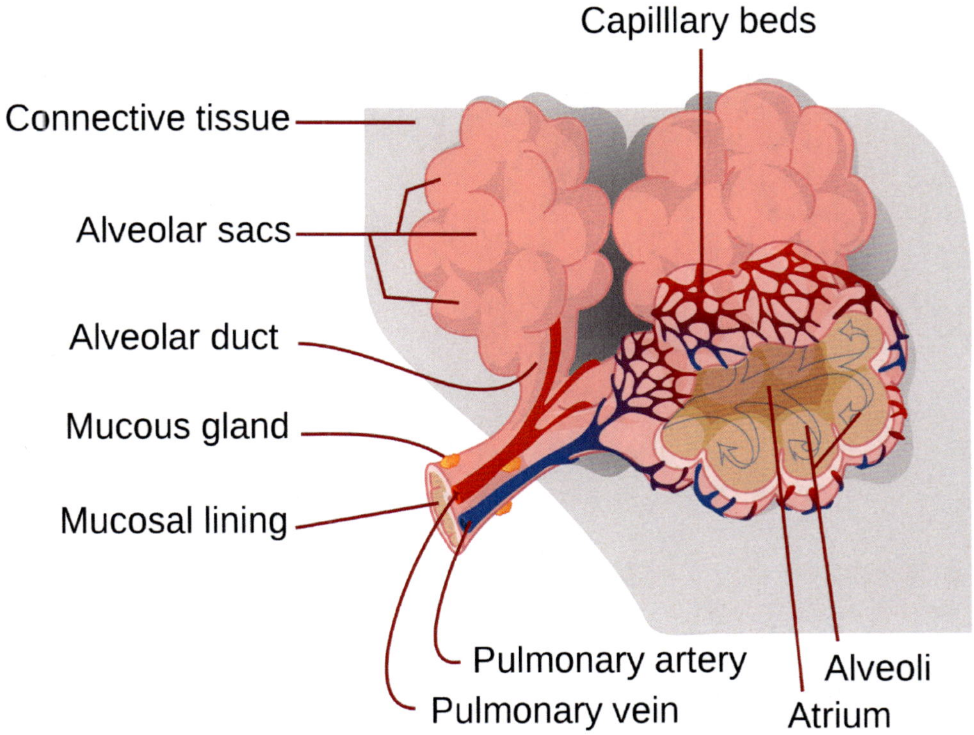

This image is by LadyofHats - self-made (extracted from Image:Respiratory system complete.svg) (duplicate of Image:Respiratory system complete en.svg), Public Domain, https://commons.wikimedia.org/w/index.php?curid=3222341. https://en.wikipedia.org/wiki/Pulmonary_alveolus#/media/File:Alveolus_diagram.svg. This work has been released into the public domain by its author, LadyofHats. No changes were made to this image.

Pulmonary toxicity

Cases of interstitial lung disease (ILD), including pneumonitis, some leading to acute respiratory distress syndrome or fatal outcome have been reported in clinical trials with KADCYLA *(Figure 33).*

Figure 33. Interstitial lung disease, as seen in the reticular markings on this AP chest x-ray caused, in this case, by Pneumocystis jiroveci pneumonia.

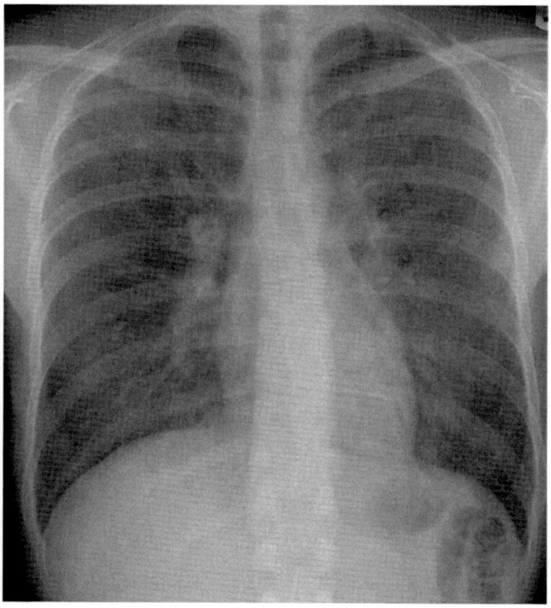

This image has been placed in the Public Domain by its creator. https://commons.wikimedia.org/w/index.php?curid=85067168. https://en.wikipedia.org/wiki/Interstitial_lung_disease#/media/File:PCP_CAP_CXR.JPG. No changes have been made to this image.

Pneumonitis at an incidence of 0.8% (7 out of 884 treated patients) has been reported, with one case of grade 3 pneumonitis. Signs and symptoms include dyspnea, cough, fatigue, and pulmonary infiltrates. These events may or may not occur as sequelae of infusion reactions. In the randomized trial (Study 1), the overall frequency of pneumonitis was 1.2%. Permanently discontinue treatment with KADCYLA in patients diagnosed with ILD or pneumonitis. Patients with dyspnea at rest due to complications of advanced malignancy and co-morbidities may be at increased risk of pulmonary toxicity.

Infusion-related reactions, hypersensitivity reactions

Treatment with KADCYLA has not been studied in patients who had trastuzumab permanently discontinued due to infusion-related reactions (IRR) and/or hypersensitivity; treatment with KADCYLA is not recommended for these patients. Infusion-related reactions, characterized by one or more of the following symptoms – flushing, chills, pyrexia, dyspnea, hypotension, wheezing, bronchospasm, and tachycardia have been reported in clinical trials of KADCYLA. In the randomized trial (Study 1), the overall frequency 203 of IRRs in patients treated with KADCYLA was 1.4%. In most patients, these reactions resolved over the course of several hours to a day after the infusion was terminated. KADCYLA treatment should be interrupted in patients with severe IRR. KADCYLA treatment should be permanently discontinued in the event of a life-threatening IRR. Patients should be observed closely for IRR reactions, especially during the first infusion. One case of a serious, allergic/anaphylactic-like reaction has been observed in clinical trials of single-agent KADCYLA. Medications to treat such reactions, as well as emergency equipment, should be available for immediate use.

Thrombocytopenia

Thrombocytopenia, or decreased platelet count, was reported in clinical trials of KADCYLA (103 of 884 treated patients with ≥ Grade 3: 283 of 884 treated patients with any Grade). The majority of these patients had Grade 1 or 2 events (< LLN to ≥ 50,000/mm^3) with the nadir occurring by day 8 and generally improving to Grade 0 or 1 (≥ 75,000 /mm^3) by the next scheduled dose. In clinical trials of KADCYLA, the incidence and severity of thrombocytopenia were higher in Asian patients. Independent of race, the incidence of severe hemorrhagic events in patients treated with KADCYLA was low. In the randomized trial (Study 1), the overall frequency of thrombocytopenia was 31.2% in the KADCYLA-treated group and 3.3% in the lapatinib plus capecitabine-treated group. The incidence of ≥ Grade 3 thrombocytopenia was 14.5% in the KADCYLA treated group and 0.4% in the lapatinib plus capecitabine-treated group. In Asian patients, the incidence of > Grade 3 thrombocytopenia was 45.1% in the KADCYLA-treated group and 1.3% in the lapatinib plus capecitabine-treated group. Monitor platelet counts prior to initiation of KADCYLA and prior to each KADCYLA dose. KADCYLA has not been studied in patients with platelet counts < 50,000/mm^3); do not administer KADCYLA until platelet counts recover to Grade 1 (≥ 75,000/mm^3). Patients with thrombocytopenia (< 100,000/mm^3) and patients on anti-coagulant treatment should be closely monitored during treatment with KADCYLA.

Neurotoxicity

Peripheral neuropathy, mainly as Grade 1 and predominantly sensory, was reported in clinical trials of KADCYLA (14 of 884 treated patients with ≥ Grade 3; 196 of 884 treated patients with any Grade) (Figure 34). In the randomized trial (Study 1), the overall frequency of peripheral neuropathy was 21.2% in the KADCYLA-treated group and 13.5% in the lapatinib plus capecitabine-treated group. The incidence of ≥ Grade 3 peripheral neuropathy was 2.2% in the KADCYLA-treated group and 0.2% in the lapatinib plus capecitabine-treated group. KADCYLA should be temporarily discontinued in patients experiencing Grade 3 or 4 peripheral neuropathy until resolution to ≤ Grade 2. Patients should be clinically monitored on an ongoing 242 basis for signs or symptoms of neurotoxicity.

Figure 34. Intermediate magnification micrograph of a vasculitic neuropathy, also neuropathy due to a vasculitis. Resin section (plastics) with toluidine blue stain. The pathologic features of vasculitic neuropathy are evident: Zonal involvement of the nerve fascicles with: Loss of myelin. Wallerian degeneration. Regeneration. Chronic active vasculitis: Active features: Perivascular and mural inflammatory infiltrate including lymphocytes and histiocytes. Plump (reactive) endothelial cells. Vessel wall cell death (necrosis). Chronic features: Vessel wall thickening due to hyperplasia. Dense fibrous tissue around the vessel. The vasculitis in this case *affects both small (< 100 micrometers) and medium vessels. Granulomas are*

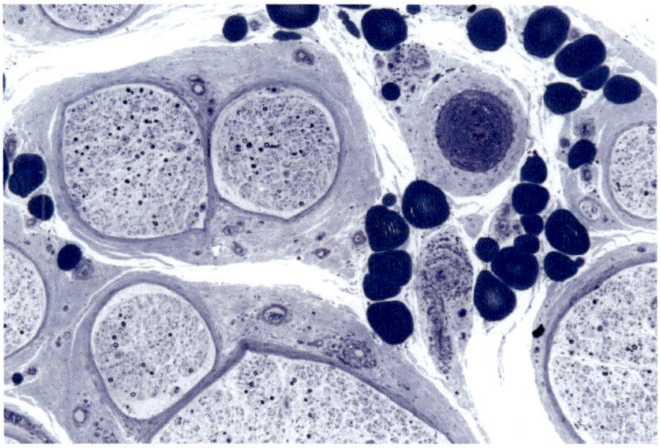

absent. Eosinophils are rare.

This image is by Nephron - Own work, CC BY-SA 3.0, https://commons.wikimedia.org/w/index.php?curid=15903807. https://en.wikipedia.org/wiki/Peripheral_neuropathy#/media/File:Vasculitic_neuropathy_-_plastics_-_intermed_mag.jpg.

HER2 testing

Detection of HER2 protein overexpression or gene amplification is necessary for selection of patients appropriate for KADCYLA therapy because these are the only patients studied for whom benefit has been shown. In the randomized study (Study 1), patients with breast cancer were required to have evidence of HER2 overexpression defined as 3+ IHC by Dako Herceptest™ or evidence of overexpression defined as FISH amplification ratio ≥ 2.0 by Dako HER2 FISH PharmDx™ test kit. Only limited data were available for patients whose breast cancer was positive by FISH and 0 or 1+ by IHC. Assessment of HER2 status should be performed by laboratories with demonstrated proficiency in the specific technology being utilized. Improper assay performance, including use of sub-optimally fixed tissue, failure to utilize specified reagents, deviation from specific assay instructions, and failure to include appropriate controls for assay validation, can lead to unreliable results.

Extravasation

In KADCYLA clinical studies, reactions secondary to extravasation have been observed. These reactions, observed more frequently within 24 hours of infusion, were usually mild and comprised erythema, tenderness, skin irritation, pain, or swelling at the infusion site. Specific treatment for KADCYLA extravasation is unknown. The infusion site should be closely monitored for possible subcutaneous infiltration during drug administration.

Immunogenicity

As with all therapeutic proteins, there is the potential for an immune response to KADCYLA. A total of 836 patients from six clinical studies were tested at multiple time points for anti-therapeutic antibody (ATA) responses to KADCYLA. Following KADCYLA dosing, 5.3% (44/836) of patients tested positive for anti-KADCYLA antibodies at one or more post-dose time points. The presence of KADCYLA in patient serum at the time of ATA sampling may interfere with the ability of this assay to detect anti-KADCYLA antibodies. As a result, data may not accurately reflect the true incidence of anti-KADCYLA antibody development. In addition, neutralizing activity of anti-KADCYLA antibodies has not been assessed. Immunogenicity data are highly dependent on the sensitivity and specificity of the test methods used. Additionally, the observed incidence of a positive result in a test method may be influenced by several factors, including sample handling, timing of sample collection, drug interference, concomitant medication and the underlying disease. Therefore, comparison of the incidence of antibodies to KADCYLA with the incidence of antibodies to other products may be misleading. Clinical significance of anti-KADCYLA antibodies is not yet known.

DRUG INTERACTIONS

No formal drug-drug interaction studies with KADCYLA have been conducted. In vitro studies indicate that DM1, the cytotoxic component of KADCYLA, is metabolized mainly by CYP3A4 and to a lesser extent by CYP3A5. Concomitant use of strong CYP3A4 inhibitors (e.g., ketoconazole, itraconazole, clarithromycin, atazanavir, indinavir, nefazodone, nelfinavir, ritonavir, saquinavir, telithromycin, and voriconazole) with KADCYLA should be avoided due to the potential for an increase in DM1 exposure and toxicity. Consider an alternate medication with no or minimal potential to inhibit CYP3A4. If concomitant use of strong CYP3A4 inhibitors is unavoidable, consider delaying KADCYLA treatment until the strong CYP3A4 inhibitors have cleared from the circulation (approximately 3 elimination half-lives of the inhibitors) when possible. If a strong CYP3A4 inhibitor is co-administered and KADCYLA treatment cannot be delayed, patients should be closely monitored for adverse reactions.

USE IN SPECIFIC POPULATIONS

Pregnancy

Pregnancy Category D

KADCYLA can cause fetal harm when administered to a pregnant woman. There are no adequate and well-controlled studies of KADCYLA in pregnant women. No reproductive and developmental toxicology studies have been conducted with ado-trastuzumab emtansine. Nevertheless, two components of KADCYLA (trastuzumab and DM1) are known or suspected to cause fetal harm or death when administered to a pregnant woman. If KADCYLA is administered during pregnancy, or if a patient becomes pregnant while receiving KADCYLA, apprise the patient of the potential hazard to the fetus. Patients should be advised to use effective contraception during treatment with KADCYLA and for 6 months following the last dose of KADCYLA. If KADCYLA is administered during pregnancy or if a patient becomes pregnant while receiving KADCYLA, immediately report exposure to the Genentech Adverse Event Line at 1-888-835 371 2555. Encourage women who may be exposed during pregnancy to enroll in the MotHER Pregnancy Registry by contacting 1-800-690-6720.

Human data

In the post-marketing setting, treatment with trastuzumab during pregnancy has resulted in cases of oligohydramnios, some associated with fatal pulmonary hypoplasia, skeletal abnormalities and neonatal death. Oligohydramnios is a condition in pregnancy characterized by a deficiency of amniotic fluid *(Figure 35)*, and can be diagnosed by ultrasound *(Figure 36)* or MRI examination.

Figure 35. A 10-week human fetus surrounded by amniotic fluid within the amniotic sac.

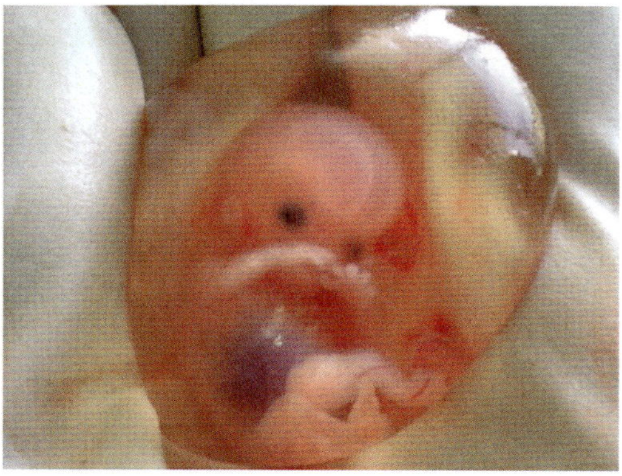

This imge is by drsuparna https://www.flickr.com/photos/74896762@N00/ - https://www.flickr.com/photos/74896762@N00/3167352760/, CC BY-SA 2.0, https://commons.wikimedia.org/w/index.php?curid=5658338. https://en.wikipedia.org/wiki/Amniotic_fluid#/media/File:Human_fetus_10_weeks_with_amniotic_sac_-_therapeutic_abortion.jpg. This file is licensed under the Creative Commons Attribution-Share Alike 2.0 Generic license. No changes have been made to this image.

Figure 36. Ultrasound image (sonogram) of a fetus in the womb, viewed at 12 weeks of pregnancy (bidimensional scan)

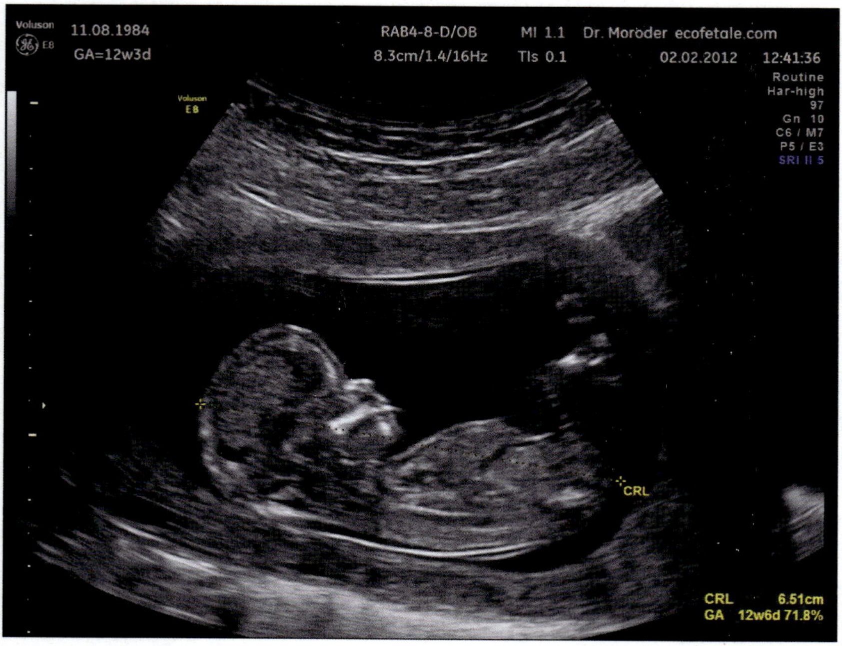

Too little amniotic fluid (oligohydramnios) can be a cause of problems for the mother and baby. In a minority of cases these include contracture of the limbs, clubbing of the feet and hands, and also hypoplastic lungs. The two pathologies (oligohydramnios and hypoplastic lungs) may be related to obstruction of the renal tract.

These case reports described oligohydramnios in pregnant women who received trastuzumab either alone or in combination with chemotherapy. In some case reports, amniotic fluid index increased after trastuzumab was stopped. In one case, trastuzumab therapy resumed after the amniotic fluid index improved, and oligohydramnios recurred.

Animal data

There were no reproductive and developmental toxicology studies conducted with ado trastuzumab emtansine. DM1, the cytotoxic component of KADCYLA, disrupts microtubule function. DM1 is toxic to rapidly dividing cells in animals and is genotoxic, suggesting it has the potential to cause embryotoxicity and teratogenicity. In studies where trastuzumab was administered to pregnant monkeys at doses up to 25 mg/kg (about 7 times the clinical dose), trastuzumab crossed the placental barrier during the early and late phases of gestation. The resulting concentrations of trastuzumab in fetal blood and amniotic fluid were approximately 33% and 25%, respectively, of those present in the maternal serum but were not associated with adverse findings.

Nursing mothers

It is not known whether KADCYLA, specifically, is excreted in human milk, but IgG is known to be excreted in human milk. In lactating monkeys, trastuzumab was excreted in small amounts (about 0.3% of maternal serum concentrations) in breast milk after post-partum doses of 25 mg/kg (about 7 times the clinical dose of KADCYLA). Because many drugs are excreted in human milk and because of the potential for serious adverse reactions in nursing infants from KADCYLA, a decision should be made whether to discontinue nursing or discontinue KADCYLA, taking into account the importance of the drug to the mother.

Pediatric use

Safety and effectiveness of KADCYLA have not been established in pediatric patients.

Geriatric use

Of 495 patients who were randomized to KADCYLA in the randomized trial (Study 1), 65 patients (13%) were ≥ 65 years of age and 11 patients (2%) were ≥ 75 years of age. In patients ≥ 65 years old (n=138 across both treatment arms) the hazard ratios for progression-free survival (PFS) and Overall Survival (OS) were 1.06 (95% CI: 0.68, 1.66) 406 and 1.05 (95% CI: 0.58, 1.91), respectively. Population pharmacokinetic analysis indicates that age does not have a clinically meaningful effect on the pharmacokinetics of ado-trastuzumab emtansine

Females of reproductive potential

KADCYLA can cause embryo-fetal harm when administered during pregnancy. Counsel patients regarding pregnancy prevention and planning. Advise females of reproductive potential to use effective contraception while receiving KADCYLA and for 6 months following the last dose of KADCYLA. If KADCYLA is administered during pregnancy or if the patient becomes pregnant while receiving KADCYLA, immediately report exposure to the Genentech Adverse Event Line at 1 417 888-835-2555. Encourage women who may be exposed during pregnancy to enroll in the 418 MotHER Pregnancy Registry by contacting 1-800-690-6720.

Renal impairment

No dedicated renal impairment trial for KADCYLA has been conducted. Based on the population pharmacokinetics, as well as analysis of Grade 3 or greater adverse drug reactions and dose modifications, dose adjustments of KADCYLA are not needed in patients with mild (creatinine clearance [CLcr] 60 to 89 mL/min) or moderate (CLcr 30 to 59 mL/min) renal impairment. No dose adjustment can be recommended for patients with severe renal impairment (CLcr less than 30 mL/min) because of the limited data available.

Hepatic impairment

In vitro studies in human liver microsomes indicates that DM1 is metabolized by CYP3A4/5. The influence of hepatic impairment on the pharmacokinetics of ado-trastuzumab emtansine conjugate has not been determined.

OVERDOSAGE

There is no known antidote for overdose of KADCYLA. In clinical trials, overdose of KADCYLA has been reported at approximately two times the recommended dose which resulted in Grade 2 thrombocytopenia (resolved 4 days later) and one death. In the fatal case, the patient incorrectly received KADCYLA at 6 mg/kg and died approximately 3 weeks following the overdose; a cause of death and a causal relationship to KADCYLA were not established.

Immunogenicity

As with all therapeutic proteins, there is the potential for an immune response to KADCYLA. A total of 836 patients from six clinical studies were tested at multiple time points for anti-therapeutic antibody (ATA) responses to KADCYLA. Following KADCYLA dosing, 5.3% (44/836) of patients tested positive for anti-KADCYLA antibodies at one or more post-dose time points. The presence of KADCYLA in patient serum at the time of ATA sampling may interfere with the ability of this assay to detect anti-KADCYLA antibodies. As a result, data may not accurately reflect the true incidence of anti-KADCYLA antibody development. In addition, neutralizing activity of anti-KADCYLA antibodies has not been assessed. Immunogenicity data are highly dependent on the sensitivity and specificity of the test methods used. Additionally, the observed incidence of a positive result in a test method may be influenced by several factors, including sample handling, timing of sample collection, drug interference, concomitant medication, and the underlying disease. Therefore, comparison of the incidence of antibodies to KADCYLA with the incidence of antibodies to other products may be misleading. Clinical significance of anti-KADCYLA antibodies is not yet known.

DESCRIPTION

KADCYLA (ado-trastuzumab emtansine) is a HER2-targeted antibody-drug conjugate (ADC) which contains the humanized anti-HER2 IgG1, trastuzumab, covalently linked to the microtubule inhibitory drug DM1 (a maytansine derivative) via the stable thioether linker MCC (4-[N-maleimidomethyl] cyclohexane-1-carboxylate). Emtansine refers to the MCC-DM1 complex. The antibody trastuzumab, is a well characterized recombinant monoclonal antibody product produced by mammalian (Chinese hamster ovary) cells, and the small molecule components (DM1 and MCC) are produced by chemical synthesis. Ado-trastuzumab emtansine contains an average of 3.5 DM1 molecules per antibody.

CLINICAL PHARMACOLOGY

Pharmacokinetics

The pharmacokinetics of KADCYLA was evaluated in a phase 1 study and in a population pharmacokinetic analysis for the ado-trastuzumab emtansine conjugate (ADC) using pooled data from 5 trials in patients with breast cancer. A linear two-compartment model with first-order elimination from the central compartment adequately describes the ADC concentration-time profile. In addition to ADC, the pharmacokinetics of total antibody (conjugated and unconjugated trastuzumab), DM1 were also determined. The pharmacokinetics of KADCYLA are summarized below.

Distribution

Maximum concentrations (Cmax) of ADC and DM1 were observed close to the end of infusion. In Study 1, mean (SD) ADC and DM1 Cycle 1 Cmax following KADCYLA administration was 83.4 (16.5) μg/mL and 4.61 (1.61) ng/mL, respectively. In vitro, the mean binding of DM1 to human plasma proteins was 93%. In vitro, DM1 was a substrate of P-glycoprotein (P-gp). Based on population pharmacokinetic analysis, the central volume of distribution of ADC was 3.13 L.

Metabolism

In vitro studies indicate that DM1, the small molecule component of KADCYLA, undergoes metabolism by CYP3A4/5. DM1 did not inhibit or induce major CYP450 enzymes in vitro. In human plasma, ado-trastuzumab emtansine catabolites MCC-DM1, Lys-MCC-DM1, and DM1 were detected at low levels.

Elimination

Based on population pharmacokinetic analysis, following intravenous infusion of KADCYLA, the clearance of the ADC was 0.68 L/day, and the elimination half-life (t1/2) was approximately 4 days. No accumulation of KADCYLA was observed after repeated dosing of intravenous infusion every 3 weeks. Based on population pharmacokinetic analysis (n=671), body weight, sum of longest diameter of target lesions by RECIST, HER2 extracellular domain (ECD) concentrations, AST, albumin, and baseline trastuzumab concentrations were identified as statistically significant covariates for ado trastuzumab emtansine clearance. However, the magnitude of effect of these covariates on ado trastuzumab emtansine exposure suggests that, with the exception of body weight, these covariates are unlikely to have a clinically meaningful effect on KADCYLA exposure. Therefore, the body weight-based dose of 3.6 mg/kg every 3 weeks without correction for other covariates is considered appropriate.

Effect of renal impairment

Based on population pharmacokinetic analysis in 668 patients, including moderate (CLcr 30 - 59 mL/min, n=53) and mild (CLcr 60 - 89 mL/min, n=254) renal impairment, indicate that pharmacokinetics of the ADC is not affected by mild to moderate renal impairment as compared to normal renal function (CLcr ≥ 90 mL/min, n=361). Data from only one patient with severe renal impairment (CLcr < 30 mL/min) is available.

Effects of age and race

Based on population pharmacokinetic analysis, age (< 65 (n=577); 65 - 75 (n=78); > 75 (n=16)) and race (Asian (n=73); non-Asian (n=598)) do not have a clinically meaningful effect on the pharmacokinetics of ado-trastuzumab emtansine.

Cardiac electrophysiology

The effect of multiple doses of KADCYLA (3.6 mg/kg every 3 weeks) on the QTc interval was evaluated in an open label, single arm study in 51 patients with HER2-

positive metastatic breast cancer. No large changes in the mean QT interval (i.e., > 20 ms) were detected in the study.

EFFICACY OF ADO-TRASTUXUMAB EMANTISINE IN THE TREATMENT OF BREAST CANCER

In patients with HER2-positive advanced breast cancer who have been heavily pretreated with anti-HER2 agents and cytotoxic chemotherapy, ADO-TRASTUXUMAB EMANTISINE was well tolerated and provided a meaningful progression-free survival of 6 months and an overall survival that has not been reached.

Yeo W, et al. Efficacy and tolerability of trastuzumab emtansine in advanced human epidermal growth factor receptor 2-positive breast cancer. Hong Kong Med J. 2018 Feb; 24: 56-62. doi: 10.12809/hkmj176808.

9.3. EVEROLIMUS (AFINITOR)

AFINITOR® (everolimus) tablets, for oral use AFINITOR DISPERZ® (everolimus tablets for oral suspension) Initial U.S. Approval: 2009

RECENT MAJOR CHANGES

Indications and Usage

Dosage and Administrations

Warnings and Precautions

INDICATIONS AND USAGE

AFINITOR is a kinase inhibitor indicated for the treatment of:

• Postmenopausal women with advanced hormone receptor-positive, HER2 negative breast cancer in combination with exemestane after failure of treatment with letrozole or anastrozole.

MECHANISM OF ACTION

Everolimus is an inhibitor of mammalian target of rapamycin (mTOR), a serine-threonine kinase, downstream of the PI3K/AKT pathway. The mTOR pathway is dysregulated in several human cancers and in tuberous sclerosis complex (TSC). Everolimus binds to an intracellular protein, FKBP-12, resulting in an inhibitory complex formation with mTOR complex 1 (mTORC1) and thus inhibition of mTOR kinase activity. Everolimus reduced the activity of S6 ribosomal protein kinase (S6K1) and eukaryotic initiation factor 4E-binding protein (4E-BP1), downstream effectors of mTOR, involved in protein synthesis. S6K1 is a substrate of mTORC1 and phosphorylates the activation domain 1 of the estrogen receptor which results in ligand-independent activation of the receptor. In addition, everolimus inhibited the expression of hypoxia-inducible factor (e.g., HIF-1) and reduced the expression of vascular endothelial growth factor (VEGF). Inhibition of mTOR by everolimus has been shown to reduce cell proliferation, angiogenesis, and glucose uptake in in vitro and/or in vivo studies. Constitutive activation of the PI3K/Akt/mTOR pathway can contribute to endocrine resistance in breast cancer. In vitro studies show that estrogen-dependent and HER2+ breast cancer cells are sensitive to the inhibitory effects of everolimus, and that combination treatment with everolimus and Akt, HER2, or aromatase inhibitors enhances the anti-tumor activity of everolimus in a synergistic manner.

DESCRIPTION

AFINITOR (everolimus) and AFINITOR DISPERZ (everolimus tablets for oral suspension) are kinase inhibitors. The chemical name of everolimus is (1R,9S,12S,15R,16E,18R,19R,21R,23S,24E,26E,28E,30S,32S,35R)-1,18-dihydroxy-12-{(1R)-2-[(1S,3R,4R)-4-(2-hydroxyethoxy)-3-methoxycyclohexyl]-1-methylethyl}-19,30-dimethoxy15,17,21,23,29,35-hexamethyl-11,36-dioxa-4-aza-tricyclo[30.3.1.04,9]hexatriaconta-16,24,26,28-tetraene-2,3,10,14,20 pentaone. The molecular formula is C53H83NO14, and the molecular weight is 958.2. The structural formula is O HO H3C O CH3 CH3 O N O O O O OH H3C CH3 O O OH 3CH O O 3CH H3C CH3 CH3.

AFINITOR for oral administration contains 2.5 mg, 5 mg, 7.5 mg, or 10 mg of everolimus and the following inactive ingredients: anhydrous lactose, butylated hydroxytoluene, crospovidone, hypromellose, lactose monohydrate, and magnesium stearate. AFINITOR DISPERZ for oral administration contains 2 mg, 3 mg, or 5 mg of everolimus and the following inactive ingredients: butylated hydroxytoluene, colloidal silicon dioxide, crospovidone, hypromellose, lactose monohydrate, magnesium stearate, mannitol, and microcrystalline cellulose.

AFINITOR is also FDA-aproved for progressive neuroendocrine tumors of pancreatic origin (PNET), adults with progressive, well-differentiated, non-functional neuroendocrine tumors (NET) of gastrointestinal (GI) or lung origin that are unresectable, locally advanced or metastatic, renal cell carcinoma (RCC) after failure of treatment with sunitinib or sorafenib, renal angiomyolipoma and tuberous sclerosis complex (TSC), TSC who have subependymal giant cell astrocytoma (SEGA) that requires therapeutic intervention but cannot be curatively resected, and as adjunctive treatment of adult and pediatric patients aged 2 years and older with TSC-associated partial-onset seizures).

However, only the breast cancer approval will be dealt with in this book.

DOSAGE AND ADMINISTRATION

Do not combine AFINITOR and AFINITOR DISPERZ to achieve the total daily dose. Modify the dose for patients with hepatic impairment or for patients taking drugs that inhibit or induce P-glycoprotein (P-gp) and CYP3A4.

Breast Cancer: • 10 mg orally once daily.

AGE FORMS AND STRENGTHS

AFINITOR: 2.5 mg, 5 mg, 7.5 mg, and 10 mg tablets

AFINITOR DISPERZ: 2 mg, 3 mg, and 5 mg tablets

CONTRAINDICATIONS: clinically significant hypersensitivity to everolimus or to other rapamycin derivatives.

- Non-infectious pneumonitis: Monitor for clinical symptoms or radiological changes. Withhold or permanently discontinue based on severity.
- Infections: monitor for signs and symptoms of infection. Withhold or permanently discontinue based on severity.

- Severe hypersensitivity reactions: permanently discontinue for clinically significant hypersensitivity.
- Angioedema: Patients taking concomitant ACE inhibitors may be at increased risk for angioedema. Permanently discontinue for angioedema.
- Stomatitis: initiate dexamethasone alcohol-free mouthwash when starting treatment.
- Renal failure: monitor renal function prior to treatment and periodically thereafter.
- Impaired wound healing: exercise caution in the peri-surgical period.
- Geriatric patients: monitor and adjust dose for adverse reactions.
- Metabolic disorders: Monitor serum glucose and lipids prior to treatment and periodically thereafter. Withhold or permanently discontinue based on severity
- Myelosuppression: monitor hematologic parameters prior to treatment and periodically thereafter. Withhold or permanently discontinue based on severity.
- Risk of infection or reduced immune response with vaccination: avoid live vaccines and close contact with those who have received live vaccines. Complete recommended childhood vaccinations prior to starting treatment.
- Embryo-fetal toxicity: can cause fetal harm. Advise patients of reproductive potential of the potential risk to a fetus and to use effective contraception.

ADVERSE REACTIONS

- Breast cancer, [NET, RCC]: Most common adverse reactions (incidence ≥ 30%) include stomatitis, infections, rash, fatigue, diarrhea, edema, abdominal pain, nausea, fever, asthenia, cough, headache, and decreased appetite.

DRUG INTERACTIONS

- P-gp and strong CYP3A4 inhibitors: avoid concomitant use.
- P-gp and moderate CYP3A4 inhibitors: reduce the dose as recommended.
- P-gp and strong CYP3A4 inducers: increase the dose as recommended

USE IN SPECIFIC POPULATIONS

• For breast cancer, [NET, RCC, or TSC-associated renal angiomyolipoma patients] with hepatic impairment, reduce the dose.

FULL PRESCRIBING INFORMATION

INDICATIONS AND USAGE

Hormone receptor-positive, HER2-negative breast cancer AFINITOR® is indicated for the treatment of postmenopausal women with advanced hormone receptor-positive, HER2 negative breast cancer in combination with exemestane, after failure of treatment with letrozole or anastrozole.

DOSAGE AND ADMINISTRATION

Important dosage information

• AFINITOR and AFINITOR DISPERZ are two different dosage forms. Select the recommended dosage form based on the indication Do not combine AFINITOR and AFINITOR DISPERZ to achieve the total dose.

• Modify the dosage for patients with hepatic impairment or for patients taking drugs that inhibit or induce Pglycoprotein (P-gp) and CYP3A4.

Recommended dosage changes because of adverse reactions are complex and the reader is advised to study the package insert carefully on contact the manufacturer if necessary.

WARNINGS AND PRECAUTIONS

- Non-infectious Pneumonitis

Non-infectious pneumonitis is a class effect of rapamycin derivatives. Non-infectious pneumonitis was reported in up to 19% of patients treated with AFINITOR/AFINITOR DISPERZ in clinical trials; some cases were reported with pulmonary hypertension (including pulmonary arterial hypertension) as a secondary event. The incidence of Grade 3 and 4 non-infectious pneumonitis was up to 4% and up to 0.2%, respectively. Fatal outcomes have been observed. Consider a diagnosis of non-infectious pneumonitis in patients presenting with non-specific respiratory signs and symptoms. Consider opportunistic infections such as *Pneumocystis jiroveci* pneumonia (PJP) in the differential diagnosis. Advise patients to report promptly any new or worsening respiratory symptoms.

Continue AFINITOR/AFINITOR DISPERZ without dose alteration in patients who develop radiological changes suggestive of non-infectious pneumonitis and have few or no symptoms. Imaging appears to overestimate the incidence of clinical pneumonitis. For Grade 2 to 4 non-infectious pneumonitis, withhold or permanently discontinue AFINITOR/AFINITOR DISPERZ based on severity. Corticosteroids may be indicated until clinical symptoms resolve. Administer prophylaxis for PJP when concomitant use of corticosteroids or other immunosuppressive agents are required. The development of pneumonitis has been reported even at a reduced dose.

- Infections

AFINITOR/AFINITOR DISPERZ has immunosuppressive properties and may predispose patients to bacterial, fungal, viral, or protozoal infections, including infections with opportunistic pathogens Localized and systemic infections, including pneumonia, mycobacterial infections, other bacterial infections, invasive fungal infections (e.g., aspergillosis, candidiasis, or PJP) and viral infections (e.g., reactivation of hepatitis B virus) have occurred *(Figures 37 and 38).*

Figure 37. Pulmonary aspergillosis histopathology.

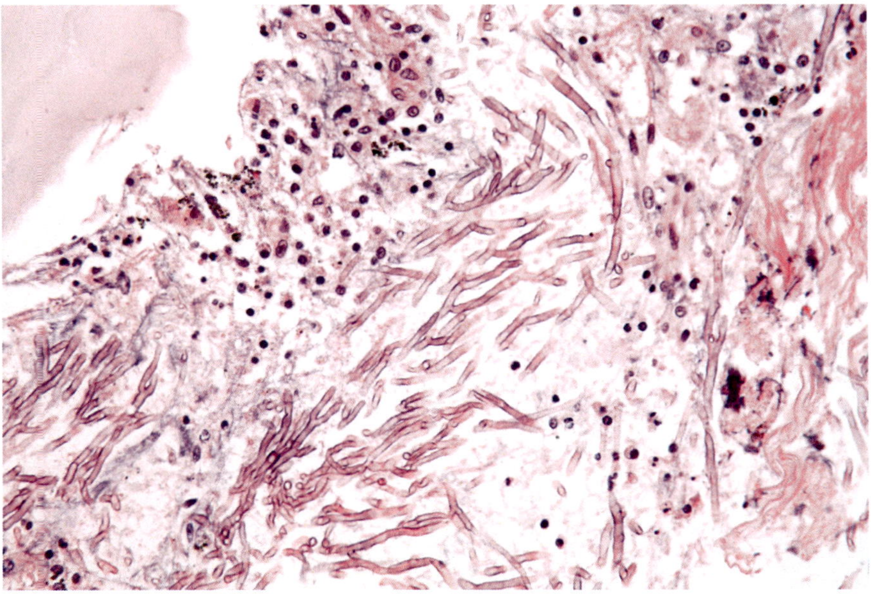

By Nephron - Own work, CC BY-SA 3.0, https://commons.wikimedia.org/w/index.php?curid=9097954. https://en.wikipedia.org/wiki/Aspergillus#/media/File:Pulmonary_aspergillosis.jpg. This file is licensed under the Creative Commons Attribution-Share Alike 3.0 Unported license. No changes have been made to this image.

Figure 38. Oral candidiasis

This image is by James Heilman, MD - Own work, CC BY-SA 3.0, https://commons.wikimedia.org/w/index.php?curid=11717223. https://en.wikipedia.org/wiki/Candidiasis#/media/File:Human_tongue_infected_with_oral_candidiasis.jpg. This file is licensed under the Creative Commons Attribution-Share Alike 3.0 Unported license. No changes were made to this image.

Figure 38. Oral candidiasis.

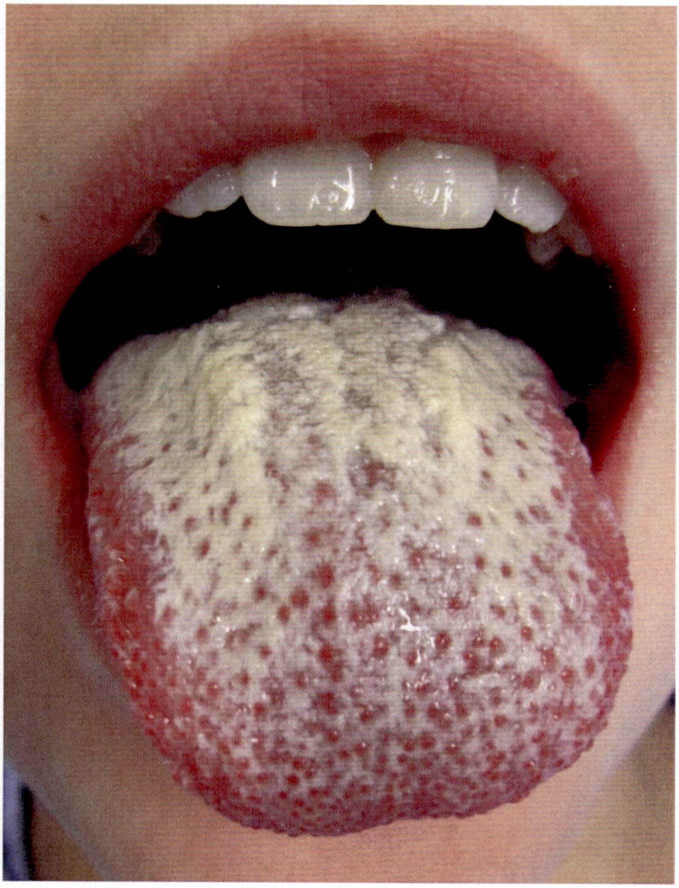

Some of these infections have been severe (e.g., sepsis, septic shock, or resulting in multisystem organ failure) or fatal. The incidence of Grade 3 and 4 infections was up to 10% and up to 3%, respectively. The incidence of serious infections was reported at a higher frequency in patients < 6 years of age. Complete treatment of preexisting invasive fungal infections prior to starting treatment. Monitor for signs and symptoms of infection. Withhold or permanently discontinue AFINITOR/AFINITOR DISPERZ based on severity of infection. Administer prophylaxis for PJP when concomitant use of corticosteroids or other immunosuppressive agents are required.

- Severe Hypersensitivity Reactions

Hypersensitivity reactions to AFINITOR/AFINITOR DISPERZ have been observed and include anaphylaxis, dyspnea, flushing, chest pain, and angioedema (e.g., swelling of the airways or tongue, with or without respiratory impairment). The incidence of Grade 3 hypersensitivity reactions was up to 1%. Permanently discontinue AFINITOR/AFINITOR DISPERZ for the development of clinically significant hypersensitivity.

- Angioedema *(Figure 39)* with concomitant use of angiotensin-converting enzyme (ACE) Inhibitors

Figure 39. Angioedema involving one half of the tongue.

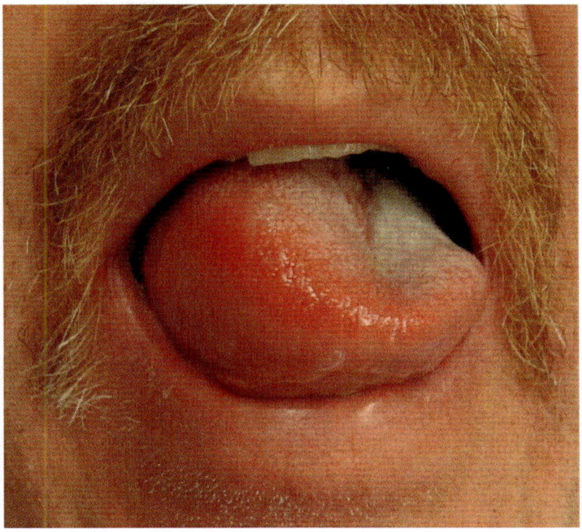

This image is by By James Heilman, MD - Own work, CC BY-SA 3.0, https://commons.wikimedia.org/w/index.php?curid=24076990.

https://en.wikipedia.org/wiki/Angioedema#/media/File:Angioedema2013.JPG. This file is licensed under the Creative Commons Attribution-Share Alike 3.0 Unported license. No changes were made to this image.

Patients taking concomitant ACE inhibitors with AFINITOR/AFINITOR DISPERZ may be at increased risk for angioedema (e.g., swelling of the airways or tongue, with or without respiratory impairment). In a pooled analysis of randomized double-blind oncology clinical trials, the incidence of angioedema in patients taking AFINITOR with an ACE inhibitor was 6.8% compared to 1.3% in the control arm with an ACE inhibitor. Permanently discontinue AFINITOR/AFINITOR DISPERZ for angioedema.

- Stomatitis

Stomatitis, including mouth ulcers and oral mucositis, has occurred in patients treated with AFINITOR/AFINITOR DISPERZ at an incidence ranging from 44% to 78% across clinical trials. Grades 3-4 stomatitis was reported in 4% to 9% of patients. Stomatitis most often occurs within the first 8 weeks of treatment. When starting AFINITOR/AFINITOR DISPERZ, initiating dexamethasone alcohol-free oral solution as a swish and spit mouthwash reduces the incidence and severity of stomatitis. If stomatitis does occur, mouthwashes and/or other topical treatments are recommended. Avoid alcohol-, hydrogen peroxide-, iodine-, or thyme-containing products, as they may exacerbate the condition. Do not administer antifungal agents unless fungal infection has been diagnosed.

- Renal failure

Cases of renal failure (including acute renal failure), some with a fatal outcome, have occurred in patients taking AFINITOR. Elevations of serum creatinine and proteinuria have been reported in patients taking AFINITOR/AFINITOR DISPERZ. The incidence of Grade 3 and 4 elevations of serum creatinine was up to 2% and up to 1%, respectively. The incidence of Grade 3 and 4 proteinuria was up to 1% and up to 0.5%, respectively. Monitor renal function at least every 6 months in patients who have additional risk factors for renal failure.

- Impaired wound healing

AFINITOR/AFINITOR DISPERZ delays wound healing and increases the occurrence of wound-related complications like wound dehiscence, *(Figure 40)* wound infection, incisional hernia, lymphocele, and seroma. These wound-related complications may require surgical intervention. Exercise caution with the use of AFINITOR/AFINITOR DISPERZ in the peri-surgical period.

Figure 40. Wound dehiscence following an inguinal hernia repair.

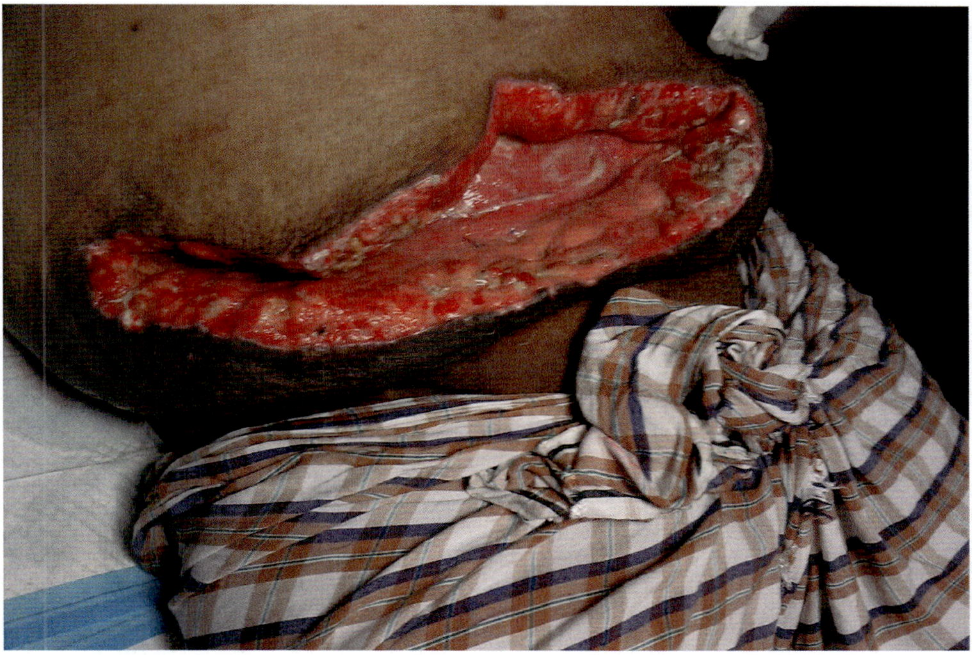

This image is by User: Phoenix119 - Own work, CC BY-SA 3.0, https://commons.wikimedia.org/w/index.php?curid=33002084. https://en.wikipedia.org/wiki/Wound_dehiscence#/media/File:Wound_Dehiscence_post_inguinal_hernia_repair_2014-05-27_00-46.jpg. This file is licensed under the Creative Commons Attribution-Share Alike 3.0 Unported license. No changes were made to this image.

Geriatric patients

In the randomized hormone receptor-positive, HER2-negative breast cancer study (BOLERO-2), the incidence of deaths due to any cause within 28 days of the last AFINITOR dose was 6% in patients ≥ 65 years of age compared to 2% in patients < 65 years of age. Adverse reactions leading to permanent treatment discontinuation occurred in 33% of patients ≥ 65 years of age compared to 17% in patients < 65 years of age. Careful monitoring and appropriate dose adjustments for adverse reactions are recommended.

- Metabolic disorders

Hyperglycemia, hypercholesterolemia, and hypertriglyceridemia have been reported in patients taking AFINITOR/AFINITOR DISPERZ at an incidence up to 75%, 86%, and 73%, respectively. The incidence of these Grade 3 and 4 laboratory abnormalities was up to 15% and up to 0.4%, respectively. In nondiabetic patients, monitor fasting serum glucose prior to starting AFINITOR/AFINITOR DISPERZ and annually thereafter. In diabetic patients, monitor fasting serum glucose more frequently as clinically indicated. Monitor lipid profile prior to starting AFINITOR/AFINITOR DISPERZ and annually thereafter. When possible, achieve optimal glucose and lipid control prior to starting AFINITOR/AFINITOR DISPERZ. For Grade 3 to 4 metabolic events, withhold or permanently discontinue AFINITOR/AFINITOR DISPERZ based on severity.

- Myelosuppression, anemia, lymphopenia, neutropenia, and

thrombocytopenia have been reported in patients taking AFINITOR/AFINITOR DISPERZ. The incidence of these Grade 3 and 4 laboratory abnormalities was up to 16% and up to 2%, respectively. Monitor complete blood count prior to starting AFINITOR/AFINITOR DISPERZ every 6 months for the first year of treatment and annually thereafter. Withhold or permanently discontinue AFINITOR/AFINITOR DISPERZ based on severity.

- Risk of infection or reduced immune response with vaccination

The safety of immunization with live vaccines during AFINITOR/AFINITOR DISPERZ therapy has not been studied. Due to the potential increased risk of infection, avoid the use of live vaccines and close contact with individuals who have received live vaccines during treatment with AFINITOR/AFINITOR DISPERZ. Due to the potential increased risk of infection or reduced immune response with vaccination, complete the recommended childhood series of vaccinations according to American Council on Immunization Practices (ACIP) guidelines prior to the start of therapy. An accelerated vaccination schedule may be appropriate.

- Embryo-fetal toxicity

Based on animal studies and the mechanism of action, AFINITOR/AFINITOR DISPERZ can cause fetal harm when administered to a pregnant woman. In animal studies, everolimus caused embryo-fetal toxicities in rats when administered during the period of organogenesis at maternal exposures that were lower than human exposures at the clinical dose of 10 mg once daily. Advise pregnant women of the potential risk to a fetus. Advise female patients of reproductive potential to avoid becoming pregnant and to use effective contraception during treatment with AFINITOR/AFINITOR DISPERZ and for 8 weeks after the last dose. Advise male patients with female partners of reproductive potential to use effective contraception during treatment with AFINITOR/AFINITOR DISPERZ and for 4 weeks after the last dose.

Postmarketing experience

The following adverse reactions have been identified during post approval use of AFINITOR/AFINITOR DISPERZ. Because these reactions are reported voluntarily from a population of uncertain size, it is not always possible to reliably estimate frequency or establish a causal relationship to drug exposure:

- Gastrointestinal: acute pancreatitis
- Hepatobiliary: cholecystitis and cholelithiasis
- Vascular: arterial thrombotic events
- Nervous system: reflex sympathetic dystrophy
- Cardiac: cardiac failure with some cases reported with pulmonary hypertension (including pulmonary arterial hypertension) as a secondary event
- Infections: sepsis and septic shock

DRUG INTERACTIONS

Effect of Other Drugs on AFINITOR/AFINITOR DISPERZ

Inhibitors

Avoid the concomitant use of P-gp and strong CYP3A4 inhibitors. Reduce the dose for patients taking AFINITOR/AFINITOR DISPERZ with a P-gp and moderate CYP3A4 inhibitor as recommended.

- Inducers

  Increase the dose for patients taking AFINITOR/AFINITOR DISPERZ with a P-gp and strong CYP3A4 inducer as recommended
- Effects of combination use of angiotensin converting enzyme (ACE) inhibitors

  Patients taking concomitant ACE inhibitors with AFINITOR/AFINITOR DISPERZ may be at increased risk for angioedema. Avoid the concomitant use of ACE inhibitors with AFINITOR/AFINITOR DISPERZ.
- **USE IN SPECIFIC POPULATIONS**

Pregnancy risk summary

Based on animal studies and the mechanism of action, AFINITOR/AFINITOR DISPERZ can cause fetal harm when administered to a pregnant woman. There are limited case reports of AFINITOR use in pregnant women; however, these reports are not sufficient to inform about risks of birth defects or miscarriage. In animal studies, everolimus caused embryo-fetal toxicities in rats when administered during the period of organogenesis at maternal exposures that were lower than human exposures at the recommended dose of AFINITOR 10 mg orally once daily. Advise pregnant women of the potential risk to the fetus. In the U.S. general population, the estimated background risk of major birth defects and miscarriage is 2% to 4% and 15% to 20% of clinically recognized pregnancies, respectively.

Data

Animal data

In animal reproductive studies, oral administration of everolimus to female rats before mating and through organogenesis induced embryo-fetal toxicities, including increased resorption, pre-implantation, and post-implantation loss, decreased numbers of live fetuses, malformation (e.g., sternal cleft), and retarded skeletal development. These effects occurred in the absence of maternal toxicities. Embryo-fetal toxicities in rats occurred at doses ≥ 0.1 mg/kg (0.6 mg/m^2) with resulting exposures of approximately 4% of the human exposure at the recommended dose of AFINITOR 10 mg orally once daily based on area under the curve (AUC). In a pre- and post-natal development study in rats, animals were dosed from implantation through lactation. At the dose of 0.1 mg/kg (0.6 mg/m^2), there were no adverse effects on delivery and lactation or signs of maternal toxicity; however, there were reductions in body weight (up to 9% reduction from the control) and in survival of offspring (~5% died or missing). There were no drug-related effects on the developmental parameters (morphological development, motor activity, learning, or fertility assessment) in the offspring.

Lactation

Risk summary

There are no data on the presence of everolimus or its metabolites in human milk, the effects of everolimus on the breastfed infant or on milk production. Everolimus and its metabolites passed into the milk of lactating rats at a concentration 3.5 times higher than in maternal serum. Because of the potential for serious adverse reactions in breastfed infants from everolimus, advise women not to breastfeed during treatment with AFINITOR/AFINITOR DISPERZ and for 2 weeks after the last dose.

Females and males of reproductive potential

Pregnancy testing

Verify the pregnancy status of females of reproductive potential prior to starting AFINITOR/AFINITOR DISPERZ.

Contraception

AFINITOR/AFINITOR DISPERZ can cause fetal harm when administered to pregnant women.

Females

Advise female patients of reproductive potential to use effective contraception during treatment with AFINITOR/AFINITOR DISPERZ and for 8 weeks after the last dose.

Males

Advise male patients with female partners of reproductive potential to use effective contraception during treatment with AFINITOR/AFINITOR DISPERZ and for 4 weeks after the last dose.

Infertility

Females

Menstrual irregularities, secondary amenorrhea, and increases in luteinizing hormone (LH) and follicle stimulating hormone (FSH) occurred in female patients taking AFINITOR/AFINITOR DISPERZ. Based on these findings, AFINITOR/AFINITOR DISPERZ may impair fertility in female patients

Males

Cases of reversible azoospermia have been reported in male patients taking AFINITOR. In male rats, sperm motility, sperm count, plasma testosterone levels and fertility were diminished at AUC similar to those of the clinical dose of AFINITOR 10 mg orally once daily. Based on these findings, AFINITOR/AFINITOR DISPERZ may impair fertility in male patients

Geriatric use

In BOLERO-2, 40% of patients with breast cancer treated with AFINITOR were ≥ 65 years of age, while 15% were ≥ 75 years of age. No overall differences in effectiveness were observed between elderly and younger patients. The incidence of deaths due to any cause within 28 days of the last AFINITOR dose was 6% in patients ≥ 65 years of age compared to 2% in patients < 65 years of age. Adverse reactions leading to permanent treatment discontinuation occurred in 33% of patients ≥ 65 years of age compared to 17% in patients < 65 years of age.

Hepatic impairment

AFINITOR/AFINITOR DISPERZ exposure may increase in patients with hepatic impairment. For patients with breast cancer, [NET, RCC, and TSC-associated renal angiomyolipoma] who have hepatic impairment, reduce the AFINITOR dose as indicated.

EFFICACY OF AFINITOR IN THE TREATMENT OF BREAST CANCER

1. The PI3K/Akt/mTOR (phosphatidylinositol 3-kinase/protein kinase B/mammalian target of rapamycin) pathway regulates several key cellular functions, and its dysregulation creates an environment that promotes tumorigenesis as well as resistance to therapy. The mTOR inhibitor everolimus has emerged as a promising agent in the treatment of breast cancer and was recently approved in combination with exemestane for advanced hormone receptor–positive disease after progression on a nonsteroidal aromatase inhibitor.

Saksena R, Wong ST. Clinical evidence of the efficacy of everolimus and its potential in the treatment of breast cancer. Breast Cancer (Dove Med Press). 2013;5:27-35. Published 2013 May 17. doi:10.2147/BCTT.S30131

2. This study suggests that everolimus plus exemestane (EE) remains an effective treatment option after prior ET or ET + CDK4/6i use. Median TTNT of EE was longer for patients who received prior ET, whereas median OS was longer for patients who received prior ET + CDK4/6i. However, this improvement in OS was not statistically significant when indexed to the start of EE therapy suggesting that OS benefit is primarily driven by prior CDK4/6i use. EE remains an effective treatment option regardless of prior treatment option.

Rozenblit, M., Mun, S., Soulos, P. et al. Patterns of treatment with everolimus exemestane in hormone receptor-positive HER2-negative metastatic breast cancer in the era of targeted therapy. Breast Cancer Res 23, 14 (2021). https://doi.org/10.1186/s13058-021-01394-y

10.4. ALPELISIB (PIQRAY®)

PIQRAY® (alpelisib) tablets, for oral use. Initial U.S. Approval: 2019.

INDICATIONS AND USAGE

PIQRAY is a kinase inhibitor indicated in combination with fulvestrant for the treatment of postmenopausal women, and men, with hormone receptor (HR)-positive, human epidermal growth factor receptor 2 (HER2)-negative, PIK3CA-mutated, advanced or metastatic breast cancer as detected by an FDA-approved test following progression on or after an endocrine-based regimen.

MECHANISM OF ACTION

Alpelisib is an inhibitor of phosphatidylinositol-3-kinase (PI3K) with inhibitory activity predominantly against PI3Kα. Gain-of-function mutations in the gene encoding the catalytic α-subunit of PI3K (PIK3CA) lead to activation of PI3Kα and Akt-signaling, cellular transformation and the generation of tumors in in vitro and in vivo models. In breast cancer cell lines, alpelisib inhibited the phosphorylation of PI3K downstream targets, including Akt and showed activity in cell lines harboring a PIK3CA mutation. In vivo, alpelisib inhibited the PI3K/Akt signaling pathway and reduced tumor growth in xenograft models, including models of breast cancer. PI3K inhibition by alpelisib treatment has been shown to induce an increase in estrogen receptor (ER) transcription in breast cancer cells. The combination of alpelisib and fulvestrant demonstrated increased antitumor activity compared to either treatment alone in xenograft models derived from ER-positive, PIK3CA mutated breast cancer cell lines.

Pharmacodynamics

Cardiac electrophysiology

Serial ECGs were collected following a single dose and at steady state to evaluate the effect of alpelisib on the QTcF interval in patients with advanced cancer. An analysis of clinical ECG data demonstrates the absence of a large effect (i.e., > 20 ms) on QTcF prolongation at the recommended 300 mg dose with or without fulvestrant.

DESCRIPTION

PIQRAY (alpelisib) is a kinase inhibitor. The chemical name of alpelisib is (2S)-N1 -[4-Methyl-5-[2-(2,2,2- trifluoro-1,1-dimethylethyl)-4-pyridinyl]-2-thiazolyl]-1,2-pyrrolidinedicarboxamide. Alpelisib is a white to almost white powder. The molecular formula for alpelisib is C19H22F3N5O2S and the relative molecular mass is 441.47 g/mol. PIQRAY film-coated tablets are supplied for oral administration with three strengths that contain 50 mg, 150 mg and 200 mg of alpelisib. The tablets also contain hypromellose, magnesium stearate, mannitol, microcrystalline cellulose, and sodium starch glycolate. The film-coating contains hypromellose, iron oxide black, iron oxide red, macrogol/polyethylene glycol (PEG) 4000, talc, and titanium dioxide.

DOSAGE AND ADMINISTRATION

• Recommended dose: 300 mg (two 150 mg tablets) taken orally once daily with food.

• For adverse reactions, consider dose interruption, dose reduction, or discontinuation.

DOSAGE FORMS AND STRENGTHS

Tablets: 50 mg, 150 mg, 200 mg

CONTRAINDICATIONS

Severe hypersensitivity to PIQRAY or to any of its components

WARNINGS AND PRECAUTIONS

• Severe hypersensitivity: permanently discontinue PIQRAY. Promptly initiate appropriate treatment.

• Severe cutaneous reactions: cases of severe cutaneous reactions, including Stevens-Johnson syndrome (SJS) and Erythema Multiforme (EM) were reported. Do not initiate treatment in patients with a history of SJS, EM, or Toxic Epidermal Necrolysis (TEN). Interrupt PIQRAY if signs or symptoms of severe cutaneous reactions are present, until etiology of the reaction has been determined. Consider consultation with a dermatologist. Permanently discontinue PIQRAY if SJS, EM, or TEN is confirmed.

• Hyperglycemia:

Severe hyperglycemia, including ketoacidosis, was reported. The safety of PIQRAY in patients with Type 1 or uncontrolled Type 2 diabetes has not been established. Before initiating treatment with PIQRAY, test fasting plasma glucose (FPG), HbA1c, and optimize blood glucose. After initiating treatment, monitor periodically. Initiate or optimize anti-hyperglycemic medications as clinically indicated. Interrupt, reduce dose, or discontinue PIQRAY if severe hyperglycemia occurs.

• Pneumonitis

Severe cases of pneumonitis and interstitial lung disease have been reported. Monitor for clinical symptoms or radiological changes. Interrupt or discontinue PIQRAY if severe pneumonitis occurs.

• Diarrhea

Severe cases of diarrhea, including dehydration and acute kidney injury, have been reported. Most patients experience diarrhea (Grade ≤ 2) during treatment with PIQRAY. Advise patients to start antidiarrheal treatment, increase oral fluids, and notify their healthcare provider if diarrhea occurs. Interrupt, reduce dose, or discontinue PIQRAY if severe diarrhea occurs.

• Embryo-fetal toxicity

PIQRAY can cause fetal harm. Advise patients of potential risk to a fetus and to use effective contraception. Also, refer to the Full Prescribing Information of fulvestrant for pregnancy and contraception information.

ADVERSE REACTIONS

The most common adverse reactions including laboratory abnormalities (all grades, incidence ≥ 20%) were glucose increased, creatinine increased, diarrhea, rash, lymphocyte count decreased, GGT increased, nausea, ALT increased, fatigue, hemoglobin decreased, lipase increased, decreased appetite, stomatitis, vomiting, weight decreased, calcium decreased, glucose decreased, aPTT prolonged, and alopecia.

INDICATIONS AND USAGE

PIQRAY is indicated in combination with fulvestrant *(Faslodex)* for the treatment of postmenopausal women, and men, with hormone receptor (HR)-positive, human epidermal growth factor receptor 2 (HER2)-negative, PIK3CA mutated, advanced or metastatic breast cancer as detected by an FDA-approved test following progression on or after an endocrine-based regimen.

DOSAGE AND ADMINISTRATION

Patient selection

Select patients for the treatment of HR-positive, HER2-negative advanced or metastatic breast cancer with PIQRAY, based on the presence of one or more PIK3CA mutations in tumor tissue or plasma specimens. If no mutation is detected in a plasma specimen, test tumor tissue. Information on FDAapproved tests for the detection of PIK3CA mutations in breast cancer is available at: http://www.fda.gov/CompanionDiagnostics.

Dosage and Administration

The recommended dose of PIQRAY is 300 mg (two 150 mg film-coated tablets) taken orally, once daily, with food. Continue treatment until disease progression or unacceptable toxicity occurs. Patients should take their dose of PIQRAY at approximately the same time each day. Swallow PIQRAY tablets whole (tablets should not be chewed, crushed or split prior to swallowing). No tablet should be ingested if it is broken, cracked, or otherwise not intact. If a dose of PIQRAY is missed, it can be taken with food within 9 hours after the time it is usually taken. After more than 9 hours, skip the dose for that day. The next day, take PIQRAY at the usual time. If the patient vomits after taking the dose, advise the patient not to take an additional dose on that day, and to resume the dosing schedule the next day at the usual time.

When given with PIQRAY, the recommended dose of fulvestrant (Faslodex) is 500 mg administered on Days 1, 15, and 29, and once monthly thereafter. Refer to the Full Prescribing Information for fulvestrant.

Dose modifications for adverse reactions

The recommended dose modifications for adverse reactions (ARs) are:

PIQRAY starting dose 300 mg once daily taken as two 150 mg tablets: First-dose reduction 250 mg once daily taken as one 200 mg tablet and one 50 mg tablet. Second-dose reduction 200 mg once daily taken as one 200 mg tablet.

Only one dose reduction is permitted for pancreatitis.

If further dose reduction below 200 mg once daily is required, discontinue PIQRAY.

PLEASE CONSULT THE FDA PRODUCT APPROVAL LABEL FOR DOSE MODIFICATIONS AND OTHER MEASURES IN THE EVENT OF GLUCOSE METABOLISM ABNORMAILTES, SEVERE CUTANEOUS REACTIONS, PNEUMONITIS AND DIARRHEA.CONTRAINDICATIONS.

PIQRAY is contraindicated in patients with severe hypersensitivity to it or any of its components

Further details on WARNINGS AND PRECAUTIONS

Severe hypersensitivity

Severe hypersensitivity reactions, including anaphylaxis and anaphylactic shock, were reported in patients treated with PIQRAY. Severe hypersensitivity reactions were manifested by symptoms including, but not limited to, dyspnea, flushing, rash, fever, or tachycardia. The incidence of Grade 3 and 4 hypersensitivity reactions was 0.7%. Advise patients of the signs and symptoms of severe hypersensitivity reactions. Permanently discontinue PIQRAY in the event of severe hypersensitivity.

Severe cutaneous reactions

Severe cutaneous reactions, including Stevens-Johnson Syndrome (SJS) and erythema multiforme (EM) were reported in patients treated with PIQRAY. SJS and EM were reported in 0.4% and 1.1% of patients, respectively. Do not initiate PIQRAY treatment in patients with a history of SJS, EM, or Toxic epidermal necrolysis (TEN). If signs or symptoms of severe cutaneous reactions occur, interrupt PIQRAY until the etiology of the reaction has been determined. Consultation with a dermatologist is recommended. If SJS, TEN, or EM is confirmed, permanently discontinue PIQRAY. Do not reintroduce PIQRAY in patients who have experienced previous severe cutaneous reactions during PIQRAY treatment. If SJS, TEN, or EM is not confirmed, PIQRAY may require dose modifications, topical corticosteroids, or oral antihistamine treatment. Advise patients of the signs and symptoms of severe cutaneous reactions (e.g., a prodrome of fever, flu-like symptoms, mucosal lesions or progressive skin rash).

Hyperglycemia

Severe hyperglycemia, including ketoacidosis, has been reported in patients treated with PIQRAY. Hyperglycemia was reported in 65% of patients treated with PIQRAY. Grade 3 (*fasting plasma glucose (FPG)* > 250-500 mg/dL) and Grade 4 (FPG > 500 mg/dL) hyperglycemia was reported in 33% and 3.9% of patients, respectively. Ketoacidosis was reported in 0.7% of patients (n = 2) treated with PIQRAY. Among the patients who experienced Grade ≥ 2 (FPG 160-250 mg/dL) hyperglycemia, the median time to first occurrence of hyperglycemia was 15 days (range: 5 to 517 days). In the 187 patients with hyperglycemia, 87% (163/187) were managed with anti-diabetic medication, and 76% (142/187) reported use of metformin as single agent or in combination with other anti-diabetic medication [i.e., insulin, dipeptidyl peptidase-4 (DPP-4) inhibitors, and sulfonylureas]. In patients with Grade ≥ 2 hyperglycemia with at least 1 grade improvement (n = 153), median time to improvement from the first event was 8 days (range: 2 to 65 days). In all patients with elevated FPG who continued fulvestrant treatment after discontinuing PIQRAY (n = 54), 96% (n = 52) of patients had FPG levels that returned to baseline. Before initiating treatment with PIQRAY, test FPG, HbA1c, and optimize blood glucose. After initiating treatment with PIQRAY, monitor blood glucose and/or FPG at least once every week for the first 2 weeks, then at least once every 4 weeks, and as clinically indicated. Monitor HbA1c every 3 months and as clinically indicated. If a patient experiences hyperglycemia after initiating treatment with PIQRAY, monitor blood glucose and/or FPG as clinically indicated, and at least twice weekly until blood glucose or FPG decreases to normal levels. During treatment with anti-diabetic medication, continue monitoring blood glucose or FPG at least once a week for 8 weeks, followed by once every 2 weeks and as clinically indicated. Consider consultation with a healthcare practitioner with expertise in the treatment of hyperglycemia and counsel patients on lifestyle changes.

The safety of PIQRAY in patients with Type 1 and uncontrolled Type 2 diabetes has not been established as these patients were excluded from the SOLAR-1 trial. Patients with a medical history of Type 2 diabetes were included. Patients with a history of diabetes mellitus may require intensified diabetic treatment. Closely monitor patients with diabetes. Based on the severity of the hyperglycemia, PIQRAY may require dose interruption, reduction, or discontinuation.

Advise patients of the signs and symptoms of hyperglycemia (e.g., excessive thirst, urinating more often than usual or higher amount of urine than usual, or increased appetite with weight loss).

Pneumonitis

Severe pneumonitis, including acute interstitial pneumonitis and interstitial lung disease, has been reported in patients treated with PIQRAY *(Figures 41 and 42).*

Figure 41. Acute interstitial pneumonia showing a marked reduction in lung capacity.

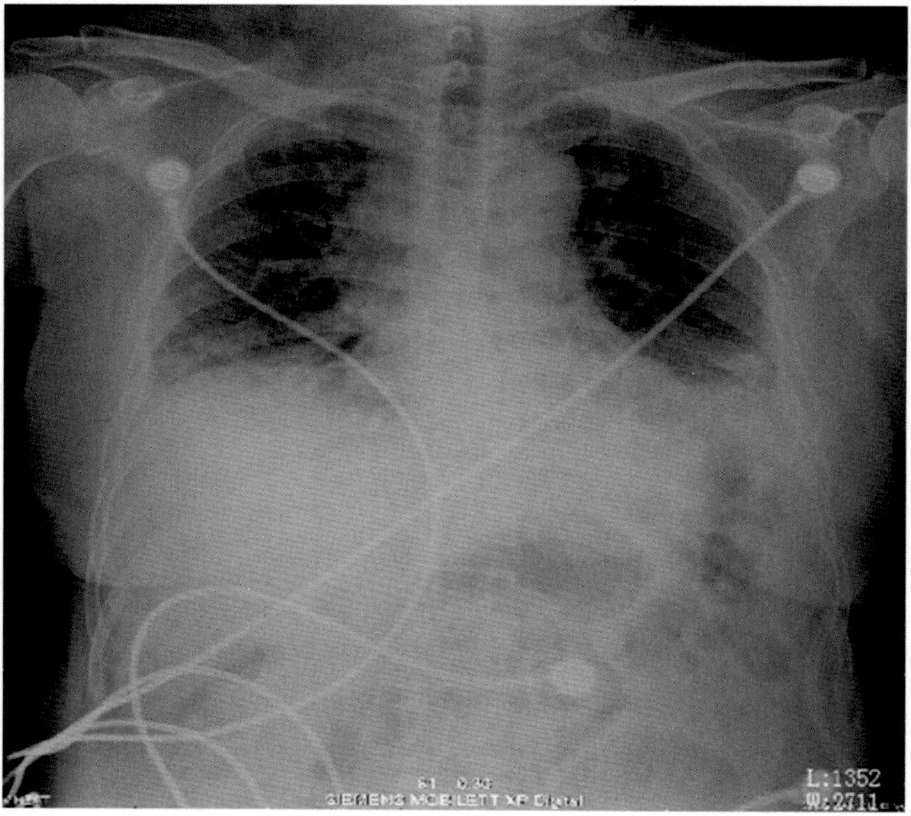

This image is by Case Rep Pulmonol - https://www.ncbi.nlm.nih.gov/pmc/articles/PMC3535733/figure/fig1/, CC BY 4.0, https://commons.wikimedia.org/w/index.php?curid=68222178. https://en.wikipedia.org/wiki/Acute_interstitial_pneumonitis#/media/File:CRIM.PULMONOLOGY2012-678249.001.jpg. This file is licensed under the Creative Commons Attribution 4.0 International license. No changes were made to this image.

Figure 42. Very high magnification micrograph of hyaline membranes, as seen in diffuse alveolar damage (DAD), the histologic correlate of acute respiratory distress syndrome (ARDS), transfusion related acute lung injury (TRALI), and acute interstitial pneumonia (AIP).

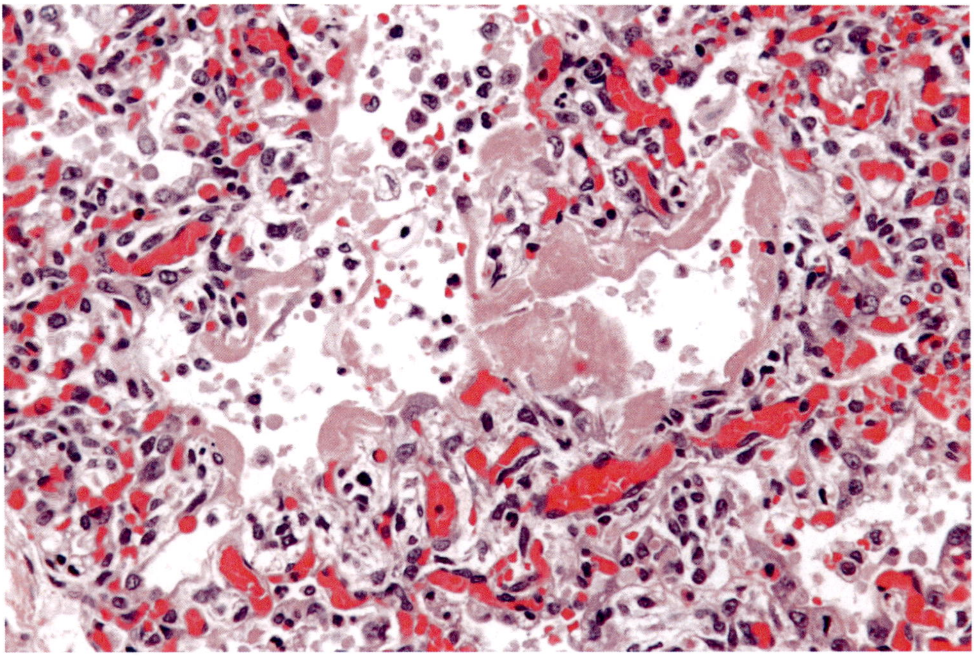

This image is by Nephron - Own work, CC BY-SA 3.0, https://commons.wikimedia.org/w/index.php?curid=14967240. https://en.wikipedia.org/wiki/Acute_interstitial_pneumonitis#/media/File:Hyaline_membranes_-_very_high_mag.jpg. This file is licensed under the Creative Commons Attribution-Share Alike 3.0 Unported license. No changes have been made to this image.

Pneumonitis was reported in 1.8% of patients treated with PIQRAY. In patients who have new or worsening respiratory symptoms or are suspected to have developed pneumonitis, interrupt PIQRAY immediately and evaluate the patient for pneumonitis. Consider a diagnosis of non-infectious pneumonitis in patients presenting with non-specific respiratory signs and symptoms such as hypoxia, cough, dyspnea, or interstitial infiltrates on radiologic exams and in whom infectious, neoplastic, and other causes have been excluded by means of appropriate investigations. Permanently discontinue PIQRAY in all patients with confirmed pneumonitis. Advise patients to immediately report new or worsening respiratory symptoms.

Diarrhea

Severe diarrhea, including dehydration and acute kidney injury *(Figure 43)* occurred in patients treated with PIQRAY.

Figure 43. Pathologic kidney specimen showing marked pallor of the cortex, contrasting to the darker areas of surviving medullary tissue. The patient died with acute kidney injury.

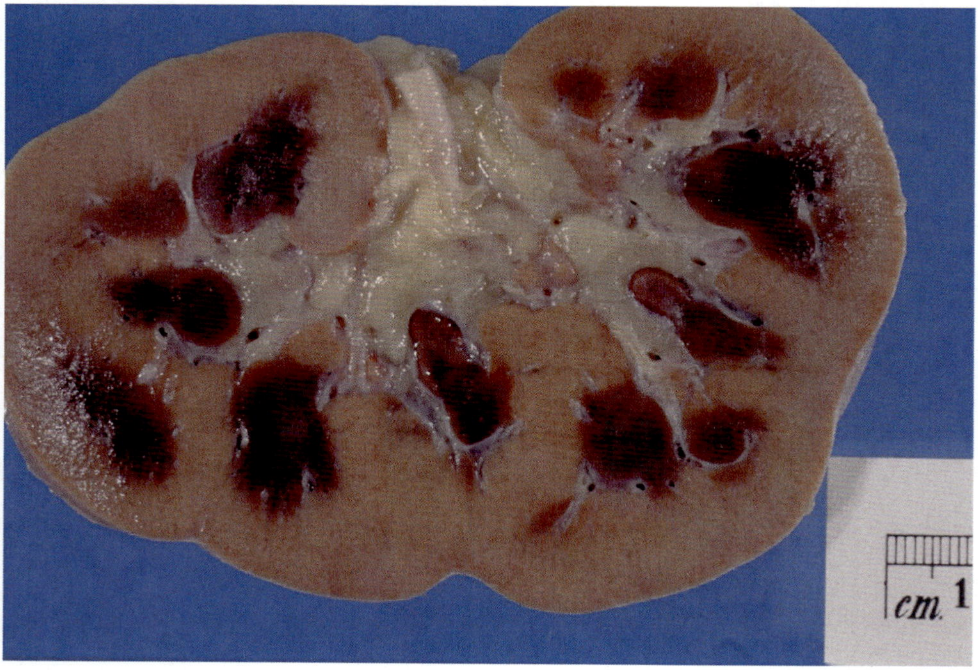

This image is by Haymanj - Self-photographed, Public Domain, https://commons.wikimedia.org/w/index.php?curid=3647869. https://en.wikipedia.org/wiki/Acute_kidney_injury#/media/File:Kidney_%E2%80%93_acute_cortical_necrosis.jpg. The creator of this image has released it into the public domain. No changes have been made to this image.

Most patients (58%) experienced diarrhea during treatment with PIQRAY. Grade 3 diarrhea occurred in 7% (n = 19) of patients. Among patients with Grade 2 or 3 diarrhea (n = 71), the median time to onset was 46 days (range: 1 to 442 days). Dose reductions of PIQRAY were required in 6% of patients and 2.8% of patients permanently discontinued PIQRAY due to diarrhea. In the 164 patients that experienced diarrhea, anti-diarrheal medications (e.g., loperamide) were required to manage symptoms in 63% (104/164) of these patients. Based on the severity of the diarrhea, PIQRAY may require dose interruption, reduction, or discontinuation.

Advise patients to start antidiarrheal treatment, increase oral fluids, and notify their healthcare provider if diarrhea occurs while taking PIQRAY.

Embryo-fetal toxicity

Based on findings in animals and its mechanism of action, PIQRAY can cause fetal harm when administered to a pregnant woman. In animal reproduction studies, oral administration of alpelisib to pregnant rats and rabbits during organogenesis caused adverse developmental outcomes including embryo-fetal mortality (postimplantation loss), reduced fetal weights, and increased incidences of fetal malformations at maternal exposures based on area under the curve (AUC) that were ≥ 0.8 times the exposure in humans at the recommended dose of 300 mg/day. Advise pregnant women and females of reproductive potential of the potential risk to a fetus. Advise females of reproductive potential to use effective contraception during treatment with PIQRAY and for 1 week after the last dose. Advise male patients with female partners of reproductive potential to use condoms and effective contraception during treatment with PIQRAY and for 1 week after the last dose Refer to the Full Prescribing Information of fulvestrant for pregnancy and contraception information.

Further information on **ADVERSE REACTIONS**

The following adverse reactions are discussed in greater detail in other sections of the labelling

- Severe hypersensitivity
- Severe cutaneous reactions
- Hyperglycemia
- Pneumonitis

DRUG INTERACTIONS

Effect of other drugs on PIQRAY

CYP3A4 Inducer

Coadministration of PIQRAY with a strong CYP3A4 inducer may decrease alpelisib concentration, which may decrease alpelisib activity. Avoid coadministration of PIQRAY with strong CYP3A4 inducers.

BCRP Inhibitors

Coadministration of PIQRAY with *a breast cancer resistance protein* (BCRP) inhibitor may increase alpelisib concentration which may increase the risk of toxicities. Avoid the use of BCRP inhibitors in patients treated with PIQRAY. If unable to use alternative drugs, when PIQRAY is used in combination with BCRP inhibitors, closely monitor for increased adverse reactions.

Effect of PIQRAY on other drugs

CYP2C9 Substrates

Coadministration of PIQRAY with CYP2C9 substrates (e.g., warfarin) may reduce plasma concentration of these drugs

Closely monitor when PIQRAY is used in combination with CYP2C9 substrates where decreases in the plasma concentration of CYP2C9 substrates may reduce activity of these drugs.

USE IN SPECIFIC POPULATIONS

Pregnancy risk summary

PIQRAY is used in combination with fulvestrant. Refer to the Full Prescribing Information of fulvestrant for pregnancy information. Based on animal data and mechanism of action, PIQRAY can cause fetal harm when administered to a pregnant woman. There are no available data in pregnant women to inform the drug-associated risk. In animal reproduction studies, oral administration of alpelisib to pregnant rats and rabbits during organogenesis caused adverse developmental outcomes including embryo-fetal mortality (postimplantation loss), reduced fetal weights, and increased incidences of fetal malformations at maternal exposures ≥ 0.8 times the exposure in humans based on AUC at the recommended dose of 300 mg/day. Advise pregnant women and females of reproductive potential of the potential risk to a fetus. The estimated background risk of major birth defects and miscarriage for the indicated population is unknown. However, the estimated background risk of major birth defects is 2% to 4% and of miscarriage is 15% to 20% of clinically recognized pregnancies in the U.S. general population.

Data

Animal data

In embryo-fetal development studies in rats and rabbits, pregnant animals received oral doses of alpelisib up to 30 mg/kg/day during the period of organogenesis. In rats, oral administration of alpelisib resulted in maternal toxicity (body weight loss, low food consumption) and no viable fetuses (post-implantation loss) at 30 mg/kg/day (approximately 3 times the exposure in humans at the recommended dose of 300 mg/day based on AUC). At a dose of 10 mg/kg/day (approximately 0.8 times the exposure in humans at the recommended dose of 300 mg/day based on AUC), toxicities included reduced fetal weight and increased incidences of skeletal malformations (bent scapula and thickened or bent long bones) and fetal variations (enlarged brain ventricle, decreased bone ossification). In a pilot embryo-fetal development study in rabbits, a dose of 30 mg/kg/day resulted in no viable fetuses (postimplantation loss). Doses ≥ 15 mg/kg/day resulted in increased embryo-fetal deaths, reduced fetal weights, and malformations, mostly related to the tail and head. At 15 mg/kg/day in rabbits, the maternal exposure was approximately 5 times the exposure achieved at the recommended human dose of 300 mg/day based on AUC.

Lactation

PIQRAY is used in combination with fulvestrant. Refer to the Full Prescribing Information of fulvestrant for lactation information. There are no data on the presence of alpelisib in human milk, its effects on milk production, or the breastfed child. Because of the potential for serious adverse reactions in the breastfed child, advise lactating women to not breastfeed during treatment with PIQRAY and for 1 week after the last dose.

Females and males of reproductive potential

PIQRAY is used in combination with fulvestrant. Refer to the Full Prescribing Information of fulvestrant for contraception and infertility information.

Pregnancy testing

Verify the pregnancy status in females of reproductive potential prior to initiating PIQRAY.

Contraception

Females

PIQRAY can cause fetal harm when administered to a pregnant woman. Advise females of reproductive potential to use effective contraception during treatment with PIQRAY and for 1 week after the last dose.

Males

Advise male patients with female partners of reproductive potential to use condoms and effective contraception during treatment with PIQRAY and for 1 week after the last dose.

Infertility

Based on findings from animal studies, PIQRAY may impair fertility in males and females of reproductive potential

Pediatric use

The safety and efficacy of PIQRAY in pediatric patients have not been established.
Geriatric use

Of 284 patients who received PIQRAY in the SOLAR-1 trial, 117 patients were ≥ 65 years of age and 34 patients were ≥ 75 years of age. In patients treated with PIQRAY plus fulvestrant, there was a higher incidence of Grade 3-4 hyperglycemia in patients ≥ 65 years of age (44%) compared to patients < 65 years of age (32%). No overall differences in effectiveness of PIQRAY were observed between patients ≥ 65 years of age compared to younger patients. There are an insufficient number of patients ≥ 75 years of age to assess whether there are differences in safety or effectiveness.

Renal impairment

The effect of severe renal impairment (CLcr < 30 mL/min) on alpelisib pharmacokinetics is unknown. No dose adjustment is recommended for patients with mild to moderate renal impairment (CLcr 30 to < 90 mL/min).

OVERDOSAGE

There is limited experience of overdose with PIQRAY in clinical trials. In the clinical studies, PIQRAY was administered at doses up to 450 mg once daily. In cases where accidental overdosage of PIQRAY was reported in the clinical studies, the adverse reactions associated with the overdose were consistent with the known safety profile of PIQRAY and included hyperglycemia, nausea, asthenia, and rash. Initiate general symptomatic and supportive measures in all cases of overdosage where necessary. There is no known antidote for PIQRAY.

The efficacy of alpelisib in the treatment of breast cancer

Treatment with alpelisib–fulvestrant prolonged progression-free survival among patients with PIK3CA-mutated, HR-positive, HER2-negative advanced breast cancer who had received endocrine therapy previously.

Fabrice André, M.D. et al. N Engl J Med 2019; 380:1929-1940
DOI: 10.1056/NEJMoa1813904

9.5. ATEZOLIZUMAB (TECENTRIQ®)

TECENTRIQ® (atezolizumab) injection, for intravenous use Initial U.S. Approval: 2016

RECENT MAJOR CHANGES

Indications and Usage, Urothelial Carcinoma

Indications and Usage, Non-Small Cell Lung Cancer

Indications and Usage, Triple-Negative Breast Cancer

Dosage and Administration

Warnings and Precautions

Please note*: although atezolizumab is also apprioved for urothelial cancer and non-small cell lung cancer, only its breast cancer approval is dealt with in this book.*

MECHANISM OF ACTION

PD-L1 may be expressed on tumor cells and/or tumor infiltrating immune cells and can contribute to the inhibition of the anti-tumor immune response in the tumor microenvironment. Binding of PD-L1 to the PD-1 and B7.1 receptors found on T cells and antigen presenting cells suppresses cytotoxic T-cell activity, T-cell proliferation and cytokine production. Atezolizumab is a monoclonal antibody that binds to PD-L1 and blocks its interactions with both PD-1 and B7.1 receptors. This releases the PD-L1/PD-1 mediated inhibition of the immune response, including activation of the anti-tumor immune response without inducing antibody-dependent cellular cytotoxicity. In syngeneic mouse tumor models, blocking PD-L1 activity resulted in decreased tumor growth.

DESCRIPTION

Atezolizumab is a programmed cell death ligand 1 (PD-L1) blocking antibody. Atezolizumab is an Fc-engineered, humanized, non-glycosylated IgG1 kappa immunoglobulin that has a calculated molecular mass of 145 kDa. TECENTRIQ (atezolizumab) injection for intravenous use is a sterile, preservative-free, colorless to slightly yellow solution in single-dose vials. Each 20 mL vial contains 1200 mg of atezolizumab and is formulated in glacial acetic acid (16.5 mg), L-histidine (62 mg), polysorbate 20 (8 mg), and sucrose (821.6 mg), with a pH of 5.8. Each 14 mL vial contains 840 mg of atezolizumab and is formulated in glacial acetic acid (11.5 mg), L-histidine (43.4 mg), polysorbate 20 (5.6 mg), and sucrose (575.1 mg) with a pH of

PHARMACOKINETICS

Patients' exposure to atezolizumab increased dose proportionally over the dose range of 1 mg/kg to 20 mg/kg, including a dose of 1200 mg administered every 3 weeks. The clearance (CV%) was 0.20 L/day (29%), the volume of distribution at steady state was 6.9 L, and the terminal half life was 27 days. Steady state was achieved after 6 to 9 weeks following multiple doses. The systemic accumulation ratio for every 2 weeks administration and every 3 weeks administration was 3.3 and 1.9 fold, respectively. Atezolizumab clearance was found to decrease over time, with a mean maximal reduction (CV%) from baseline value of approximately 17% (41%); however, the decrease in clearance was not considered clinically relevant.

Specific Populations

Age (21 to 89 years), body weight, sex, albumin levels, tumor burden, region or race, mild or moderate renal impairment [estimated glomerular filtration rate (eGFR) 30 to 89 mL/min/1.73 m^2], mild hepatic impairment (bilirubin ≤ ULN and AST > ULN or bilirubin > 1 to 1.5 × ULN and any AST), level of PD-L1 expression, or performance status had no clinically significant effect on the systemic exposure of atezolizumab. In OAK, IMpower150 (TECENTRIQ, bevacizumab, paclitaxel, carboplatin arm only), and IMpassion130 (TECENTRIQ and paclitaxel protein-bound) atezolizumab clearance in patients who tested positive for treatment-emergent anti-drug antibodies (ADA) was 25%, 18%, and 22% higher, respectively, as compared to clearance in patients who tested negative for treatment-emergent ADA. The effect of severe renal impairment or moderate or severe hepatic impairment on the pharmacokinetics of atezolizumab is unknown.

Drug interaction studies

The drug interaction potential of atezolizumab is unknown.

INDICATIONS AND USAGE

TECENTRIQ is a programmed death-ligand 1 (PD-L1) blocking antibody *(Figure 44)* indicated in:

Triple-Negative Breast Cancer (TNBC)

• in combination with paclitaxel protein-bound for the treatment of adult patients with unresectable locally advanced or metastatic TNBC whose tumors express PD-L1 (PD-L1 stained tumor-infiltrating immune cells [IC] of any intensity covering ≥ 1% of the tumor area), as determined by an FDA approved test. This indication is approved under accelerated approval based on progression-free survival. Continued approval for this indication may be contingent upon verification and description of clinical benefit in a confirmatory trial(s).

Figure 44. Cancer therapy by inhibition of negative immune regulation (CTLA4, PD1). This image is by Guido4 - Own work, CC BY-SA 3.0, https://commons.wikimedia.org/w/index.php?curid=73319886. https://en.wikipedia.org/wiki/Immune_checkpoint#/media/File:11_Hegasy_CTLA4_P

D1_Immunotherapy.png. This file is licensed under the Creative Commons Attribution-Share Alike 3.0 Unported license. No changes were made to this image.

Figure 44. Cancer therapy by inhibition of negative immune regulation (CTLA4, PD1)

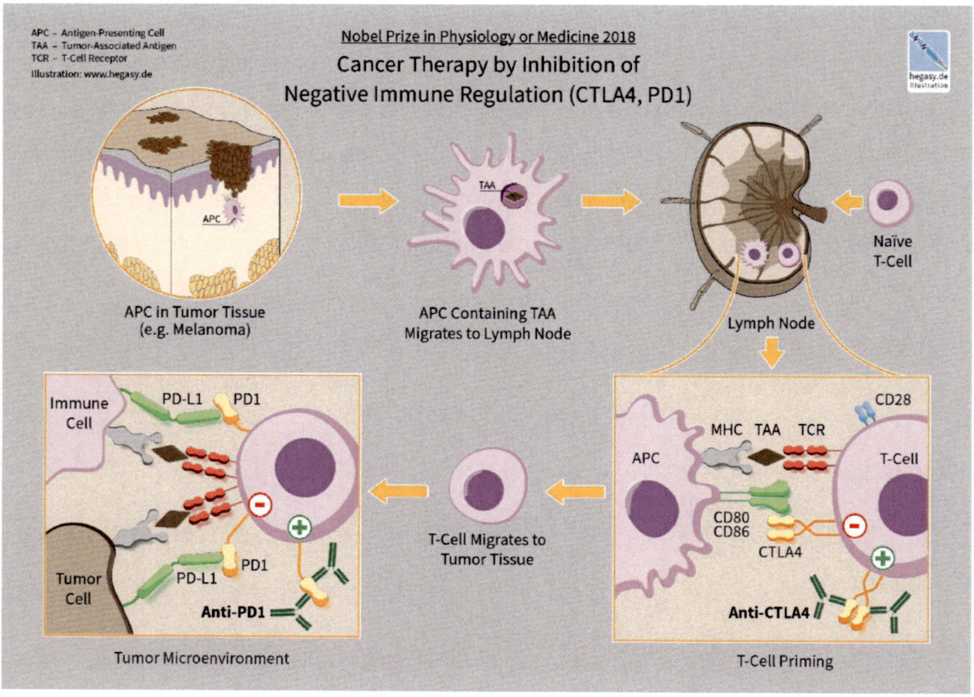

DOSAGE AND ADMINISTRATION

Metastatic

Treatment of triple-negative breast cancer (TNBC)

•TECENTRIQ 840 mg IV over 60 minutes, followed by 100 mg/m^2 paclitaxel protein-bound. For each 28 day cycle, TECENTRIQ is administered on days 1 and 15, and paclitaxel protein-bound is administered on days 1, 8, and 15. If the first infusion is tolerated, all subsequent infusions may be delivered over 30 minutes.

DOSAGE FORMS AND STRENGTHS

840 mg/14 mL (60 mg/mL) solution in a single-dose vial

CONTRAINDICATIONS: none

WARNINGS AND PRECAUTIONS

• Immune-mediated pneumonitis: withhold or permanently discontinue based on severity of pneumonitis.

• Immune-mediated hepatitis *(Figure 45):* Monitor for changes in liver function. Withhold or permanently discontinue based on severity of transaminase or total bilirubin elevation.

Figure 45. Micrograph showing a lymphoplasmacytic interface hepatitis - the characteristic histomorphologic finding of autoimmune hepatitis. Liver biopsy. H&E stain.

.

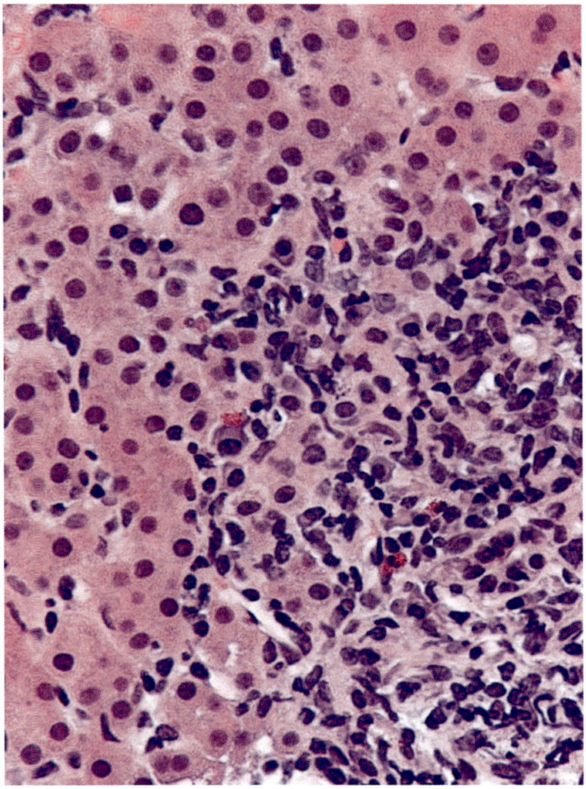

This image is by Nephron - Own work, CC BY-SA 3.0, https://commons.wikimedia.org/w/index.php?curid=15981350. https://en.wikipedia.org/wiki/Autoimmune_hepatitis#/media/File:Autoimmune_hepatitis_-_cropped_-_very_high_mag.jpg. This file is licensed under the Creative

• Immune-Mediated Colitis *(Figure 46).*

Figure 46. Intermediate magnification micrograph of collagenous colitis. H&E stain.

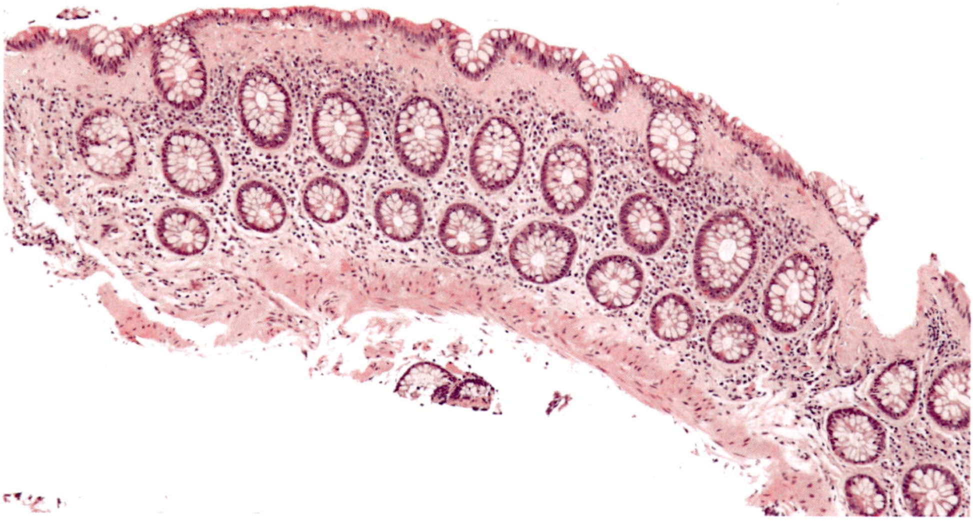

Withhold or permanently discontinue based on severity of colitis.

• Immune-mediated endocrinopathies

o Hypophysitis: withhold based on severity of hypophysitis.

o Thyroid disorders: Monitor for changes in thyroid function. Withhold based on severity of hyperthyroidism *(Figure 47).*

o Adrenal insufficiency: withhold based on severity of adrenal insufficiency.

o Type 1 Diabetes mellitus *(Figures 48 and 49)*: withhold based on severity of hyperglycemia.

Figure 47. The classic findings of exophthalmos and lid retraction in Grave's disease. Grave's disease is the commonest cause of hyperthyroidism.

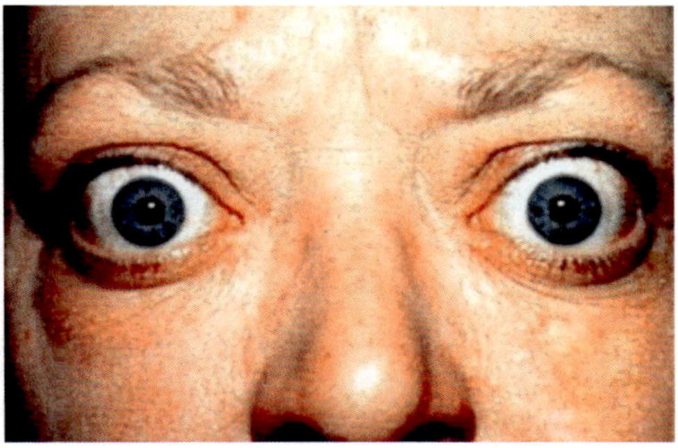

This image is by Jonathan Trobe, M.D. - University of Michigan Kellogg Eye Center - The Eyes Have It, CC BY 3.0, https://commons.wikimedia.org/w/index.php?curid=16115992. https://en.wikipedia.org/wiki/Graves%27_disease#/media/File:Proptosis_and_lid_retraction_from_Graves'_Disease.jpg. This file is licensed under the Creative Commons Attribution 3.0 Unported license. No changes have been made to this image.

Figure 48. Overview of the main symptoms of diabetes mellitus.

This image is by By Mikael Häggström - See above. All used images are in public domain. Public Domain, https://commons.wikimedia.org/w/index.php?curid=6055528. https://en.wikipedia.org/wiki/Diabetes#/media/File:Main_symptoms_of_diabetes.svg. The copyright holder of this image has released it into the public domain. No changes were made to this image.

Figure 48. Overview of the main symptoms of diabetes mellitus.

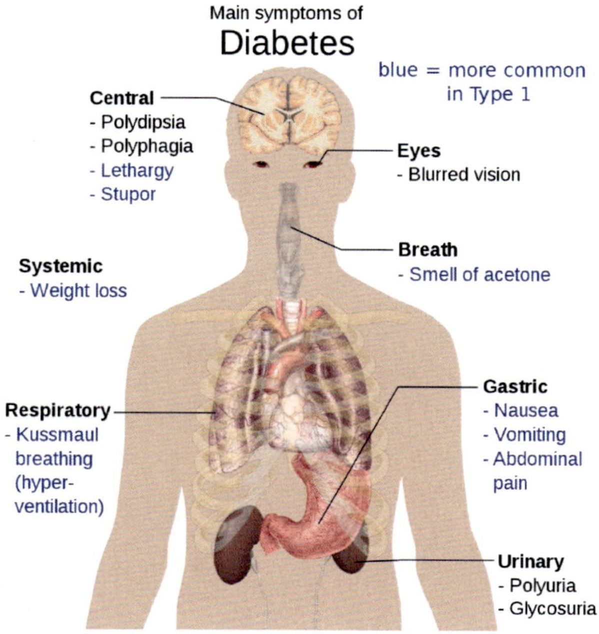

Figure 49. Retinopathy, nephropathy, and neuropathy are potential complications of diabetes mellitus.

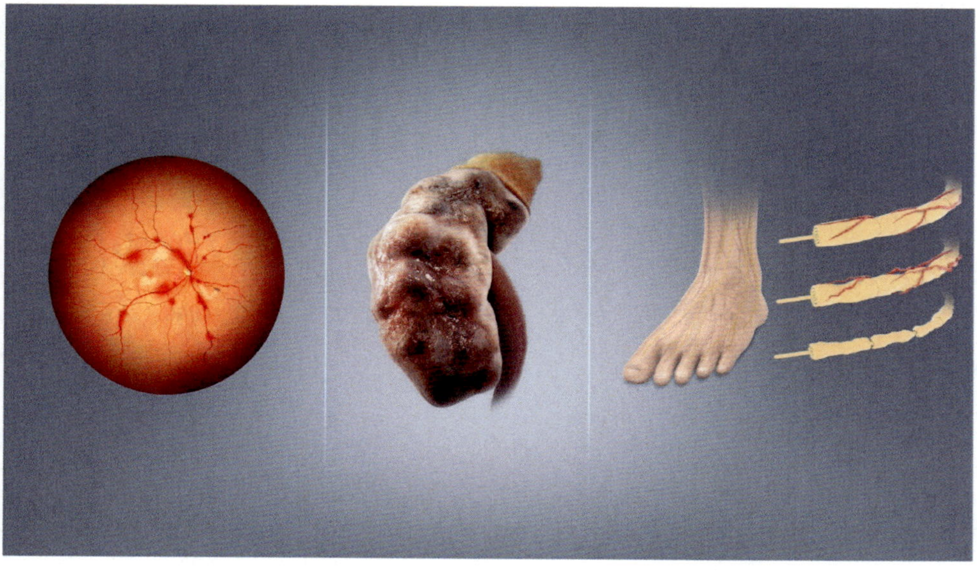

- Infections: withhold for severe or life-threatening infection.

• Infusion-related Reactions: interrupt, slow the rate of infusion, or permanently discontinue based on severity of infusion reactions.

• Embryo-fetal toxicity: can cause fetal harm. Advise females of reproductive potential of the potential risk to a fetus and use of effective contraception.

ADVERSE REACTIONS

The most common adverse reactions (reported in ≥ 20% of patients) with TECENTRIQ as a single agent were fatigue, nausea, constipation, cough, dyspnea, and decreased appetite.

• The most common adverse reactions (reported in ≥ 20% of patients) with TECENTRIQ in combination with bevacizumab, paclitaxel, and carboplatin were fatigue/asthenia, alopecia, nausea, diarrhea, constipation, decreased appetite, arthralgia, hypertension, and peripheral neuropathy.

• The most common adverse reactions (reported in ≥ 20% of patients) with TECENTRIQ in combination with paclitaxel protein-bound were alopecia, peripheral neuropathies, fatigue, nausea, diarrhea, anemia, constipation, cough, headache, neutropenia, vomiting, and decreased appetite.

FULL PRESCRIBING INFORMATION

INDICATIONS AND USAGE

Locally advanced or metastatic triple-negative breast cancer

TECENTRIQ in combination with paclitaxel protein-bound is indicated for the treatment of adult patients with unresectable locally advanced or metastatic triple-negative breast cancer (TNBC) whose tumors express PD-L1 (PD-L1 stained tumor-infiltrating immune cells [IC] of any intensity covering ≥ 1% of the tumor area), as determined by an FDA-approved test. This indication is approved under accelerated approval based on progression free survival. Continued approval for this indication may be contingent upon verification and description of clinical benefit in a confirmatory trial(s).

DOSAGE AND ADMINISTRATION

Patient selection for treatment of triple-negative breast cancer

Select patients with locally advanced or metastatic triple-negative breast cancer for treatment with TECENTRIQ in combination with paclitaxel protein-bound based on the PD-L1 expression on tumor infiltrating immune cells. Information on FDA-approved tests for the determination of PD-L1 expression in triple-negative breast cancer are available at: http://www.fda.gov/CompanionDiagnostics

Recommended dosage for TECENTRIQ for locally advanced or metastatic TNBC

The recommended dosage of TECENTRIQ is 840 mg administered as an intravenous infusion over 60 minutes, followed by 100 mg/ m^2paclitaxel protein bound. For each 28-day cycle, TECENTRIQ is administered on days 1 and 15, and paclitaxel proteinbound is administered on days 1, 8, and 15 until disease progression or unacceptable toxicity. TECENTRIQ and paclitaxel protein-bound may be discontinued for toxicity independently of each other. If the first infusion is tolerated, all subsequent infusions of TECENTRIQ may be delivered over 30 minutes. See also the prescribing information for paclitaxel protein-bound prior to initiation.

DOSAGE MODIFICATIONS FOR ADVERSE REACTIONS

Pneumonitis: reaction grade 2: withhold dose until Grade 1 or resolved and corticosteroid dose is less than or equal to prednisone 10 mg per day (or equivalent)

Reaction grade 3 or 4: permanently discontinue

Hepatitis:

AST or ALT more than 3 and up to 8 times the upper limit of normal or total bilirubin more than 1.5 and up to 3 times the upper limit of normal: withhold dose until Grade

1 or resolved and corticosteroid dose is less than or equal to prednisone 10 mg per day (or equivalent).

AST or ALT more than 8 times the upper limit of normal or total bilirubin more than 3 times the upper limit of normal: permanently discontinue

Colitis or diarrhea

Grade 2 or 3: withhold dose until Grade 1 or resolved and corticosteroid dose is less than or equal to prednisone 10 mg per day (or equivalent)

Grade 4: permanently discontinue

Endocrinopathies (including but not limited to hypophysitis, adrenal insufficiency, hyperthyroidism, and type 1 diabetes mellitus)

Grade 2, 3, or 4: withhold dose until Grade 1 or resolved and clinically stable on hormone replacement therapy.

Other immune-mediated adverse reactions involving a major organ

Withhold dose until Grade 1 or resolved and corticosteroid dose is less than or equal to prednisone 10 mg per day (or equivalent)

Grade 4: permanently discontinue

Infections Grade 3 or 4

Withhold dose until Grade 1 or resolved

Infusion-Related Reactions

Grade 1 or 2: Interrupt or slow the rate of infusion

Grade 3 or 4: permanently discontinue

Persistent Grade 2 or 3 adverse reaction (excluding endocrinopathies)

Grade 2 or 3 adverse reaction that does not recover to Grade 0 or 1 within 12 weeks after last TECENTRIQ dose: permanently discontinue.

Inability to taper corticosteroid

Inability to reduce to less than or equal to prednisone 10 mg per day (or equivalent) within 12 weeks after last TECENTRIQ dose: permanently discontinue

Recurrent Grade 3 or 4 (severe or lifethreatening) adverse reaction: permanently discontinue

CONTRAINDICATIONS: none.

Further information on **WARNINGS AND PRECAUTIONS**

Immune-mediated pneumonitis

TECENTRIQ can cause immune-mediated pneumonitis or interstitial lung disease, defined as requiring use of corticosteroids, including fatal cases. Monitor patients for signs and symptoms of pneumonitis. Evaluate patients with suspected pneumonitis with radiographic imaging. Administer corticosteroids, prednisone 1–2 mg/kg/day or equivalents, followed by a taper; for Grade 2 or higher pneumonitis: withhold or permanently discontinue TECENTRIQ based on the severity. In clinical studies enrolling 2616 patients with various cancers who received TECENTRIQ as a single agent pneumonitis occurred in 2.5% of patients, including Grade 3 (0.6%), Grade 4 (0.1%), and Grade 5 (< 0.1%) immune-mediated pneumonitis. The median time to onset of pneumonitis was 3.6 months (3 days to 20.5 months) and median duration of pneumonitis was 1.4 months (1 day to 15.1 months). Pneumonitis resolved in 67% of patients. Pneumonitis led to discontinuation of TECENTRIQ in 0.4% of the 2616 patients. Systemic corticosteroids were required in 1.5% of patients, including 0.8% who received high-dose corticosteroids (prednisone ≥ 40 mg per day or equivalent) for a median duration of 4 days (1 day to 45 days) followed by a corticosteroid taper. The incidence of pneumonitis in 793 TECENTRIQ-treated patients in *(the clinical trial)* IMpower150 was 4.5%, including Grade 3-4 (1.8%) events. Systemic corticosteroids were required in 4% of patients, including 2.8% who received high-dose corticosteroids (prednisone ≥ 40 mg per day or equivalent) for a median duration of 3 days (1 day to 43 days) followed by a corticosteroid taper.

Immune-mediated hepatitis

TECENTRIQ can cause liver test abnormalities and immune-mediated hepatitis, defined as requiring use of corticosteroids. Fatal cases have been reported. Monitor patients for signs and symptoms of hepatitis, during and after discontinuation of TECENTRIQ, including clinical chemistry monitoring. Administer corticosteroids, prednisone 1–2 mg/kg/day or equivalents, followed by a taper for Grade 2 or higher elevations of ALT, AST and/or total bilirubin. Interrupt or permanently discontinue TECENTRIQ based on the severity. In clinical studies enrolling 2616 patients with various cancers who received TECENTRIQ, hepatitis occurred in 9% of paients, including Grade 3 (2.3%), Grade 4 (0.6%), and Grade 5 (< 0.1%). The median time to onset of hepatitis was 1.4 months (1 day to 25.8 months) and median duration was 24 days (1 day to 13 months). Hepatitis resolved in 71% of patients. Hepatitis led to discontinuation of TECENTRIQ in 0.4% of 2616 patients. Systemic corticosteroids were required in 2% of the patients, with 1.3% requiring high-dose corticosteroids for a median duration of 3 days (1 day to 35 days) followed by a corticosteroid taper. The incidence of hepatitis in 793 TECENTRIQ-treated patients in IMpower150 was 12.1%, including Grade 3-4 (4.0%) events. Systemic corticosteroids were required in 3.8% of the patients, with 2.6% requiring high-dose corticosteroids for a median duration of 7 days (1 day to 68 days) followed by a corticosteroid taper.

Immune-mediated colitis

TECENTRIQ can cause immune-mediated colitis or diarrhea, defined as requiring use of corticosteroids. Monitor patients for signs and symptoms of diarrhea or colitis. Withhold treatment with TECENTRIQ for Grade 2 or 3 diarrhea or colitis. If symptoms persist for longer than 5 days or recur, administer corticosteroids, prednisone 1–2 mg/kg/day or equivalents, followed by a taper.

For Grade 2 diarrhea or colitis, interrupt or permanently discontinue TECENTRIQ based on the severity. In clinical studies enrolling 2616 patients with various cancers who received TECENTRIQ as a single agent diarrhea or colitis occurred in 20%, including Grade 3 (1.4%) events. The median time to onset of diarrhea or colitis was 1.5 months (1 day to 41 months). Diarrhea and colitis resolved in 85% of the patients. Diarrhea or colitis led to discontinuation of TECENTRIQ in 0.2% of 2616 patients. Systemic corticosteroids were required in 1.1% of patients and high-dose corticosteroids was required in 0.4% patients with a median duration of 3 days (1 day to 11 days) followed by a corticosteroid taper. The incidence of diarrhea or colitis in 793 TECENTRIQ-treated patients in IMpower150 was 27%, including Grade 3-4 (4.3%) events. Systemic corticosteroids were required in 4.5% of patients and high-dose corticosteroids was required in 3.2% patients with a median duration of 5 days (1 day to 103 days) followed by a corticosteroid taper.

Immune-mediated endocrinopathies

TECENTRIQ can cause immune-mediated endocrinopathies, including thyroid disorders, adrenal insufficiency, and type 1 diabetes mellitus, including diabetic ketoacidosis, and hypophysitis/hypopituitarism.

Thyroid disorders

Monitor thyroid function prior to and periodically during treatment with TECENTRIQ. Initiate hormone replacement therapy or medical management of hyperthyroidism as clinically indicated. Continue TECENTRIQ for hypothyroidism and interrupt for hyperthyroidism based on the severity. In clinical studies enrolling 2616 patients who received TECENTRIQ, hypothyroidism occurred in 4.6% of patients, and 3.8% of patients required the use of hormone replacement therapy. Hyperthyroidism occurred in 1.6% of patients. One patient experienced acute thyroiditis. The incidence of hypothyroidism in 793 TECENTRIQ-treated patients in IMpower150 was 11.3%, and 8.6% of patients required hormone replacement therapy. Hyperthyroidism occurred in 3.4% of patients and 0.1% experienced thyroiditis.

Adrenal insufficiency

Monitor patients for clinical signs and symptoms of adrenal insufficiency. For Grade 2 or higher adrenal insufficiency, initiate prednisone 1 to 2 mg/kg/day or equivalents, followed by a taper and hormone replacement as clinically indicated. Interrupt TECENTRIQ based on the severity. In clinical studies enrolling 2616 patients who received TECENTRIQ as a single agent, adrenal insufficiency occurred in 0.4% of patients, including Grade 3 (< 0.1%) adrenal insufficiency. Median time to onset was 5.7 months (3 days to 19 months). There was insufficient information to adequately characterize the median duration of adrenal insufficiency. Adrenal insufficiency resolved in 27% of patients. Systemic corticosteroids were required in 0.3% of 2616 patients, including 0.1% who required high-dose corticosteroids. The incidence of adrenal insufficiency in 793 TECENTRIQ-treated patients in Study IMpower150 was 0.8%.

Type 1 Diabetes mellitus

Monitor patients for hyperglycemia or other signs and symptoms of diabetes. Initiate treatment with insulin as clinically indicated. Interrupt TECENTRIQ based on the severity. In clinical studies enrolling 2616 patients who received TECENTRIQ as a single agent, type 1 diabetes mellitus occurred in < 0.1% of patients. Insulin was required in one patient. The incidence of new onset diabetes mellitus in 698 TECENTRIQ-treated patients in Study IMpower150 was 0.1%.

Hypophysitis

For Grade 2 or higher hypophysitis, initiate prednisone 1−2 mg/kg/day or equivalents, followed by a taper and hormone replacement therapy as clinically indicated. Interrupt TECENTRIQ based on the severity. In clinical studies enrolling 2616 patients who received TECENTRIQ as a single agent, Grade 2 hypophysitis occurred in < 0.1% of patients. The incidence of hypophysitis in 793 TECENTRIQ-treated patients in IMpower150 was 0.4%, including Grade 2 (0.1%) and Grade 3 (0.1%) events.

Other immune-mediated adverse reactions

TECENTRIQ can cause severe and fatal immune-mediated adverse reactions. These immunemediated reactions may involve any organ system. While immune-mediated reactions usually manifest during treatment with TECENTRIQ, immune-mediated adverse reactions can also manifest *after discontinuation* of TECENTRIQ. For suspected Grade 2 immune-mediated adverse reactions, exclude other causes and initiate corticosteroids as clinically indicated. For severe (Grade 3 or 4) adverse reactions, administer corticosteroids, prednisone 1 to 2 mg/kg/day or equivalents, followed by a taper. Interrupt or permanently discontinue TECENTRIQ, based on the severity of the reaction.

If uveitis occurs in combination with other immune-mediated adverse reactions, evaluate for Vogt-Koyanagi-Harada syndrome *(Figure 50)*, which has been observed with other products in this class and may require treatment with systemic steroids to reduce the risk of permanent vision loss. *Vogt–Koyanagi–Harada disease (VKH) is a multisystem disease of presumed autoimmune cause that affects pigmented tissues, which have melanin. The most significant manifestation is bilateral, diffuse uveitis, which affects the eyes. VKH may variably also involve the inner ear, with effects on hearing, the skin and the meninges of the central nervous system.*

Figure 50. The diagnostic clue in this patient is the telltale loss of hair coloring in the left eyebrow and eyelashes (poliosis) with contiguous vitiligo. Additional features of this syndrome - all of which this patient had - include panuveitis, retinal detachment, pinpoint retinal leaks on fluorescein angiography, and evidence of auditory and central nervous system dysfunction, including aseptic meningitis. Decreased visual acuity is the rule. The cause is uncertain, but immune-mediated damage of melanocyte-containing tissue seems likely. Long-term corticosteroid therapy usually halts further ocular damage and often improves vision.

Figure 50. Vogt–Koyanagi–Harada disease.

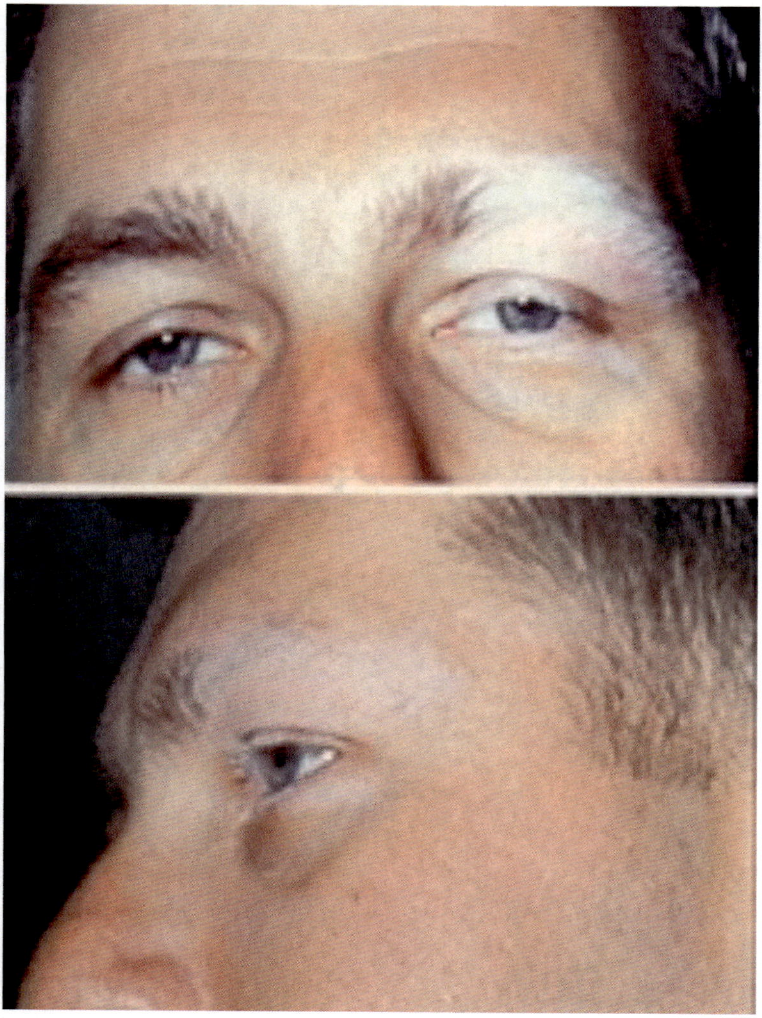

This image is by Herbert L. Fred, MD, Hendrik A. van Dijk - http://cnx.org/content/m14919/latest/, CC BY 2.0, https://commons.wikimedia.org/w/index.php?curid=2801350. https://en.wikipedia.org/wiki/Vogt%E2%80%93Koyanagi%E2%80%93Harada_disease#/media/File:VKHS.jpg. This file is licensed under the Creative Commons Attribution 2.0 Generic license. No changes have been made to this image.

The following clinically significant, immune-mediated adverse reactions occurred at an incidence of < 1% in 2616 patients who received TECENTRIQ or were reported in other products in this class

Cardiac: myocarditis (*Figure 51)*

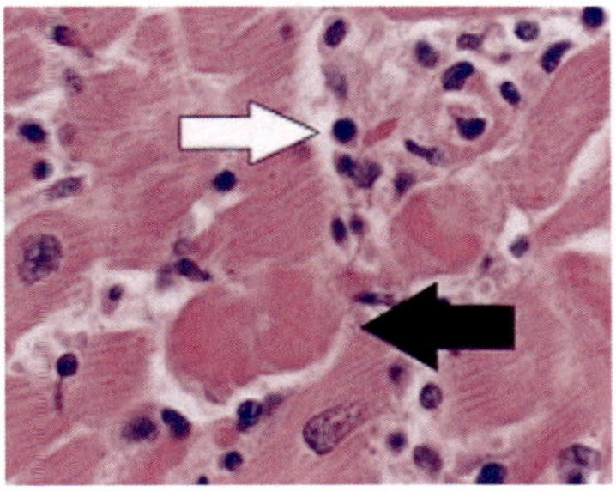

Figure 51. Lymphocytic myocarditis (white arrow points to a lymphocyte), commonly showing myocyte necrosis (black arrow), seen as hypereosinophilic cytoplasm with loss of striations. This image is by B Mikael Häggström, M.D.- Author info- Reusing imagesMikael HäggströmConsent note:Consent from the patient or patient's relatives is regarded as redundant, because of absence of identifiable features (List of HIPAA identifiers) in the media and case information (See also HIPAA case reports guidance). - Own work, CC0, https://commons.wikimedia.org/w/index.php?curid=103645821. https://en.wikipedia.org/wiki/Myocarditis#/media/File:Histopathology_of_lymphocytic_myocarditis_with_myocyte_necrosis,_annotated.jpg. This file is made available under the Creative Commons CC0 1.0 Universal Public Domain Dedication. No changes have been made to this image.

Dermatologic: bullous dermatitis bullous pemphigoid (*Figure 52)*, erythema multiforme, Stevens Johnson Syndrome (SJS)/toxic epidermal necrolysis (TEN).

Figure 52. Bullous pemphigoid. The blisters are tense, about 1–4 cm in diameter, leaving eroded and crusted areas. This image is by Jubward - Own work, CC BY-SA

4.0, https://commons.wikimedia.org/w/index.php?curid=70038371.
https://en.wikipedia.org/wiki/Pemphigoid#/media/File:Legs_Bullous_Pemphigoid.jpg.
This file is licensed under the Creative Commons Attribution-Share Alike 4.0 International license. No changes have been to this image.

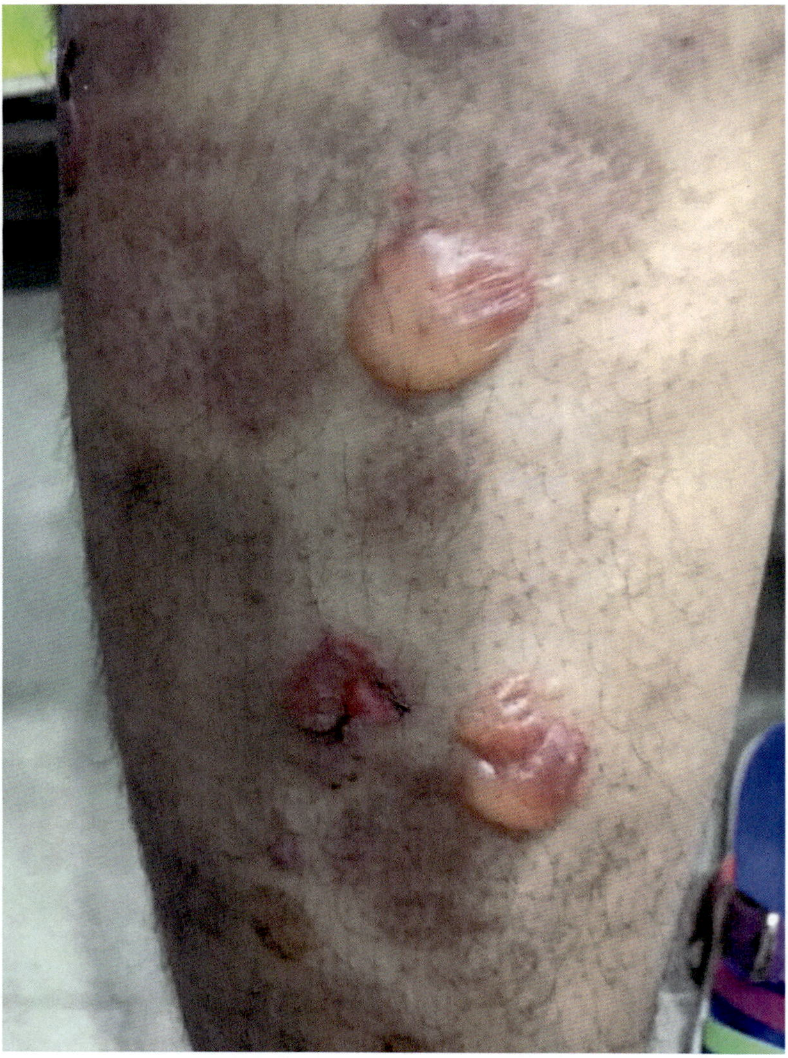

Gastrointestinal: pancreatitis, including increases in serum amylase or lipase levels
General: systemic inflammatory response syndrome, histiocytic necrotizing lymphadenitis

Hematological: autoimmune hemolytic anemia, immune thrombocytopenic purpura *(Figure 53).*

Figure 53. Immune thrombocytopenic purpura (ITP). This blood film shows giant

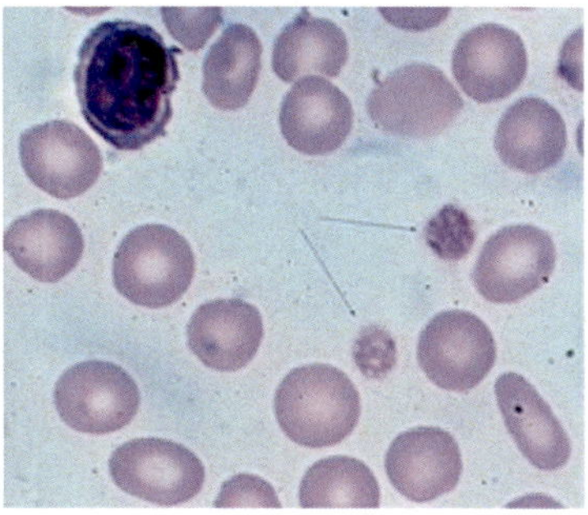

platelets - arrows - in a person with ITP (Giemsa stain). This image is by Dr Graham Beards - Own work, CC BY-SA 4.0, https://commons.wikimedia.org/w/index.php?curid =104497433. https://en.wikipedia.org/wiki/Immune_thrombocyto penic_purpura#/media/File:Giant_platelets_in_ITP .jpg. This file is licensed under the Creative Commons Attribution-Share Alike 4.0 International license. No changes have been made to this image.

Musculoskeletal: myositis, rhabdomyolysis *(Figure 54)*.

Figure 54. A container half-full with brown-stained urine, characteristic for rhabdomyolysis

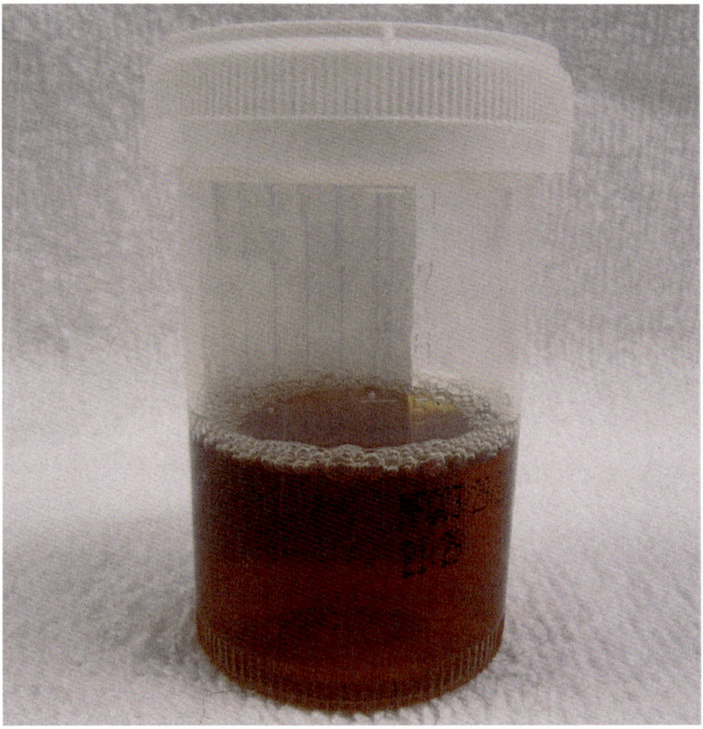

This image is by James Heilman, MD - Own work, CC BY-SA 3.0, https://commons.wikimedia.org/w/index.php?curid=11309876.

https://en.wikipedia.org/wiki/Rhabdomyolysis#/media/File:RhabdoUrine.JPG. This file is licensed under the Creative Commons Attribution-Share Alike 3.0 Unported license. No changes have been made to this image.

Neurological: *Guillain-Barre syndrome, myasthenia syndrome/myasthenia gravis, demyelination, immune-related meningoencephalitis, aseptic meningitis, encephalitis, facial and abducens nerve paresis (Figure 55), polymyalgia rheumatica, autoimmune neuropathy, and Vogt-KoyanagiHarada syndrome (Figure 50).*

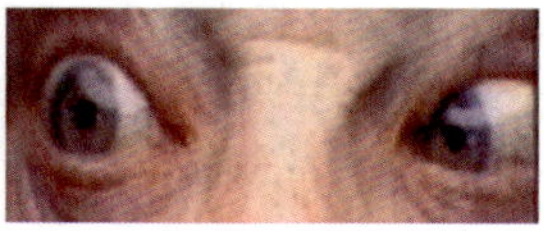

Figure 55. Sixth nerve (abducens) palsy. Limitation of abduction of the right eye. This individual tries to look to his right, but the right eye fails to turn to the side. This image is by Mohammad T Masoud, Ajmal Rehman and Yusuf Shaikh - Lateral rectus metastasis from an occult systemic malignancy masquerading as abducens palsy: a case report, Journal of Medical Case Reports 2008, 2:194 doi:10.1186/1752-1947-2-194, CC BY 2.0, https://commons.wikimedia.org/w/index.php?curid=4290390. https://en.wikipedia.org/wiki/Sixth_nerve_palsy#/media/File:Abducens_palsy.jpg. This file is licensed under the Creative Commons Attribution 2.0 Generic license. No changes were made to this image.

Ophthalmological: uveitis, iritis.

Renal: nephrotic syndrome (*Figure 56),* nephritis.

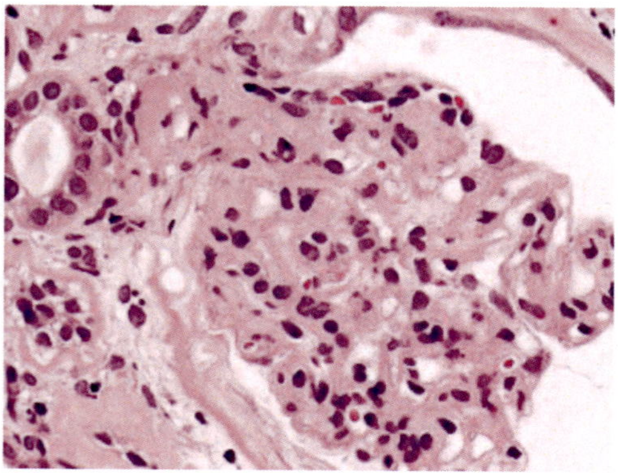

Figure 56. Microscopic image of diabetic glomerulosclerosis, the main cause of nephrotic syndrome in adults. This image is by No machine-readable author provided. KGH assumed (based on copyright claims). - No machine-readable source provided. Own work assumed (based on copyright claims).CC BY-SA 3.0, https://commons.wikimedia.org/w/index.php?curid=523856. https://en.wikipedia.org/wiki/Nephrotic_syndrome#/media/File:Diabetic_glomeruloscl

erosis_(1)_HE.jpg. This file is licensed under the Creative Commons Attribution-Share Alike 3.0 Unported license. No changes were made to this image

Vascular: vasculitis

Infections

TECENTRIQ can cause severe infections including fatal cases. Monitor patients for signs and symptoms of infection. For Grade 3 or higher infections, withhold TECENTRIQ and resume once clinically stable. In clinical studies enrolling 2616 patients with various cancers who received TECENTRIQ infections occurred in 42% of patients, including Grade 3 (8.7%), Grade 4 (1.5%), and Grade 5 (1%). The incidence of infections in 793 TECENTRIQ-treated patients in IMpower150 was 50.1%, including Grade 3 (12%), Grade 4 (1.9%), and Grade 5 (0.4%). The most common Grade 3 or higher infection was pneumonia, occurring in 4.8% of patients.

Infusion-related reactions

TECENTRIQ can cause severe or life-threatening infusion-related reactions. Monitor for signs and symptoms of infusion-related reactions. Interrupt, slow the rate of, or permanently discontinue TECENTRIQ based on the severity. For Grade 1 or 2 infusion-related reactions, consider using pre-medications with subsequent doses. In clinical studies enrolling 2616 patients with various cancers who received TECENTRIQ as a single agent, infusion-related reactions occurred in 1.3% of patients, including Grade 3 (0.2%). The incidence of infusion-related reactions in 793 TECENTRIQ-treated patients in IMpower150 was 3.8%, including Grade 3-4 (0.8%).

Embryo-fetal toxicity

Based on its mechanism of action, TECENTRIQ can cause fetal harm when administered to a pregnant woman. There are no available data on the use of TECENTRIQ in pregnant women. Animal studies have demonstrated that inhibition of the PD-L1/PD-1 pathway can lead to increased risk of immune-related rejection of the developing fetus resulting in fetal death. Verify pregnancy status of females of reproductive potential prior to initiating TECENTRIQ. Advise females of reproductive potential of the potential risk to a fetus. Advise females of reproductive potential to use effective contraception during treatment with TECENTRIQ and for at least 5 months after the last dose

EFFICACY OF ATEZOLIZUMAB IN THE TREATMENT OF BREAST CANCER

1. Atezolizumab for the treatment of triple-negative breast cancer

Atezolizumab, a novel immune checkpoint inhibitors targeting PD-L1, is an effective and well-tolerated treatment option for metastatic TNBC. In general, TNBC has a high unmet medical need, hence the clinical development of atezolizumab should continue, particularly for TNBC. Indeed, atezolizumab has the potential to substantially augment the therapeutic armamentarium for TNBC. This should lead to improved immunotherapeutic strategies and the enhancement of the outcome for this group of breast cancer patients.

Anne-Sophie Heimes &Marcus Schmidt

Drug Evaluation Pages 1-5 | Accepted 21 Nov 2018.

2. Atezolizumab plus nab-paclitaxel as first-line treatment for unresectable, locally advanced or metastatic triple-negative breast cancer (IMpassion130): updated efficacy results from a randomised, double-blind, placebo-controlled, phase 3 trial

Peter Schmid MD et al.

Interpretation

Consistent with the first interim analysis, this second interim overall survival analysis of IMpassion130 indicates no significant difference in overall survival between the treatment groups in the intention-to-treat population but suggests a clinically meaningful overall survival benefit with atezolizumab plus nab-paclitaxel in patients with PD-L1 immune cell-positive disease. However, this positive result could not be formally tested due to the prespecified statistical testing hierarchy. For patients with PD-L1 immune cell-positive metastatic triple-negative breast cancer, atezolizumab plus nab-paclitaxel is an important therapeutic option in a disease with high unmet need.

The Lancet Oncology, 44-59, 2020.

9.6. FAM-TRASTUZUMAB DERUXLICAN-NXKI (ENHERTU®)

ENHERTU® (fam-trastuzumab deruxtecan-nxki) for injection, for intravenous use. Initial U.S. Approval: 2019.

MECHANISM OF ACTION

Fam-trastuzumab deruxtecan-nxki is a HER2-directed antibody-drug conjugate. The antibody is a humanized anti-HER2 IgG1. The small molecule, DXd, is a topoisomerase I inhibitor attached to the antibody by a cleavable linker. Following binding to HER2 on tumor cells, fam-trastuzumab deruxtecan-nxki undergoes internalization and intracellular linker cleavage by lysosomal enzymes. Upon release, the membrane-permeable DXd causes DNA damage and apoptotic cell death.

WARNING: INTERSTITIAL LUNG DISEASE and EMBRYO-FETAL TOXICITY See full prescribing information for complete boxed warning.

• Interstitial lung disease (ILD) and pneumonitis, including fatal cases, have been reported with ENHERTU. Monitor for and promptly investigate signs and symptoms including cough, dyspnea, fever, and other new or worsening respiratory symptoms. Permanently discontinue ENHERTU in all patients with Grade 2 or higher ILD/pneumonitis. Advise patients of the risk and to immediately report symptoms.

• Exposure to ENHERTU during pregnancy can cause embryo-fetal harm. Advise patients of these risks and the need for effective contraception.

PHARMACODYNAMICS

Cardiac electrophysiology

The administration of multiple doses of ENHERTU (6.4 mg/kg every 3 weeks, which is 1.2 times the recommended dosage) did not show large mean effect (i.e. >20 ms) on the QTc interval in an open label, single-arm study in 51 patients with HER2-expressing metastatic breast cancer.

INDICATIONS AND USAGE

ENHERTU is a HER2-directed antibody and topoisomerase inhibitor conjugate indicated for the treatment of adult patients with unresectable or metastatic HER2-positive breast cancer who have received two or more prior anti-HER2-based regimens in the metastatic setting. This indication is approved under accelerated approval based on tumor response rate and duration of response. Continued approval for this indication may be contingent upon verification and description of clinical benefit in a confirmatory trial.

DOSAGE AND ADMINISTRATION

• Do not substitute ENHERTU for or with trastuzumab or adotrastuzumab emtansine.
• For intravenous infusion only. Do not administer as an intravenous push or bolus. Do not use Sodium Chloride Injection, USP.

• The recommended dosage of ENHERTU is 5.4 mg/kg given as an intravenous infusion once every 3 weeks (21-day cycle) until disease progression or unacceptable toxicity.

• Management of adverse reactions (ILD, neutropenia, or left ventricular dysfunction) may require temporary interruption, dose reduction, or discontinuation of ENHERTU.
DOSAGE FORMS AND STRENGTHS

For injection: 100 mg lyophilized powder in a single-dose vial
CONTRAINDICATIONS: None.

WARNINGS AND PRECAUTIONS

• Neutropenia

Monitor complete blood counts prior to initiation of ENHERTU and prior to each dose, and as clinically indicated. Manage through treatment interruption or dose reduction.

• Left ventricular dysfunction

Assess LVEF prior to initiation of ENHERTU and at regular intervals during treatment as clinically indicated. Manage through treatment interruption or discontinuation. Permanently discontinue ENHERTU in patients with symptomatic congestive heart failure (CHF) *(Figures 57, 58 and 59).*

Figure 57. A person with congestive heart failure who presented with an exceedingly elevated JVP, the arrow is pointing to the external jugular vein (marked by the arrow) however, JVD is measured by the internal jugular vein which can also be seen here

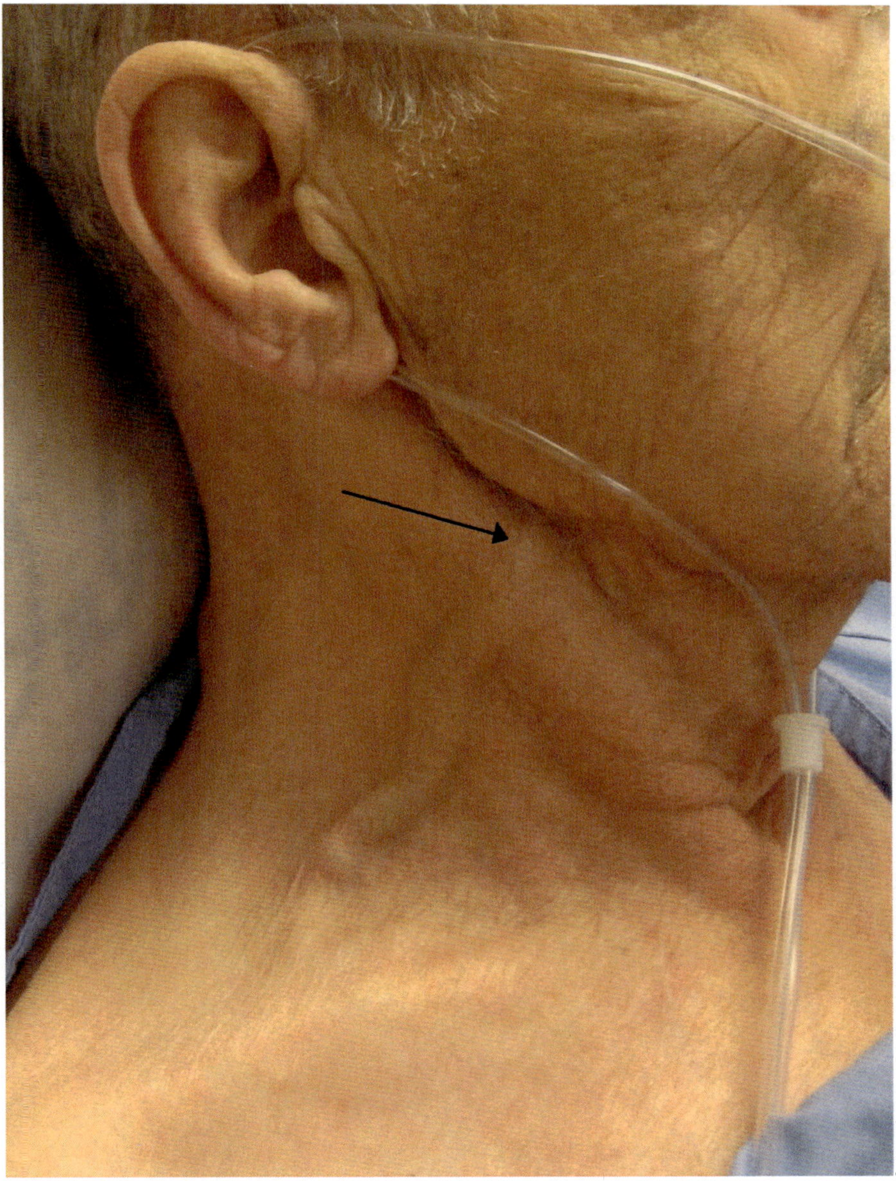

This image is by By James Heilman, MD - Own work, CC BY-SA 3.0, https://commons.wikimedia.org/w/index.php?curid=11509072. https://en.wikipedia.org/wiki/Heart_failure#/media/File:Elevated_JVP.JPG. This file is licensed under the Creative Commons Attribution-Share Alike 3.0 Unported license. No changes have been made to this image.

Figure 58. Severe peripheral pitting edema

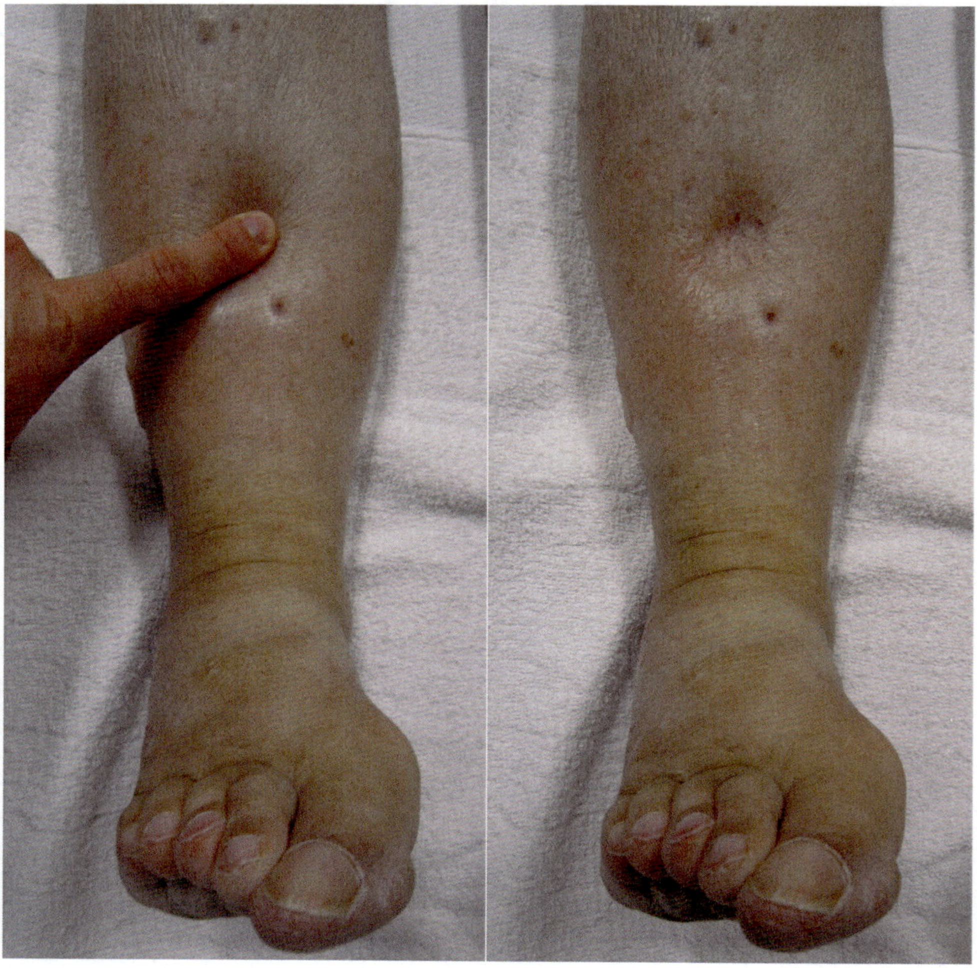

By James Heilman, MD - Own work, CC BY-SA 3.0, https://commons.wikimedia.org/w/index.php?curid=11787530. https://en.wikipedia.org/wiki/Heart_failure#/media/File:Combinpedal.jpg. This file is licensed under the Creative Commons Attribution-Share Alike 3.0 Unported license. No changes have been made to this image.

Figure 59. Congestive heart failure with small bilateral effusions.

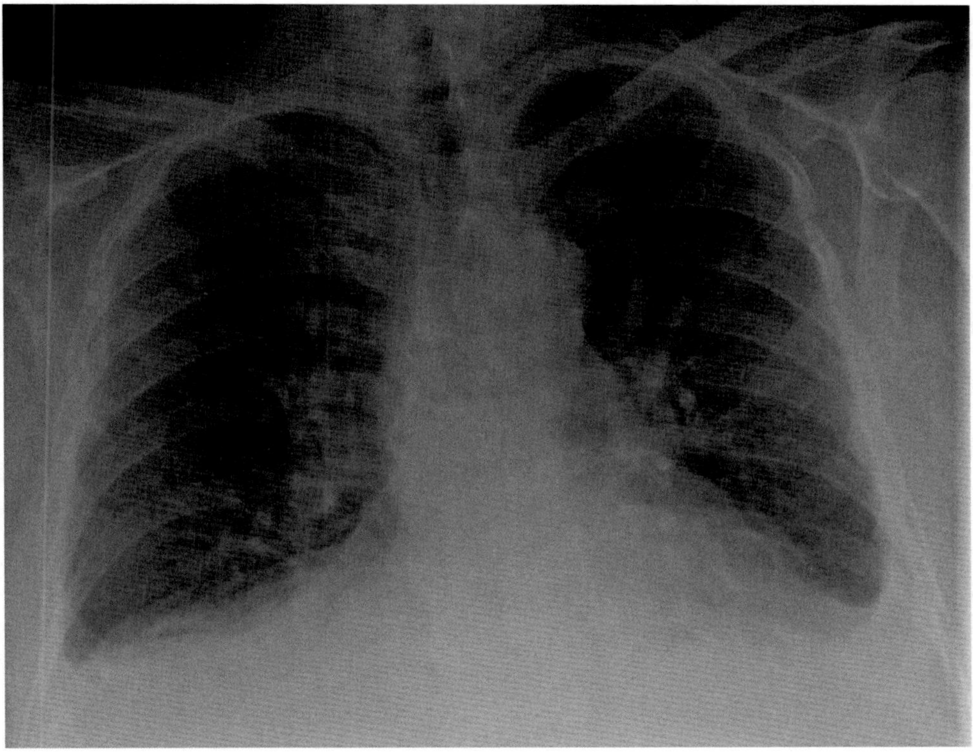

This image is by By James Heilman, MD - Own work, CC BY-SA 4.0, https://commons.wikimedia.org/w/index.php?curid=49086911. https://en.wikipedia.org/wiki/Heart_failure#/media/File:CHF2016.png. This file is licensed under the Creative Commons Attribution-Share Alike 4.0 International license. No changes were made to this image.

ADVERSE REACTIONS

The most common adverse reactions (≥20%) were nausea, fatigue, vomiting, alopecia, constipation, decreased appetite, anemia, neutropenia, diarrhea, leukopenia, cough, and thrombocytopenia.

USE IN SPECIFIC POPULATIONS

• Lactation: advise not to breastfeed.

• Females and males of reproductive potential: verify pregnancy status of females prior to initiation of ENHERTU.

FULL PRESCRIBING INFORMATION

WARNING: INTERSTITIAL LUNG DISEASE and EMBRYO-FETAL TOXICITY

• Interstitial lung disease (ILD) and pneumonitis, including fatal cases, have been reported with ENHERTU *(Figures 60 and 61).* Monitor for and promptly investigate signs and symptoms including cough, dyspnea, fever, and other new or worsening respiratory symptoms. Permanently discontinue ENHERTU in all patients with Grade 2 or higher ILD/pneumonitis. Advise patients of the risk and the need to immediately report symptoms.

Figure 60. Interstitial lung disease affects gas flow in the alveoli.

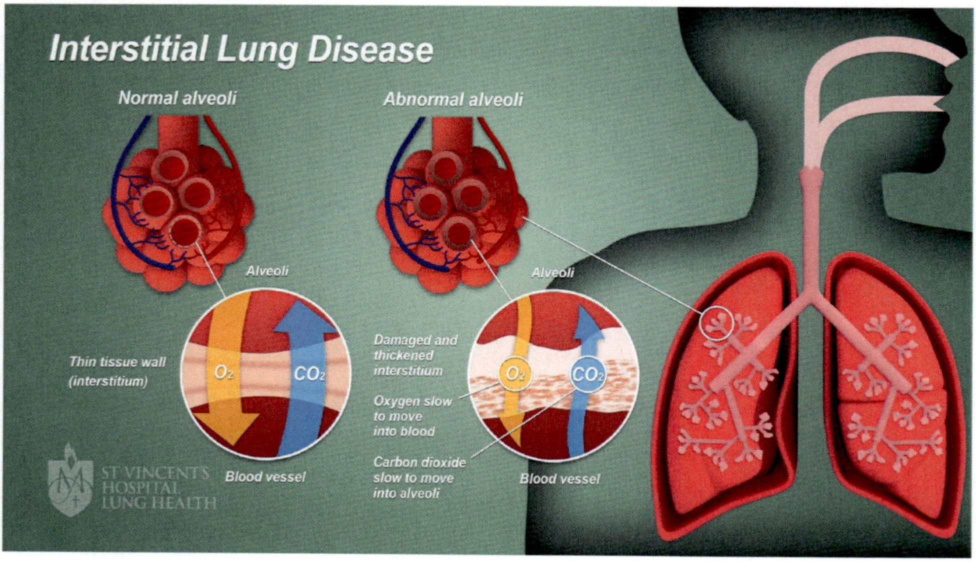

This image is by By Anatomyclassproj1 - Own work, CC BY-SA 4.0, https://commons.wikimedia.org/w/index.php?curid=97172556. https://en.wikipedia.org/wiki/Interstitial_lung_disease#/media/File:2_SVH_Lung_Health_Interstitial_Lung_Disease_final_1080.jpg. This file is licensed under the Creative Commons Attribution-Share Alike 4.0 International license. No changes have been made to this image.

Figure 61. Micrograph of usual interstitial pneumonia (UIP). UIP is the most common pattern of idiopathic interstitial pneumonia (a type of interstitial lung disease) and usually represents idiopathic pulmonary fibrosis. H&E stain. Autopsy specimen.

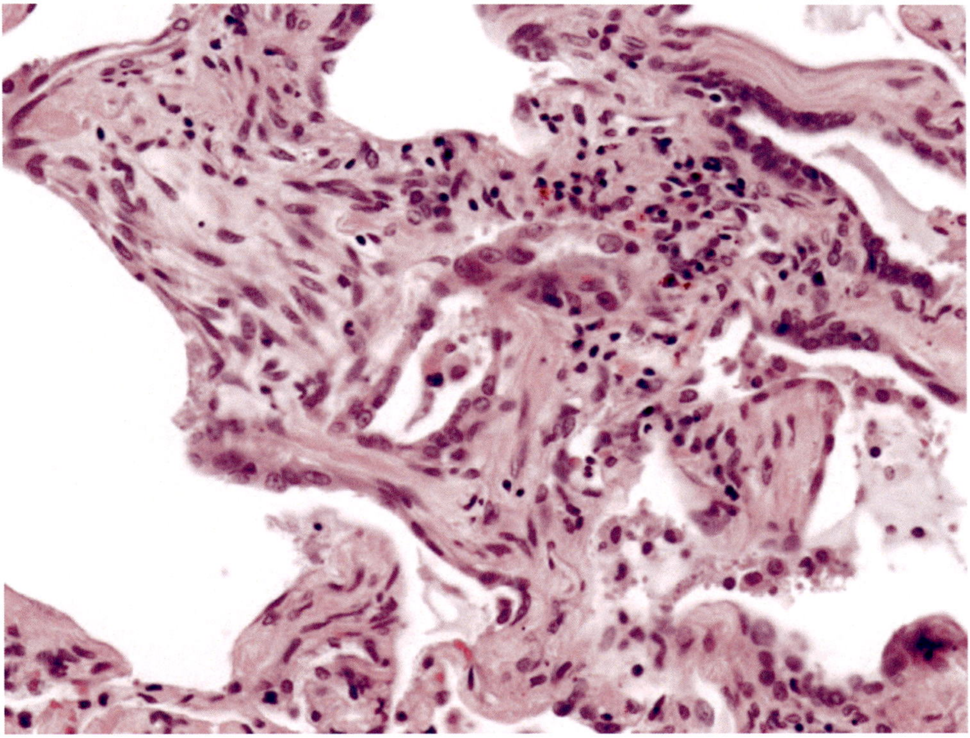

• Embryo-fetal toxicity: exposure to ENHERTU during pregnancy can cause embryo-fetal harm. Advise patients of these risks and the need for effective contraception.

INDICATIONS AND USAGE

ENHERTU is indicated for the treatment of adult patients with unresectable or metastatic HER2-positive breast cancer who have received two or more prior anti-

HER2-based regimens in the metastatic setting. This indication is approved under accelerated approval based on tumor response rate and duration of response. Continued approval for this indication may be contingent upon verification and description of clinical benefit in a confirmatory trial.

DOSAGE AND ADMINISTRATION

Recommended dosage and schedules

Do not substitute ENHERTU for or with trastuzumab or ado-trastuzumab emtansine. The recommended dosage of ENHERTU is 5.4 mg/kg given as an intravenous infusion once every 3 weeks (21-day cycle) until disease progression or unacceptable toxicity.

First infusion: administer infusion over 90 minutes. Subsequent infusions: administer over 30 minutes if prior infusions were well tolerated. Slow or interrupt the infusion rate if the patient develops infusion-related symptoms. Permanently discontinue ENHERTU in case of severe infusion reactions.

Dose modifications

Management of adverse reactions may require temporary interruption, dose reduction, or treatment discontinuation of ENHERTU.

Do not re-escalate the ENHERTU dose after a dose reduction is made. If a planned dose is delayed or missed, administer as soon as possible; do not wait until the next planned cycle. Adjust the schedule of administration to maintain a 3-week interval between doses. Administer the infusion at the dose and rate the patient tolerated in the most recent infusion.

First dose reduction: 4.4 mg/kg

Second dose reduction: 3.2 mg/kg

Requirement for further dose reduction: discontinue treatment

Dose modifications for adverse reactions

Interstitial Lung Disease (ILD)/pneumonitis

Asymptomatic ILD/pneumonitis (Grade 1)

- Interrupt ENHERTU until resolved to Grade 0, then:

• if resolved in 28 days or less from date of onset, maintain dose.

• if resolved in greater than 28 days from date of onset, reduce dose one level

• consider corticosteroid treatment as soon as ILD/pneumonitis is suspected

Symptomatic ILD/pneumonitis

• Permanently discontinue ENHERTU. (Grade 2 or greater)

• Promptly initiate corticosteroid treatment as soon as ILD/pneumonitis is suspected

Neutropenia Grade 3 (less than 1.0 to 0.5 x 10^9/L)

- Interrupt ENHERTU until resolved to Grade 2 or less, then maintain dose.
- Grade 4 (less than 0.5 x 10^9/L)
  - Interrupt ENHERTU until resolved to Grade 2 or less.
  - Reduce dose by one level

Febrile neutropenia: absolute neutrophil count of less than 1.0x10^9/L andtemperature greater than 38.3°C or a sustained temperature of 38°C or greater for more than one hour:

• Interrupt ENHERTU until resolved

and

Reduce dose by one level

Thrombocytopenia Grade 3 (platelets less than 50 to 25 x 10^9/L

- Interrupt ENHERTU until resolved to Grade 1 or less, then maintain dose

Thrombocytopenia Grade 4 (platelets less than 25 x 10^9/L

- Interrupt ENHERTU until resolved to Grade 1 or less
- Reduce dose by one level

Left ventricular dysfunction

- LVEF greater than 45% and absolute decrease from baseline is less than 10%

  • Continue treatment with ENHERTU.

- LVEF 40% to 45% and absolute decrease from baseline is less than 10%
  • Continue treatment with ENHERTU.
  • Repeat LVEF assessment within 3 weeks.
- LVEF 40% to 45% and absolute decrease from baseline is 10% to 20%
  • Interrupt ENHERTU.
  • Repeat LVEF assessment within 3 weeks.
  • If LVEF has not recovered to within 10% from baseline, permanently discontinue ENHERTU.
  • If LVEF recovers to within 10% from baseline, resume treatment with ENHERTU at the same dose.
- LVEF less than 40% or absolute decrease from baseline is greater than 20%
  • Interrupt ENHERTU.
  • Repeat LVEF assessment within 3 weeks.
  • If LVEF of less than 40% or absolute decrease from baseline of greater than 20% is confirmed, permanently discontinue ENHERTU.

Symptomatic congestive heart failure (CHF)

• Permanently discontinue ENHERTU.

Toxicity grades are in accordance with National Cancer Institute Common Terminology Criteria for Adverse Events Version 4.03 (NCI-CTCAE v.4.03).

Data

Human data

There are no available data on the use of ENHERTU in pregnant women. In postmarketing reports in pregnant women receiving a HER2-directed antibody, cases of oligohydramnios manifesting as fatal pulmonary hypoplasia, skeletal abnormalities, and neonatal death have been reported. These case reports described oligohydramnios in pregnant women who received a HER2-directed antibody either alone or in combination with chemotherapy. In some case reports, amniotic fluid index increased after use of a HER2-directed antibody was stopped.

Animal data

There were no animal reproductive or developmental toxicity studies conducted with fam-trastuzumab deruxtecan-nxki.

Lactation risk summary

There are no data regarding the presence of fam-trastuzumab deruxtecan-nxki in human milk, the effects on the breastfed child, or the effects on milk production. Because of the potential for serious adverse reactions in a breastfed child, advise women not to breastfeed during treatment with ENHERTU and for 7 months after the last dose.

Females and males of reproductive potential

Pregnancy

Testing

Verify pregnancy status of females of reproductive potential prior to initiation of ENHERTU.

Contraception

Females

ENHERTU can cause fetal harm when administered to a pregnant woman Advise females of reproductive potential to use effective contraception during treatment with ENHERTU and for at least 7 months following the last dose.

Males

Because of the potential for genotoxicity, advise male patients with female partners of reproductive potential to use effective contraception during treatment with ENHERTU and for at least 4 months following the last dose Infertility.

Based on findings in animal toxicity studies, ENHERTU may impair male reproductive function and fertility

Pediatric use

Safety and effectiveness of ENHERTU have not been established in pediatric patients.

Geriatric use

Of the 234 patients with HER2-positive breast cancer treated with ENHERTU 5.4 mg/kg, 26% were 65 years or older and 5% were 75 years or older. No overall differences in efficacy were observed between patients ≥65 years of age compared to younger patients. There was a higher incidence of Grade 3-4 adverse reactions observed in patients aged 65 years or older (53%) as compared to younger patients (42%).

Renal impairment

No dose adjustment of ENHERTU is required in patients with mild (creatinine clearance (CLcr) ≥60 and ULN or total bilirubin >1 to 1.5 times ULN and any AST) or moderate (total bilirubin >1.5 to 3 times ULN and any AST) hepatic impairment. In patients with moderate hepatic impairment, due to potentially increased exposure, closely monitor for increased toxicities related to the topoisomerase inhibitor, DXd.

Hepatic imparment

No dose adjustment of ENHERTU is required in patients with mild (total bilirubin ≤ULN and any AST >ULN or total bilirubin >1 to 1.5 times ULN and any AST) or moderate (total bilirubin >1.5 to 3 times ULN and any AST) hepatic impairment. In patients with moderate hepatic impairment, due to potentially increased exposure, closely monitor for increased toxicities related to the topoisomerase inhibitor, DXd. No data are available in patients with severe (total bilirubin >3 to 10 times ULN and any AST) hepatic impairment.

Efficacy of ENHERTU as adjuvant treatment for early breast cancer

On November 2nd 2020 Daiichi Sankyo Company, Limited and AstraZeneca announced the initiation of DESTINY-Breast05, a global phase 3, head-to-head trial of ENHERTU® (fam-trastuzumab deruxtecan-nxki) versus ado-trastuzumab emtansine (T-DM1) as adjuvant therapy in patients with HER2 positive early breast cancer with high risk of disease recurrence who have residual invasive disease in the breast or axillary lymph nodes after receiving neo-adjuvant therapy. DESTINY-Breast05 will be conducted in collaboration with the National Surgical Adjuvant Breast and Bowel Project Foundation (NSABP), the German Breast Group (GBG),

Arbeitsgemeinschaft Gynäkologische Onkologie (AGO-B) and the SOLTI Breast Cancer Research Group.

No information is yet available on the role of ENHERTU in the treatment of eary breast cancer.

Efficacy of ENHURTU as treatment for metastatic breast cancer

Trastuzumab-deruxtecan (Enhertu® or DS-8201a) is a novel antibody-drug conjugate (ADC) that connects the humanized monoclonal antibody, trastuzumab, via a tetrapeptide linkage to the topoisomerase 1 inhibitor, deruxtecan. The peptide linkage is stable throughout the bloodstream and cleaved selectively in HER2+ tumor cells that upregulate lysosomal proteases, leading to the targeted distribution of chemotherapy within cells. In comparison to the previously-approved ADC, T-DM1, DS-8201a offers a drug-to-antibody ratio of 8 vs. 3-4 and a payload that more easily crosses the cell membrane for greater cytotoxic effect to neighboring cells within the tumor microenvironment. Since its inception, DS-8201a has been granted Fast Track Designation in 2016 and Breakthrough Therapy Designation in 2017 by the FDA for the treatment of patients with locally-advanced or metastatic HER2+ BC previously treated with either trastuzumab or pertuzumab and resistance to T-DM1. Most recently, DS-8201a received FDA accelerated approval in December 2019 for unresectable or metastatic HER2+ BC, who have received two or more prior anti-HER therapies.

Kreutzfeldt, Jordyn et al. "The trastuzumab era: current and upcoming targeted HER2+ breast cancer therapies." American journal of cancer research vol. 10, 1045-1067. 1 Apr. 2020.

9.7. TRASTUZUMAB (HERCEPTIN®)

Herceptin (Trastuzumab) Intravenous Infusion. Initial U.S. Approval: 1998.

WARNING: CARDIOMYOPATHY, INFUSION REACTIONS, and PULMONARY TOXICITY See full prescribing information for complete boxed warning.

Cardiomyopathy: Herceptin can result in sub-clinical and clinical cardiac failure manifesting as CHF, and decreased LVEF, with greatest risk when administered concurrently with anthracyclines. Evaluate cardiac function prior to and during treatment. Discontinue Herceptin for cardiomyopathy.

Infusion reactions, pulmonary toxicity: Discontinue Herceptin for anaphylaxis, angioedema, interstitial pneumonitis, or acute respiratory distress syndrome.

MECHANISM OF ACTION

The HER2 (or c-erbB2) proto-oncogene encodes a transmembrane receptor protein of 185 kDa, which is structurally related to the epidermal growth factor receptor. Herceptin has been shown, in both in vitro assays and in animals, to inhibit the proliferation of human tumor cells that overexpress HER2. Herceptin is a mediator of antibody-dependent cellular cytotoxicity (ADCC). In vitro, Herceptin-mediated ADCC has been shown to be preferentially exerted on HER2 overexpressing cancer cells compared with cancer cells that do not overexpress HER2.

DESCRIPTION

Herceptin (trastuzumab) is a humanized IgG1 kappa monoclonal antibody that selectively binds with high affinity to the extracellular domain of the human epidermal growth factor receptor 2 protein, HER2. Trastuzumab is produced by recombinant DNA technology in a mammalian cell (Chinese Hamster Ovary) culture containing the antibiotic gentamicin. Gentamicin is not detectable in the final product. Herceptin is a sterile, white to pale yellow, preservative-free lyophilized powder for intravenous administration. Each multi-use vial of Herceptin contains 440 mg trastuzumab, 400 mg α,,α-trehalose dihydrate, 9.9 mg L-histidine HCl, 6.4 mg L-histidine, and 1.8 mg polysorbate 20, USP. Reconstitution with 20 mL of the appropriate diluent (BWFI or SWFI) yields a solution containing 21 mg/mL trastuzumab, at a pH of approximately 6.

RECENT MAJOR CHANGES

Note: while Herceptin has also been approved for treatment of HER2-overexpressing metastatic gastric or gastroesophageal junction adenocarcinoma, this book deals only with its role in breast cancer.

INDICATIONS AND USAGE

Herceptin is a HER2/neu receptor antagonist indicated for:

• the treatment of HER2 overexpressing breast cancer

DOSAGE AND ADMINISTRATION

For intravenous (IV) infusion only. Do not administer as an IV push or bolus.

Treatment of HER2-Overexpressing Breast Cancer

Administer at either:

- Initial dose of 4 mg/kg over 90-minute IV infusion, then 2 mg/kg over 30 minute IV infusion weekly for 52 weeks, or
- Initial dose of 8 mg/kg over 90 minutes IV infusion, then 6 mg/kg over 30−90 minutes IV infusion every three weeks for 52 weeks.

Metastatic HER2-Overexpressing Breast Cancer

- Initial dose of 4 mg/kg as a 90-minute IV infusion followed by subsequent weekly doses of 2 mg/kg as 30 minute IV infusions.

DOSAGE FORMS AND STRENGTHS

- Multidose vial nominally containing 440 mg Herceptin as a lyophilized, sterile powder.

CONTRAINDICATIONS: None.

WARNINGS AND PRECAUTIONS

- Cardiomyopathy
- Infusion Reactions
- Exacerbation of chemotherapy-induced neutropenia
- Pulmonary toxicity
- HER2 testing should be performed using FDA-approved tests by laboratories with demonstrated proficiency.
- Embryo-fetal toxicity

ADVERSE REACTIONS

Adjuvant Breast Cancer

- The most common adverse reactions (≥5%) are headache, diarrhea, nausea, and chills.

Metastatic Breast Cancer

- The most common adverse reactions (> 10%) are fever, chills, headache, infection, congestive heart failure, insomnia, cough, and rash.

USE IN SPECIFIC POPULATIONS

Nursing others

Discontinue nursing or discontinue Herceptin.

FULL PRESCRIBING INFORMATION

WARNING: CARDIOMYOPATHY, INFUSION REACTIONS, and PULMONARY TOXICITY

Cardiomyopathy

Herceptin administration can result in sub-clinical and clinical cardiac failure. The incidence and severity was highest in patients receiving Herceptin with anthracycline-containing chemotherapy regimens. Evaluate left ventricular function in all patients prior to and during treatment with Herceptin. Discontinue Herceptin treatment in patients receiving adjuvant therapy and withold Herceptin in patients with metastatic disease for clinically significant decrease in left ventricular function.

Infusion reactions; pulmonary toxicity

Herceptin administration can result in serious and fatal infusion reactions and pulmonary toxicity. Symptoms usually occur during or within 24 hours of Herceptin administration. Interrupt Herceptin infusion for dyspnea or clinically significant hypotension. Monitor patients until symptoms completely resolve. Discontinue Herceptin for anaphylaxis, angioedema, interstitial pneumonitis, or acute respiratory distress syndrome.

INDICATIONS AND USAGE

Adjuvant breast cancer

Herceptin is indicated for adjuvant treatment of HER2 overexpressing node positive or node negative (ER/PR negative or with one high risk feature breast cancer

• as part of a treatment regimen consisting of doxorubicin, cyclophosphamide, and either paclitaxel or docetaxel

• with docetaxel and carboplatin

• as a single agent following multi-modality anthracycline-based therapy.

Metastatic breast cancer

Herceptin is indicated

• In combination with paclitaxel for first-line treatment of HER2-overexpressing metastatic breast cancer

• As a single agent for treatment of HER2-overexpressing breast cancer in patients who have received one or more chemotherapy regimens for metastatic disease.

DOSAGE AND ADMINISTRATION

Recommended doses and schedules

Do not administer as an intravenous push or bolus.

Do not mix Herceptin with other drugs.

Adjuvant Treatment,

Breast Cancer

Administer according to one of the following doses and schedules for a total of 52 weeks of Herceptin therapy: During and following paclitaxel, docetaxel, or docetaxel/carboplatin.

• Initial dose of 4 mg/kg as an intravenous infusion over 90 minutes then at 2 mg/kg as an intravenous infusion over 30 minutes weekly during chemotherapy for the first 12 weeks (paclitaxel or docetaxel) or 18 weeks (docetaxel/carboplatin).

• One week following the last weekly dose of Herceptin, administer Herceptin at mg/kg as an intravenous infusion over 30−90 minutes every three weeks.

As a single agent within three weeks following completion of multi-modality, anthracycline-based chemotherapy regimens.

• Initial dose at 8 mg/kg as an intravenous infusion over 90 minutes

• Subsequent doses at 6 mg/kg as an intravenous infusion over 30−90 minutes every three weeks.

• Administer Herceptin, alone or in combination with paclitaxel, at an initial dose of 4 mg/kg as a 90-minute intravenous infusion followed by subsequent once weekly doses of 2 mg/kg as 30-minute intravenous infusions until disease progression.

• Decrease the rate of infusion for mild or moderate infusion reactions

• Interrupt the infusion in patients with dyspnea or clinically significant hypotension

• Discontinue Herceptin for severe or life-threatening infusion reactions.

Cardiomyopathy

Assess left ventricular ejection fraction (LVEF) prior to initiation of Herceptin and at regular intervals during treatment. Withhold Herceptin dosing for at least 4 weeks for either of the following:

• ≥ 16% absolute decrease in LVEF from pre-treatment values

• LVEF below institutional limits of normal and ≥ 10% absolute decrease in LVEF from pretreatment values. Herceptin may be resumed if, within 4−8 weeks, the LVEF returns to normal limits and the absolute decrease from baseline is ≤ 15%. Permanently discontinue Herceptin for a persistent (> 8 weeks) LVEF decline or for suspension of Herceptin dosing on more than 3 occasions for cardiomyopathy.

Preparation for administration reconstitution

Reconstitute each 440 mg vial of Herceptin with 20 mL of Bacteriostatic Water for Injection (BWFI), USP, containing 1.1% benzyl alcohol as a preservative to yield a multi-dose solution containing 21 mg/mL trastuzumab. In patients with known hypersensitivity to benzyl alcohol, reconstitute with 20 mL of Sterile Water for Injection (SWFI) without preservative to yield a single use solution. Use appropriate aseptic technique when performing the following reconstitution steps: Using a sterile syringe, slowly inject the 20 mL of diluent into the vial containing the lyophilized cake of Herceptin. The stream of diluent should be directed into the lyophilized cake. Swirl the vial gently to aid reconstitution. DO NOT SHAKE. Slight foaming of the product may be present upon reconstitution. Allow the vial to stand undisturbed for approximately 5 minutes.

• Parenteral drug products should be inspected visually for particulate matter and discoloration prior to administration, whenever solution and container permit. Inspect visually for particulates and discoloration. The solution should be free of visible particulates, clear to slightly opalescent and colorless to pale yellow.

• Store reconstituted Herceptin at 2−8°C; discard unused Herceptin after 28 days. If Herceptin is reconstituted with SWFI without preservative, use immediately and discard any unused portion.

• Determine the dose (mg) of Herceptin. Calculate the volume of the 21 mg/mL reconstituted Herceptin solution needed, withdraw this amount from the vial and add it to an infusion bag containing 250 mL of 0.9% Sodium Chloride Injection, USP. DO NOT USE DEXTROSE (5%) SOLUTION.

• Gently invert the bag to mix the solution.

DOSAGE FORMS AND STRENGTHS: 440 mg lyophilized powder per multi-use vial.

CONTRAINDICATIONS: None

WARNINGS AND PRECAUTIONS

Cardiomyopathy

Herceptin can cause left ventricular cardiac dysfunction, arrhythmias, hypertension, disabling cardiac failure, cardiomyopath, and cardiac death [see Boxed Warning: Cardiomyopathy].

Figure 62. Kerley B lines in acute cardiac decompensation. The short, horizontal lines can be found everywhere in the right lung. This image is by By Hellerhoff - Own work, CC BY-SA 3.0, https://commons.wikimedia.org/w/index.php?curid=37883875. https://en.wikipedia.org/wiki/Heart_failure#/media/File:Kerley-B-Linien.jpg. This file is licensed under the Creative Commons Attribution-Share Alike 3.0 Unported license. No changes have been made to this image.

Figure 62. Kerley B lines

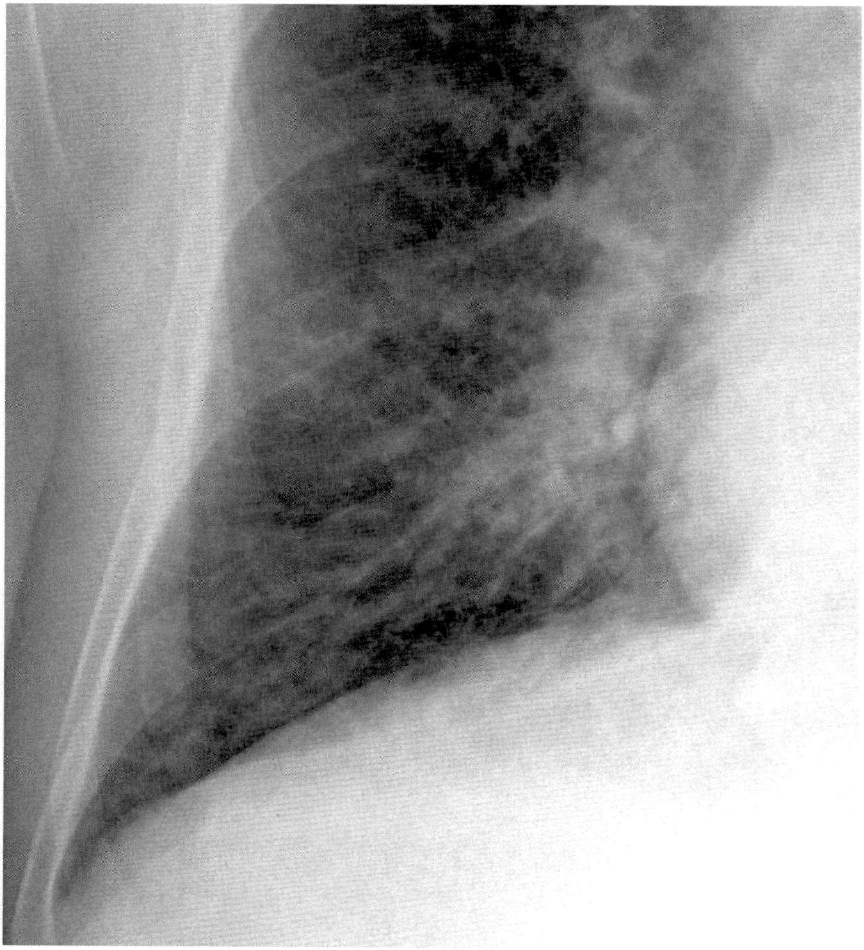

Figure 63. Ventricular fibrillation.

Figure 63. Ventricular fibrillation

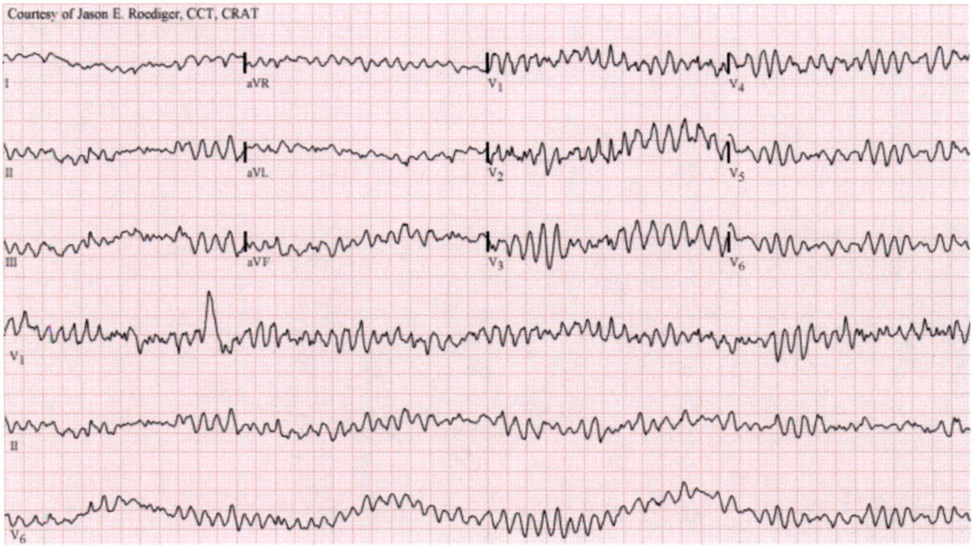

Figure 64. Automated arm blood pressure meter showing arterial hypertension (shown by a systolic blood pressure 158 mmHg, diastolic blood pressure 99 mmHg and heart rate of 80 beats per minute).

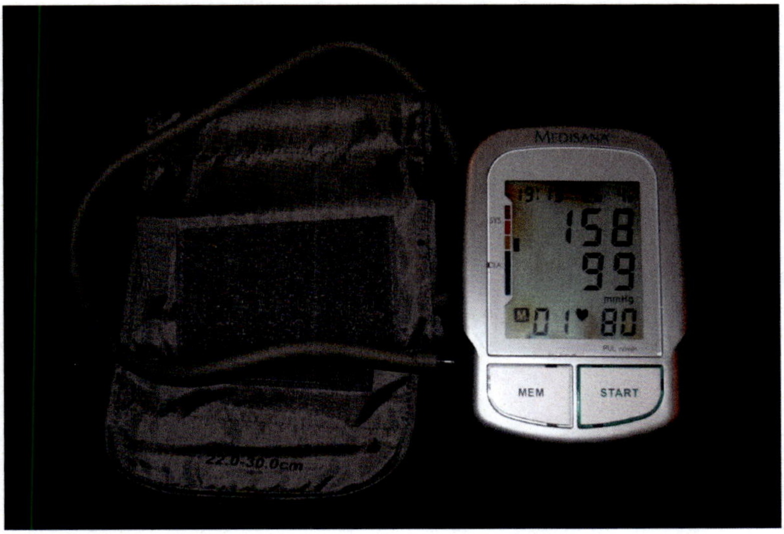

This image is by By Steven Fruitsmaak - Own work, CC BY 3.0, https://commons.wikimedia.org/w/index.php?curid=5866201.

https://en.wikipedia.org/wiki/Hypertension#/media/File:Grade_1_hypertension.jpg. This file is licensed under the Creative Commons Attribution 3.0 Unported license. No changes have been made to this image.

Figure 65. Coronary bypass surgery for ischemic cardiomyopathy.

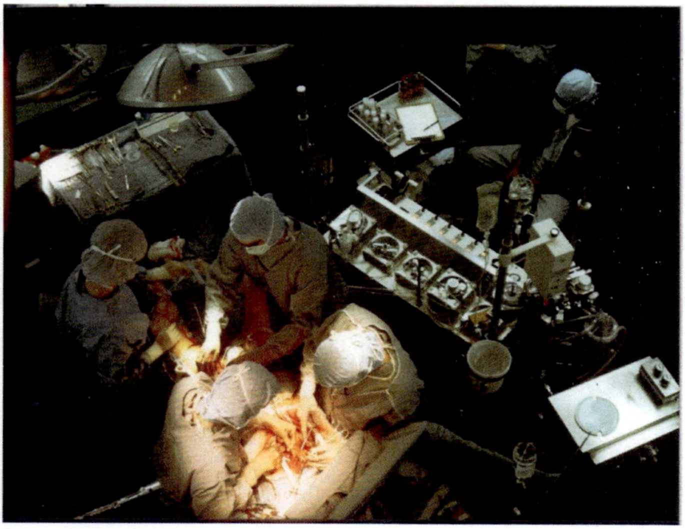

This image is by Jerry Hecht - http://fmp.cit.nih.gov/hi/ - Image ID: 657 C, Public Domain, https://commons.wikimedia.org/w/index.php?curid=780261. https://en.wikipedia.org/wiki/Ischemic_cardiomyopathy#/media/File:Coronary_artery_bypass_surgery_Image_657C-PH.jpg. This image is a work of the National Institutes of Health, part of the United States Department of Health and Human Services. As a work of the U.S. federal government, the image is in the public domain. No changes have been made to this image.

Herceptin can also cause asymptomatic decline in left ventricular ejection fraction (LVEF). There is a 4 to 6-fold increase in the incidence of symptomatic myocardial dysfunction among patients receiving Herceptin as a single agent or in combination therapy compared with those not receiving Herceptin. The highest absolute incidence occurs when Herceptin is administered with an anthracycline. Withhold Herceptin for ≥ 16% absolute decrease in LVEF from pre-treatment values or an

LVEF value below institutional limits of normal and ≥ 10% absolute decrease in LVEF from pretreatment values.

The safety of continuation or resumption of Herceptin in patients with Herceptin-induced left ventricular cardiac dysfunction has not been studied.

Cardiac monitoring

Conduct thorough cardiac assessment, including history, physical examination, and determination of LVEF by echocardiogram or MUGA scan. The following schedule is recommended:

• Baseline LVEF measurement immediately prior to initiation of Herceptin

• LVEF measurements every 3 months during and upon completion of Herceptin

• Repeat LVEF measurement at 4-week intervals if Herceptin is withheld for significant left ventricular cardiac dysfunction

• LVEF measurements every 6 months for at least 2 years following completion of Herceptin as a component of adjuvant therapy.

In Study 1, 16% (136/844) of patients discontinued Herceptin due to clinical evidence of myocardial dysfunction or significant decline in LVEF. In Study 3, the number of patients who discontinued Herceptin due to cardiac toxicity was 2.6% (44/1678). In Study 4, a total of 2.9% (31/1056) patients in the TCH arm (1.5% during the chemotherapy phase and 1.4% during the monotherapy phase) and 5.7% (61/1068) patients in the AC-TH arm (1.5% during the chemotherapy phase and 4.2% during the monotherapy phase) discontinued Herceptin due to cardiac toxicity.

Among 32 patients receiving adjuvant chemotherapy (Studies 1 and 2) who developed congestive heart failure, one patient died of cardiomyopathy and all other patients were receiving cardiac medication at last follow-up. Approximately half of the surviving patients had recovery to a normal LVEF (defined as ≥ 50%) on continuing medical management at the time of last follow-up. The safety of continuation or resumption of Herceptin in patients with Herceptin-induced left ventricular cardiac dysfunction has not been studied.

The incidence of congestive heart failure in adjuvant breast cancer studies was as follows: in Studies 1 and 2 it was 2%in the Herceptin arm and 0.4% in the control arm. In Study 3 it was 2% in the Herceptin arm and 0.3% in the control arm. In Study 4 it was 2% in the Herceptin arm and 0.3% in the control arm. In Study 4 a total of 2.9%of patients in the TCH arm and 5.7% in the AC-TH arm discontinued Herceptin due to cardiac toxicity.

The incidence of cardiac dysfunction in metatastatic breast cancer studies was as follows: in Study 5 utilizing AC, using NYHA criteria I-IV it was 28% in the Herceptin arm and 7% in the control arm. In Study 5 using paclitaxel it was11% in the Herceptin arm and 1% in the control arm. In Study 6 it wa 7% in the Herceptin arm and N/A in the control arm. Using NYHA criteria III-IV the corresponding figures in Study 5 using AC were 19% in the Herceptin arm and 3% in the control arm. In Study 5 using pactitaxel it was 4 % in the Herceptin arm and 1% in the control arm. In Study 6 it was 5% in the Herceptin arm and N/A in the control arm.

In Study 4, the incidence of NCI-CTC Grade 3/4 cardiac ischemia/infarction was higher in the Herceptin containing regimens: (AC-TH: 0.3% (3/1068) and TCH 0.2% (2/1056)) as compared to none in AC-T.

Infusion reactions consist of a symptom complex characterized by fever and chills, and on occasion included nausea, vomiting, pain (in some cases at tumor sites), headache, dizziness, dyspnea, hypotension, rash, and asthenia.

In postmarketing reports, serious and fatal infusion reactions have been reported. Severe reactions which include bronchospasm, anaphylaxis *(Figure 66)*, angioedema *(Figure 67)*, hypoxia, and severe hypotension, were usually reported during or immediately following the initial infusion. However, the onset and clinical course were variable including progressive worsening, initial improvement followed by clinical deterioration, or delayed post-infusion events with rapid clinical deterioration.

Figure 66. Signs and symptoms of anaphylaxis.

This image is by By Mikael Häggström - Own work, CC0, https://commons.wikimedia.org/w/index.php?curid=17700404. https://en.wikipedia.org/wiki/Anaphylaxis#/media/File:Signs_and_symptoms_of_anap

hylaxis.svg. This file is made available under the Creative Commons CC0 1.0 Universal Public Domain Dedication. No changes have been made to this image.

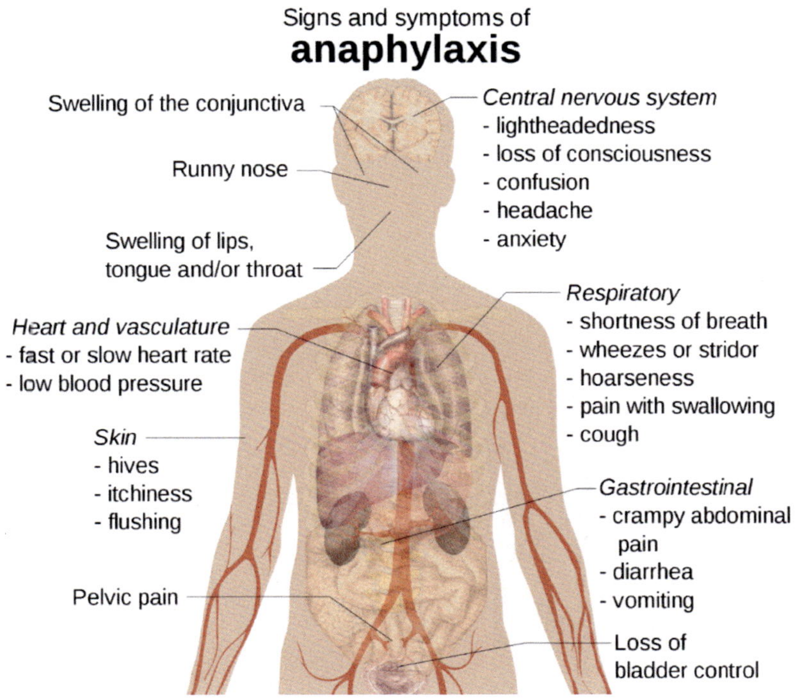

For fatal events, death occurred within hours to days following a serious infusion reaction. Interrupt Herceptin infusion in all patients experiencing dyspnea, clinically significant hypotension, and intervention of medical therapy should *be* administered, which may include: epinephrine, corticosteroids, diphenhydramine, bronchodilators, and oxygen. Patients should be evaluated and carefully monitored until complete resolution of signs and symptoms. Permanent discontinuation should be strongly considered in all patients with severe infusion reactions.

There are no data regarding the most appropriate method of identification of patients who may safely be retreated with Herceptin after experiencing a severe infusion reaction. Prior to resumption of Herceptin infusion, the majority of patients who experienced a severe infusion reaction were pre-medicated with antihistamines and/or corticosteroids. While some patients tolerated Herceptin infusions, others had recurrent severe infusion reactions despite pre-medications.

Figure 67. Angioedema of the face.

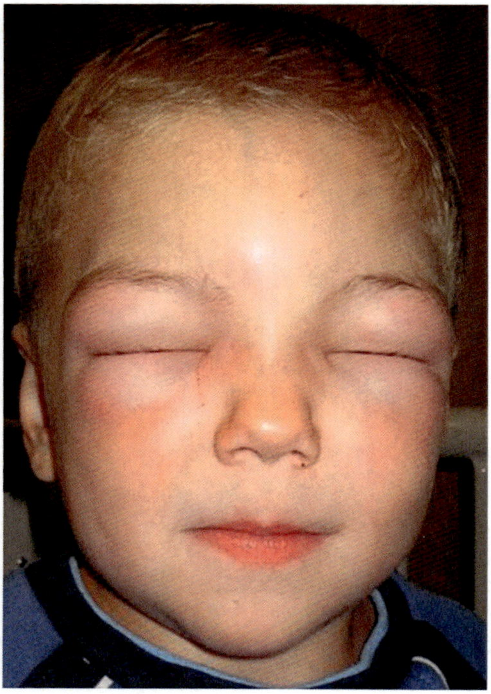

This image is by By James Heilman, MD - Own work, CC BY-SA 3.0, https://commons.wikimedia.org/w/index.php?curid=9445432. https://en.wikipedia.org/wiki/Anaphylaxis#/media/File:Angioedema2010.JPG. This file is licensed under the Creative Commons Attribution-Share Alike 3.0 Unported license. The uploader asserts the following regarding consent of identifiable persons: I personally created this media. All identifiable persons shown specifically consented to publication of this photograph or video. No changeshave been made to this image.

Exacerbation of chemotherapy-induced neutropenia

In randomized, controlled clinical trials the per-patient incidences of NCI CTC Grade 3−4 neutropenia and of febrile neutropenia were higher in patients receiving Herceptin in combination with myelosuppressive chemotherapy as compared to those who received chemotherapy alone. The incidence of septic death was similar among patients who received Herceptin and those who did not.

Pulmonary toxicity

Herceptin use can result in serious and fatal pulmonary toxicity. Pulmonary toxicity includes dyspnea, interstitial pneumonitis, pulmonary infiltrates, pleural effusions *(Figure 68)*, non-cardiogenic pulmonary edema, pulmonary insufficiency and hypoxia, acute respiratory distress syndrome *(Figure 69),* and pulmonary fibrosis. Such events can occur as sequelae of infusion reactions.

Figure 68. CT scan of the chest showing a left-sided pleural effusion. The fluid usually settles at the lowest space due to gravity; in this case, at the back because the patient is supine.

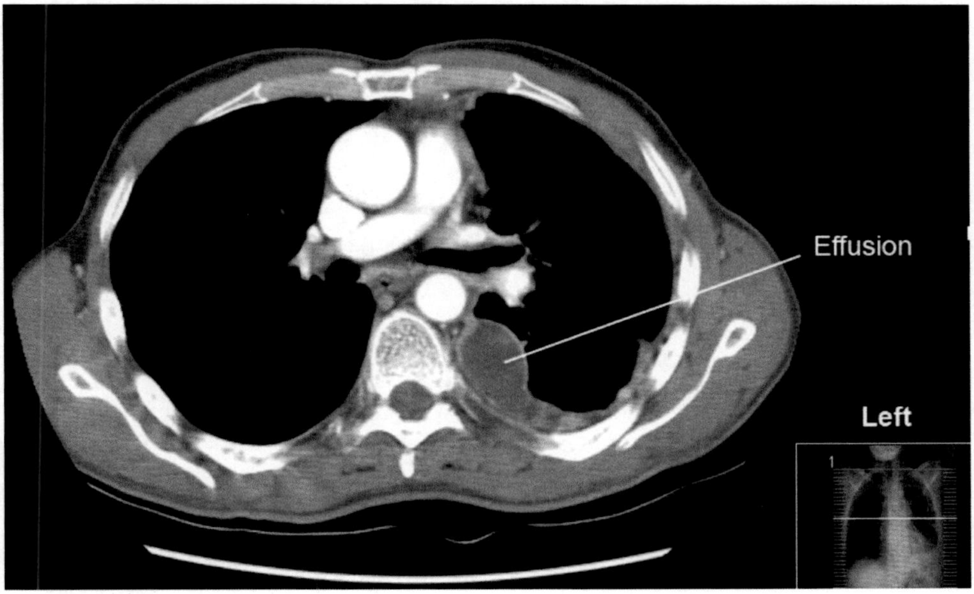

Figure 69. Severe acute respiratory distress syndrome (ARDS). Person is intubated with an oro-gastric tube (OG) in place.

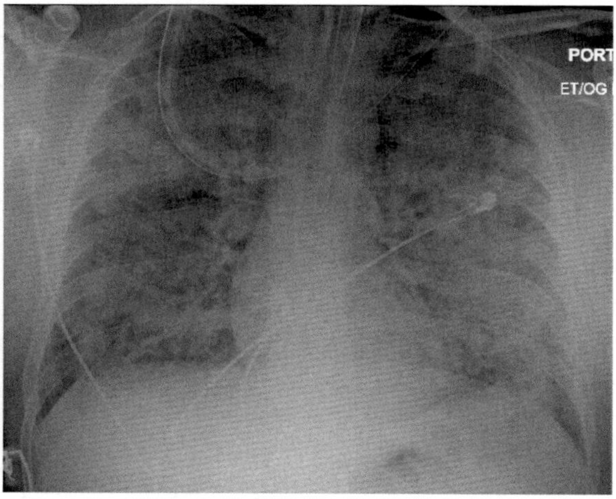

This image is by By James Heilman, MD - Own work, CC BY-SA 4.0, https://commons.wikimedia.org/w/index.php?curid=62501459. https://en.wikipedia.org/wiki/Acute_respiratory_distress_syndrome#/media/File:ARDSSevere.png. This file is licensed under the Creative Commons Attribution-Share Alike 4.0 International license. No changes have been made to this image.

Patients with symptomatic intrinsic lung disease or with extensive tumor involvement of the lungs, resulting in dyspnea at rest, appear to have more severe toxicity.

HER2 testing

Detection of HER2 protein overexpression is necessary for selection of patients appropriate for Herceptin therapy because these are the only patients studied and for whom benefit has been shown. Due to differences in tumor histopathology, use FDA-approved tests for the specific tumor type (breast or gastric/gastroesophageal adenocarcinoma) to assess HER2 protein overexpression and HER2 gene amplification. Tests should be performed by laboratories with demonstrated proficiency in the specific technology being utilized. Improper assay performance, including use of suboptimally fixed tissue, failure to utilize specified reagents, deviation from specific assay instructions, and failure to include appropriate controls for assay validation, can lead to unreliable results. Several FDA-approved commercial assays are available to aid in the selection of breast cancer and metastatic gastric cancer patients for Herceptin therapy. Users should refer to the package inserts of specific assay kits for information on the Intended Use, and the validation and performance of each U.S. BL 103792 Supplement: Trastuzumab–Genentech, Inc.

Limitations in assay precision make it inadvisable to rely on a single method to rule out potential Herceptin benefit.

Embryo-fetal toxicity

Herceptin can cause fetal harm when administered to a pregnant woman. Post-marketing case reports suggest that Herceptin use during pregnancy increases the risk of oligohydramnios during the second and third trimesters. If Herceptin is used during pregnancy or if a woman becomes pregnant while taking Herceptin, she should be apprised of the potential hazard to a fetus.

Immunogenicity

As with all therapeutic proteins, there is a potential for immunogenicity. Among 903 women with metastatic breast cancer, human anti-human antibody (HAHA) to Herceptin was detected in one patient using an enzyme-linked immunosorbent assay (ELISA). This patient did not experience an allergic reaction. Samples for assessment of HAHA were not collected in studies of adjuvant breast cancer. The incidence of antibody formation is highly dependent on the sensitivity and the specificity of the assay. Additionally, the observed incidence of antibody (including neutralizing antibody) positivity in an assay may be influenced by several factors including assay methodology, sample handling, timing of sample collection, concomitant medications, and underlying disease. For these reasons, comparison of the incidence of antibodies to Herceptin with the incidence of antibodies to other products may be misleading.

Post-marketing experience

The following adverse reactions have been identified during post approval use of Herceptin. Because these reactions are reported voluntarily from a population of uncertain size, it is not always possible to reliably estimate their frequency or establish a causal relationship to drug exposure.

- Infusion reaction
- Oligohydramnios

DRUG INTERACTIONS

In Study 5, the mean serum trough concentration of trastuzumab was consistently elevated approximately 1.5-fold, when administered in combination with paclitaxel as compared to trough concentrations of trastuzumab when administered in combination with an anthracycline and cyclophosphamide. In other pharmacokinetic studies, where Herceptin was administered in combination with paclitaxel, docetaxel or doxorubicin, Herceptin did not alter the plasma concentrations of these chemotherapeutic agents, or the metabolites that were analyzed. In a drug interaction substudy conducted in patients in Study 7, the pharmacokinetics of cisplatin, capecitabine and their metabolites were not altered when administered in combination with Herceptin.

PHARMACOKINETICS

The pharmacokinetics of trastuzumab were studied in women with metastatic breast cancer. Short duration intravenous infusions of 10 to 500 mg Herceptin once weekly demonstrated dose-dependent pharmacokinetics. Mean half-life increased and clearance decreased with increasing dose level. The half-life averaged 2 and 12 days at the 10 and 500 mg dose levels, respectively. The volume of distribution of trastuzumab was approximately that of serum volume (44 mL/kg). At the highest weekly dose studied (500 mg), mean peak serum concentrations were 377 mcg/mL. In studies using an initial dose of 4 mg/kg followed by a weekly dose of 2 mg/kg, a mean half-life of 6 days (range 1−32 days) was observed. Between weeks 16 and 32, trastuzumab serum concentrations reached a steady state with mean trough and peak concentrations of approximately 79 mcg/mL and 123 mcg/mL, respectively. In a study of women receiving adjuvant therapy for breast cancer, a mean half-life of trastuzumab of 16 days (range: 11−23 days) was observed after an initial dose of 8 mg/kg followed by a dose of 6 mg/kg every three weeks. Between weeks 6 and 37, trastuzumab serum concentrations reached a steady-state with mean trough and peak concentrations of 63 mcg/mL and 216 mcg/mL, respectively. In patients with metastatic gastric cancer (Study 7), mean serum trastuzumab trough concentrations at steady state were 24 to 63% lower as compared to the concentrations observed in patients with breast cancer receiving treatment for metastatic disease in combination with paclitaxel, as monotherapy for metastatic disease, or as adjuvant monotherapy. Sixty-four percent (286/447) of women with metastatic breast cancer had detectable circulating extracellular domain of the HER2 receptor (shed antigen), which ranged as high as 1880 ng/mL (median 11 ng/mL). Patients with higher baseline shed antigen levels were more likely to have lower serum trough concentrations. Data suggest that the disposition of trastuzumab is not altered based on age or serum creatinine (≤2.0 mg creatinine/dL).

USE IN SPECIFIC POPULATIONS

Pregnancy Category D

(Pregnancy Category D indicates that there is positive evidence of human fetal risk based on adverse reaction data from investigational or marketing experience or studies in humans, but potential benefits may warrant use of the drug in pregnant women despite potential risks).

Herceptin can cause fetal harm when administered to a pregnant woman. Post-marketing case reports suggest that Herceptin use during pregnancy increases the risk for oligohydramnios during the second and third trimester. If Herceptin is used during pregnancy or if a woman becomes pregnant while taking Herceptin, she should be apprised of the potential hazard to a fetus. In the postmarketing setting, oligohydramnios was reported in women who received Herceptin during pregnancy, either alone or in combination with chemotherapy. In half of these women, amniotic fluid index increased after Herceptin was stopped. In one case, Herceptin was resumed after the amniotic fluid index improved, and oligohydramnios recurred. Women using Herceptin during pregnancy should be monitored for oligohydramnios. If oligohydramnios occurs, fetal testing should be done that is appropriate for gestational age and consistent with community standards of care. Additional intravenous (IV) hydration has been helpful when oligohydramnios has occurred following administration of other chemotherapy agents, however the effects of additional IV hydration with Herceptin treatment are not known.

No teratogenic effects were observed in offspring from reproduction studies in cynomolgus monkeys at doses up to 25 times the recommended weekly human dose of 2 mg/kg trastuzumab. In mutant mice lacking HER2, embryos died in early gestation. Trastuzumab exposure was reported at delivery in offspring of cynomolgus monkeys treated during the early (Days 20-50 of gestation) or late (Days 120-150 of gestation) fetal development periods, at levels of 15 to 28% of the maternal blood levels.

Registry

Pregnant women with breast cancer who are using Herceptin are encouraged to enroll in MotHERthe Herceptin Pregnancy Registry: phone 1-800-690-6720.

Nursing mothers

It is not known whether Herceptin is excreted in human milk, but human IgG is excreted in human milk. Published data suggest that breast milk antibodies do not enter the neonatal and infant circulation in substantial amounts. Trastuzumab was present in the breast milk of lactating cynomolgus monkeys given 12.5 times the recommended weekly human dose of 2 mg/kg of Herceptin. Infant monkeys with detectable serum levels of trastuzumab did not have any adverse effects on growth or development from birth to 3 months of age; however, trastuzumab levels in animal breast milk may not accurately reflect human breast milk levels. Because many drugs are secreted in human milk and because of the potential for serious adverse reactions in nursing infants from Herceptin, a decision should be made whether to discontinue nursing, or discontinue drug, taking into account the elimination half-life of trastuzumab and the importance of the drug to the mother.

Pediatric use

The safety and effectiveness of Herceptin in pediatric patients has not been established.

Geriatric use

Herceptin has been administered to 386 patients who were 65 years of age or over (253 in the adjuvant treatment and 133 in metastatic breast cancer treatment settings). The risk of cardiac dysfunction was increased in geriatric patients as compared to younger patients in both those receiving treatment for metastatic disease in Studies 5 and 6, or adjuvant therapy in Studies 1 and 2. Limitations in data collection and differences in study design of the 4 studies of Herceptin in adjuvant treatment of breast cancer preclude a determination of whether the toxicity profile of Herceptin in older patients is different from younger patients. The reported clinical experience is not adequate to determine whether the efficacy improvements (ORR, TTP, OS, DFS) of Herceptin treatment in older patients is different from that observed in patients.

OVERDOSAGE

There is no experience with overdosage in human clinical trials. Single doses higher than 8 mg/kg have not been tested.

1. Efficacy of Herceptin as adjuvant treatment for primary breast cancer

The addition of 1 year of adjuvant trastuzumab significantly improved disease-free and overall survival among women with HER2-positive breast cancer. The risk–benefit ratio favored the nonanthracycline TCH regimen over AC-T plus trastuzumab, given its similar efficacy, fewer acute toxic effects, and lower risks of cardiotoxicity and leukemia.

Slamon, D et al. N Engl J Med 2011; 365:1273-1283
DOI: 10.1056/NEJMoa0910383.

2. Efficacy of Herceptin as adjuvant treatment for metastatic breast cancer

Authors' conclusions:

Trastuzumab improved overall survival and progression-free survival in HER2-positive women with metastatic breast cancer, but it also increased the risk of cardiac toxicities, such as congestive heart failure and LVEF decline. The available subgroup analyses are limited by the small number of studies. Studies that administered trastuzumab as first-line treatment, or along with a taxane-based regimen, improved mortality outcomes. The evidence to support the use of trastuzumab beyond progression is limited. The recruitment in three out of seven studies was stopped early and in three trials more than 50% of patients in the control groups were permitted to switch to the trastuzumab arms at progression, making it more difficult to understand the real net benefit of trastuzumab.

Balduzzi S, et al. Trastuzumab-containing regimens for metastatic breast cancer. Cochrane Database of Systematic Reviews 2014, Issue 6. Art. No.: CD006242. DOI: 10.1002/14651858.CD006242.pub2.

10.8. HERCEPTIN HYLECTA (TRASTUZUMAB and HYALURONIC ACID)

HERCEPTIN HYLECTA™ (trastuzumab and hyaluronidase-oysk) injection, for subcutaneous use. Initial U.S. Approval: 2019.

WARNING: CARDIOMYOPATHY, EMBRYO-FETAL TOXICITY, and PULMONARY TOXICITY See full prescribing information for complete boxed warning.

MECHANISM OF ACTION

The HER2 (or c-erbB2) proto-oncogene encodes a transmembrane receptor protein of 185 kDa, which is structurally related to the epidermal growth factor receptor. Trastuzumab has been shown, in both in vitro assays and in animals, to inhibit the proliferation of human tumor cells that overexpress HER2. Trastuzumab is a mediator of antibody-dependent cellular cytotoxicity (ADCC). In vitro, trastuzumab-mediated ADCC has been shown to be preferentially exerted on HER2 overexpressing cancer cells compared with cancer cells that do not overexpress HER2. Hyaluronan is a polysaccharide found in the extracellular matrix of the subcutaneous tissue. It is depolymerized by the naturally occurring enzyme hyaluronidase. Unlike the stable structural components of the interstitial matrix, hyaluronan has a half-life of approximately 0.5 days. Hyaluronidase increases permeability of the subcutaneous tissue by depolymerizing hyaluronan. In the doses administered, hyaluronidase in HERCEPTIN HYLECTA acts transiently and locally. The effects of hyaluronidase are reversible and permeability of the subcutaneous tissue is restored within 24 to 48 hours. Hyaluronidase has been shown to increase the absorption rate of a trastuzumab product into the systemic circulation when given in the subcutis of Göttingen Minipigs (Figure 127).

DESCRIPTION

HERCEPTIN HYLECTA is a combination of trastuzumab and hyaluronidase. Trastuzumab is a humanized IgG1 kappa monoclonal antibody that selectively binds with high affinity to the extracellular domain of the human epidermal growth factor receptor 2 protein, HER2. Trastuzumab is produced by recombinant DNA technology in a mammalian cell (Chinese Hamster Ovary) culture. Trastuzumab has a molecular weight of approximately 148 kDa. Hyaluronidase (recombinant human) is an endoglycosidase used to increase the dispersion and absorption of coadministered drugs when administered subcutaneously. It is a glycosylated single-chain protein produced by mammalian (Chinese Hamster Ovary) cells containing a DNA plasmid encoding for a soluble fragment of human hyaluronidase (PH20). Hyaluronidase (recombinant human) has a molecular weight of approximately 61 kDa. HERCEPTIN HYLECTA (trastuzumab and hyaluronidase) injection is a sterile, preservative-free, colorless to yellowish, clear to opalescent solution supplied in single-dose vials for subcutaneous administration. HERCEPTIN HYLECTA is supplied as 600 mg trastuzumab and 10,000 units hyaluronidase per 5 mL in singledose vials. Each mL of solution contains trastuzumab (120 mg), hyaluronidase (2,000 units), L-histidine (0.39 mg), L-histidine hydrochloride monohydrate (3.67 mg), L-methionine (1.49 mg), polysorbate 20 (0.4 mg), α, αtrehalose dihydrate (79.45 mg), and Water for Injection.

Cardiomyopathy

HERCEPTIN HYLECTA can result in subclinical and clinical cardiac failure manifesting as CHF, and decreased LVEF, with greatest risk when administered concurrently with anthracyclines. Evaluate cardiac function prior to and during treatment. Discontinue HERCEPTIN HYLECTA for cardiomyopathy.

Pulmonary toxicity: discontinue HERCEPTIN HYLECTA for anaphylaxis, angioedema, interstitial pneumonitis or acute respiratory distress syndrome.

Embryo-fetal toxicity: exposure to HERCEPTIN HYLECTA during pregnancy can result in oligohydramnios, in some cases complicated by pulmonary hypoplasia and neonatal death. Advise patients of these risks and the need for effective contraception.

PHARMACODYNAMICS

Cardiac electrophysiology

The effects of trastuzumab on electrocardiographic (ECG) endpoints, including QTc interval duration, were evaluated in patients with HER2-positive solid tumors. Trastuzumab had no clinically relevant effect on the QTc interval duration and there was no apparent relationship between serum trastuzumab concentrations and change in QTcF interval duration in patients with HER2-positive solid tumors.

INDICATIONS AND USAGE

HERCEPTIN HYLECTA is a combination of trastuzumab, a HER2/neu receptor antagonist, and hyaluronidase, an endoglycosidase, indicated in adults for:

• The treatment of HER2-overexpressing breast cancer. Select patients for therapy based on an FDA-approved companion diagnostic for trastuzumab.

DOSAGE AND ADMINISTRATION

For **subcutaneous use only**. HERCEPTIN HYLECTA has different dosage and administration instructions than intravenous trastuzumab products. Do **not** administer intravenously. Do not substitute HERCEPTIN HYLECTA for or with ado-trastuzumab emtansine.

Perform HER2 testing using FDA-approved tests by laboratories with demonstrated proficiency.

The recommended dose of HERCEPTIN HYLECTA is 600 mg/10,000 units (600 mg trastuzumab and 10,000 units hyaluronidase) administered subcutaneously over approximately 2-5 minutes once every three weeks.

DOSAGE FORMS AND STRENGTHS

• Injection: 600 mg trastuzumab and 10,000 units hyaluronidase per 5 mL (120 mg/2,000 units per mL) solution in a single-dose vial.

CONTRAINDICATIONS

• None.

WARNINGS AND PRECAUTIONS

• Exacerbation of chemotherapy-induced neutropenia.

• Hypersensitivity and administration-related reactions (ARRs)

Severe ARRs, including anaphylaxis, have been reported with HERCEPTIN HYLECTA. Monitor patients for systemic hypersensitivity reactions. Permanently discontinue HERCEPTIN HYLECTA in patients who experience anaphylaxis or severe hypersensitivity reactions.

ADVERSE REACTIONS

Adjuvant breast cancer

• The most common adverse reactions (≥10%) for HERCEPTIN HYLECTA are fatigue, arthralgia, diarrhea, injection site reaction, upper respiratory tract infection, rash, myalgia, nausea, headache, edema, flushing, pyrexia, cough, and pain in extremity.

Metastatic breast cancer (based on intravenous trastuzumab)

• The most common adverse reactions (≥10%) are fever, chills, headache, infection, congestive heart failure, insomnia, cough, and rash. To report SUSPECTED ADVERSE REACTIONS, contact Genentech at 1-888-835-2555 or FDA at 1-800-FDA-1088 or www.fda.gov/medwatch.

USE IN SPECIFIC POPULATIONS

Females and Males of Reproductive Potential

Verify the pregnancy status of females prior to initiation of HERCEPTIN HYLECTA.

Revised: 2/2019 **FULL PRESCRIBING INFORMATION WARNING: CARDIOMYOPATHY, EMBRYO-FETAL TOXICITY, and PULMONARY TOXICITY**

Cardiomyopathy

HERCEPTIN HYLECTA administration can result in sub-clinical and clinical cardiac failure. The incidence and severity were highest in patients receiving HERCEPTIN HYLECTA with anthracycline-containing chemotherapy regimens. Evaluate left ventricular function in all patients prior to and during treatment with HERCEPTIN HYLECTA. Discontinue HERCEPTIN HYLECTA treatment in patients receiving adjuvant therapy and withhold HERCEPTIN HYLECTA in patients with metastatic disease for clinically significant decrease in left ventricular function.

Pulmonary toxicity

HERCEPTIN HYLECTA administration can result in serious and fatal pulmonary toxicity. Symptoms usually occur during or within 24 hours of HERCEPTIN

HYLECTA administration. Discontinue HERCEPTIN HYLECTA for anaphylaxis, angioedema, interstitial pneumonitis, or acute respiratory distress syndrome. Monitor patients until symptoms completely resolve.

Embryo-fetal toxicity

Exposure to HERCEPTIN HYLECTA during pregnancy can result in oligohydramnios and oligohydramnios sequence manifesting as pulmonary hypoplasia, skeletal abnormalities, and neonatal death. Advise patients of these risks and the need for effective contraception.

INDICATIONS AND USAGE

Adjuvant breast cancer

HERCEPTIN HYLECTA is indicated for adjuvant treatment of adults with HER2 overexpressing node positive or node negative (ER/PR negative or with one high risk feature breast cancer

• as part of a treatment regimen consisting of doxorubicin, cyclophosphamide, and either paclitaxel or docetaxel

• as part of a treatment regimen with docetaxel and carboplatin

• as a single agent following multi-modality anthracycline-based therapy.

Select patients for therapy based on an FDA-approved companion diagnostic for trastuzumab.

Metastatic breast cancer

HERCEPTIN HYLECTA is indicated in adults

• In combination with paclitaxel for first-line treatment of HER2-overexpressing metastatic breast cancer

• As a single agent for treatment of HER2-overexpressing breast cancer in patients who have received one or more chemotherapy regimens for metastatic disease. Select patients for therapy based on an FDA-approved companion diagnostic for trastuzumab

DOSAGE AND ADMINISTRATION

Patient selection

Select patients based on HER2 protein overexpression or HER2 gene amplification in tumor specimens. Assessment of HER2 protein overexpression and HER2 gene amplification should be performed using FDA-approved tests specific for breast cancer by laboratories with demonstrated proficiency. Information on the FDA-approved tests for the detection of HER2 protein overexpression and HER2 gene amplification is available at: http://www.fda.gov/CompanionDiagnostics. Improper assay performance, including use of suboptimally fixed tissue, failure to utilize specified reagents, deviation from specific assay instructions, and failure to include appropriate controls for assay validation, can lead to unreliable results.

Recommended Doses and Schedules

HERCEPTIN HYLECTA is for subcutaneous use only. HERCEPTIN HYLECTA has different dosage and administration instructions than intravenous trastuzumab products. Do not administer intravenously. Do not substitute HERCEPTIN HYLECTA for or with ado-trastuzumab emtansine. The recommended dose of HERCEPTIN HYLECTA is 600 mg/10,000 units (600 mg trastuzumab and 10,000 units hyaluronidase) administered subcutaneously over approximately 2-5 minutes once every three weeks. No loading dose is required. No dose adjustments for patient body weight or for different concomitant chemotherapy regimens are required.

Duration of treatment

Patients with adjuvant breast cancer should be treated with HERCEPTIN HYLECTA for 52 weeks or until disease recurrence, whichever occurs first; extending treatment in adjuvant breast cancer beyond one year is not recommended. Patients with metastatic breast cancer (MBC) should be treated with HERCEPTIN HYLECTA until progression of disease.

Missed dose

If one dose is missed, it is recommended to administer the next 600 mg/10,000 units dose (i.e. the missed dose) as soon as possible. The interval between subsequent HERCEPTIN HYLECTA doses should not be less than three weeks.

Dosage Modification for Adverse Reactions Cardiomyopathy [see Boxed Warning, Warnings and Precautions

Assess left ventricular ejection fraction (LVEF) prior to initiation of HERCEPTIN HYLECTA and at regular intervals during treatment. Withhold HERCEPTIN HYLECTA dosing for at least 4 weeks for either of the following

• ≥16% absolute decrease in LVEF from pre-treatment values

• LVEF below institutional limits of normal and ≥10% absolute decrease in LVEF from pretreatment values. HERCEPTIN HYLECTA may be resumed if, within 4−8 weeks, the LVEF returns to normal limits and the absolute decrease from baseline is ≤15%.

Permanently discontinue HERCEPTIN HYLECTA for a persistent (>8 weeks) LVEF decline or for suspension of HERCEPTIN HYLECTA dosing on more than 3 occasions for cardiomyopathy.

Administration and storage

To prevent medication errors, it is important to check the vial labels to ensure that the drug being prepared and administered is HERCEPTIN HYLECTA and not ado-trastuzumab emtansine or intravenous trastuzumab.

HERCEPTIN HYLECTA should be administered by healthcare professional. Parenteral drug products should be inspected visually for particulate matter and discoloration prior to administration, whenever solution and container permit. Do **not** use vial if particulates or discoloration is present. Discard any unused portion remaining in the vial.

HERCEPTIN HYLECTA is for single use only. The 600 mg/10,000 units (600 mg trastuzumab and 10,000 units hyaluronidase) solution are a ready to use solution for injection which does not need to be diluted. To avoid needle clogging, attach the hypodermic injection needle to the syringe immediately prior to administration followed by volume adjustment to 5 mL. HERCEPTIN HYLECTA is compatible with polypropylene and polycarbonate syringe material and stainless-steel transfer and injection needles.

Prepare the dosing syringe in controlled and validated aseptic conditions. After the solution of HERCEPTIN HYLECTA is withdrawn from the vial and into the syringe, replace the transfer needle with a syringe closing cap. Label the syringe with the peel-off sticker.

Administration

The injection site should be alternated between the left and right thigh. New injections should be given at least 2.5 cm from the old previous site on healthy skin and never into areas where the skin is red, bruised, tender, or hard, or areas where there are moles or scars. During the treatment course with HERCEPTIN HYLECTA other medicinal products for subcutaneous administration should preferably be injected at different sites. The dose should be administered subcutaneously over approximately 2 to 5 minutes.

Storage

If the syringe containing HERCEPTIN HYLECTA is not used immediately, then the syringe can be stored in the refrigerator (2°C to 8°C) for up to 24 hours and subsequently at room temperature (20°C to 25°C) for up to 4 hours. Protect from light. Do not shake or freeze.

DOSAGE FORMS AND STRENGTHS

HERCEPTIN HYLECTA is a colorless to yellowish, clear to opalescent solution for subcutaneous injection:

- Injection: 600 mg trastuzumab and 10,000 units hyaluronidase per 5 mL (120 mg/2,000 units per mL) in a single-dose vial.

CONTRAINDICATIONS: None.

WARNINGS AND PRECAUTIONS

Cardiomyopathy

HERCEPTIN HYLECTA can cause left ventricular cardiac dysfunction, arrhythmias, hypertension, disabling cardiac failure *(Figure 70)*, cardiomyopathy, and cardiac death [see Boxed Warning: Cardiomyopathy]. HERCEPTIN HYLECTA can also cause asymptomatic decline in LVEF. There is a 4 to 6-fold increase in the incidence of symptomatic myocardial dysfunction among patients receiving trastuzumab as a single agent or in combination therapy compared with those not receiving trastuzumab. The highest absolute incidence occurs when trastuzumab is administered with an anthracycline. The incidence of symptomatic myocardial dysfunction for intravenous trastuzumab and HERCEPTIN HYLECTA was similar in clinical trials.

Withhold HERCEPTIN HYLECTA for ≥16% absolute decrease in LVEF from pre-treatment values or an LVEF value below institutional limits of normal and ≥10% absolute decrease in LVEF from pretreatment values

The safety of continuation or resumption of HERCEPTIN in patients with HERCEPTIN HYLECTA-induced left ventricular cardiac dysfunction has not been studied. Patients who receive anthracycline after stopping HERCEPTIN HYLECTA may also be at increased risk of cardiac dysfunction.

Cardiac monitoring

Conduct thorough cardiac assessment, including history, physical examination, and determination of LVEF by echocardiogram *(Figure 70)* or MUGA scan *(Figure 71)*

Figure 70. Ultrasound showing severe systolic heart failure.

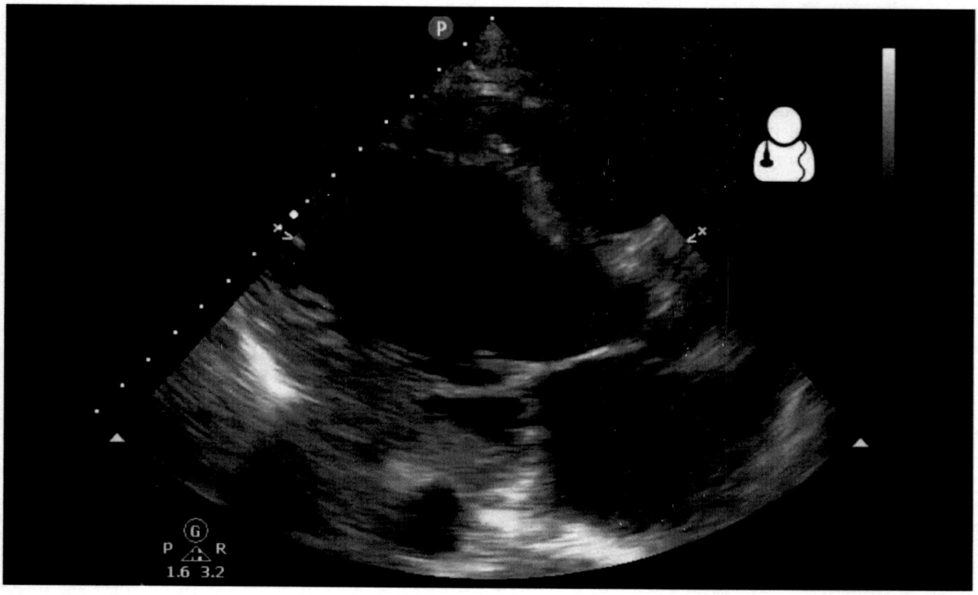

This image is by By Ben Smith https://www.ultrasoundoftheweek.com, CC BY-SA 4.0, https://commons.wikimedia.org/w/index.php?curid=58647880. https://en.wikipedia.org/wiki/Heart_failure#/media/File:UOTW_48_-

_Ultrasound_of_the_Week_5.jpg. This file is licensed under the Creative Commons Attribution-Share Alike 4.0 International license. Attribution: Ben Smith https://www.ultrasoundoftheweek.com No changes have been made to this image.

Figure 71. A normal MUGA scan.

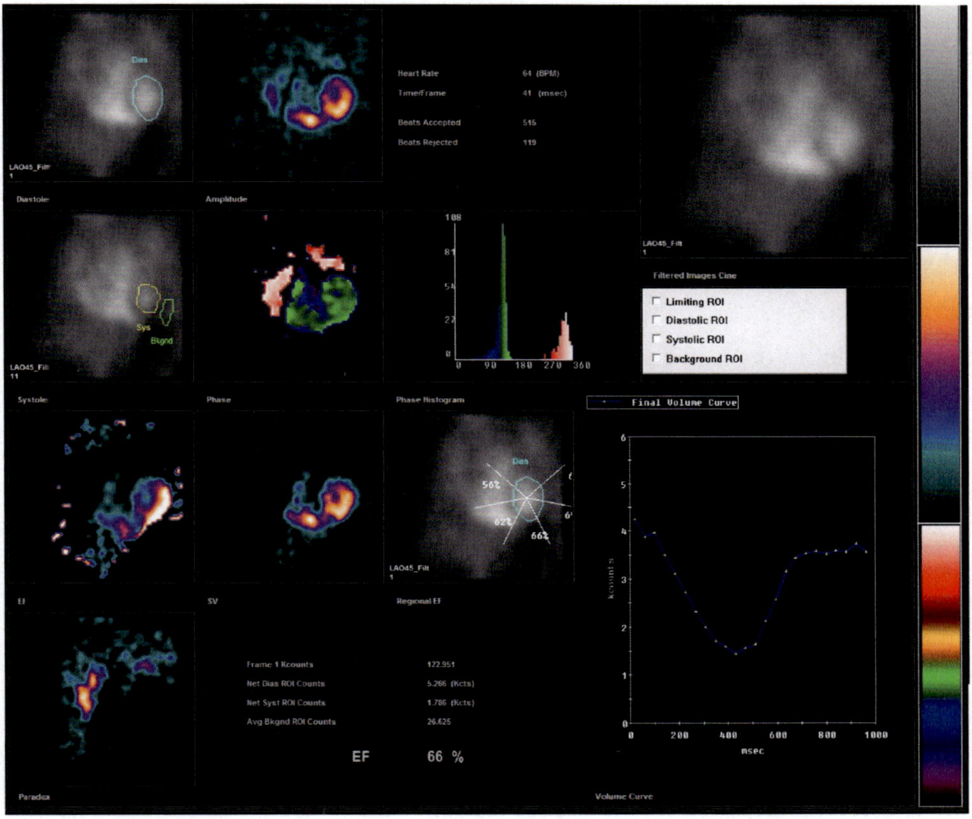

This image is by By Jmarchn - Own work, CC BY-SA 3.0, https://commons.wikimedia.org/w/index.php?curid=105264974. https://en.wikipedia.org/wiki/Radionuclide_angiography#/media/File:Normal_MUGA_scan_1.png. This file is licensed under the Creative Commons Attribution-Share Alike 3.0 Unported license. No changes were made to this image.

The following schedule is recommended

• Baseline LVEF measurement immediately prior to initiation of HERCEPTIN HYLECTA

• LVEF measurements every 3 months during and upon completion of HERCEPTIN HYLECTA

• Repeat LVEF measurement at 4 week intervals if HERCEPTIN HYLECTA is withheld for significant left ventricular cardiac dysfunction

• LVEF measurements every 6 months for at least 2 years following completion of HERCEPTIN HYLECTA as a component of adjuvant therapy.

In the HannaH study, the overall percentage of patients with at least one cardiac disorder was similar in both study arms: 15% (44/297) of patients in the HERCEPTIN HYLECTA arm and 14% (42/298) of patients in the intravenous trastuzumab arm. The most frequent cardiac adverse reactions were left ventricular dysfunction [3.4% (10/297) and 4.0% (12/298)], tachycardia [2% (6/297) and 3% (9/298)] and palpitations [2% (6/297) and 1.3% (4/298)] in the HERCEPTIN HYLECTA arm and the intravenous trastuzumab arm, respectively. The incidence of cardiac failure and congestive cardiac failure was 1% (3/297) in the HERCEPTIN HYLECTA arm and <1% (1/298) in the intravenous trastuzumab arm. The proportion of patients in each treatment arm with a significant decrease in LVEF defined as a drop of ≥10% points to a LVEF of <50% was comparable between treatment arms [3.8% (11/297) in the HERCEPTIN HYLECTA arm and 4.2% (12/298) in the intravenous trastuzumab arm. In patients with lower body weights (<59 kg, the lowest body weight quartile) the fixed dose used in the HERCEPTIN HYLECTA arm was not associated with an increased risk of cardiac events or significant drop in LVEF.

In the SafeHER study, in patients treated with HERCEPTIN HYLECTA, 17% (323/1864) reported a cardiac disorder during the treatment period. Decreased ejection fraction, reported in 4.5% (84/1864) of the patients was the most frequently reported cardiac disorder. Congestive cardiac failure was reported in <1% (10/1864) of patients and <1% (4/1864) of patients reported cardiac failure during the treatment period. One patient reported congestive cardiac failure during the follow-up period. Six percent (111/1864) of the patients treated with HERCEPTIN HYLECTA had an LVEF <50% with a decrease of ≥10 points in LVEF from baseline.

Trastuzumab (intravenous formulation)

In study NSABP B31 (NCT00004067), 15% (158/1031) of patients discontinued intravenous trastuzumab due to clinical evidence of myocardial dysfunction or significant decline in LVEF after a median follow-up duration of 8.7 years in the AC-TH arm. In the HERA study (one-year intravenous trastuzumab treatment; NCT00045032), the number of patients who discontinued intravenous trastuzumab due to cardiac toxicity at 12.6 months median duration of follow-up was 2.6% (44/1678). In the BCIRG006 study (NCT00021255), a total of 2.9% (31/1056) of patients in the TCH arm (1.5% during the chemotherapy phase and 1.4% during the monotherapy phase) and 5.7% (61/1068) of patients in the AC-TH arm (1.5% during the chemotherapy phase and 4.2% during the monotherapy phase) discontinued intravenous trastuzumab due to cardiac toxicity.

Among 64 patients receiving adjuvant chemotherapy (studies NSABP B31 and NCCTG N9831; NCT00005970) who developed congestive heart failure (CHF), one patient died of cardiomyopathy, one patient died suddenly without documented etiology, and 33 patients were receiving cardiac medication at last follow-up. Approximately 24% of the surviving patients had recovery to a normal LVEF (defined as ≥ 50%) and no symptoms on continuing medical management at the time of last follow-up. The safety of continuation or resumption of intravenous trastuzumab in patients with trastuzumab-induced left ventricular cardiac dysfunction has not been studied.

In the HERA study (one-year intravenous trastuzumab treatment), at a median follow-up duration of 8 years, the incidence of severe CHF (NYHA III & IV) was 0.8%, and the rate of mild symptomatic and asymptomatic left ventricular dysfunction was 4.6%.

In the BCIRG006 study, the incidence of NCI-CTC Grade 3/4 cardiac ischemia/infarction was higher in the intravenous trastuzumab containing regimens [AC-TH: 0.3% (3/1068) and TCH: 0.2% (2/1056)] as compared to none in AC-T.

Embryo-fetal toxicity

HERCEPTIN HYLECTA can cause fetal harm when administered to a pregnant woman. In post-marketing reports, use of trastuzumab during pregnancy resulted in cases of oligohydramnios and oligohydramnios sequence manifesting as pulmonary hypoplasia, skeletal abnormalities, and neonatal death. Verify the pregnancy status of females of reproductive potential prior to the initiation of HERCEPTIN HYLECTA. Advise pregnant women and females of reproductive potential that exposure to HERCEPTIN HYLECTA during pregnancy or within 7 months prior to conception can result in fetal harm. Advise females of reproductive potential to use effective contraception during treatment and for 7 months following the last dose of HERCEPTIN.

Pulmonary toxicity

HERCEPTIN HYLECTA can result in serious and fatal pulmonary toxicity. Pulmonary toxicity includes dyspnea, interstitial pneumonitis, pulmonary infiltrates *(Figure 72)*, pleural effusions, non-cardiogenic pulmonary edema, pulmonary insufficiency and hypoxia, acute respiratory distress syndrome, and pulmonary fibrosis. Patients with symptomatic intrinsic lung disease or with extensive tumor involvement of the lungs, resulting in dyspnea at rest, appear to have more severe toxicity. A pulmonary infiltrate is a substance denser than air, such as pus, blood, or protein, which lingers within the parenchyma of the lungs. Pulmonary infiltrates are often associated with pneumonia *(Figure 72)*.

Figure 72. A pulmonary infiltrate is a substance denser than air, such as pus, blood, or protein, which lingers within the parenchyma of the lungs. Pulmonary infiltrates are associated with pneumonia. This chest x-ray shows patchy infiltrates, mainly in the right upper lobe.

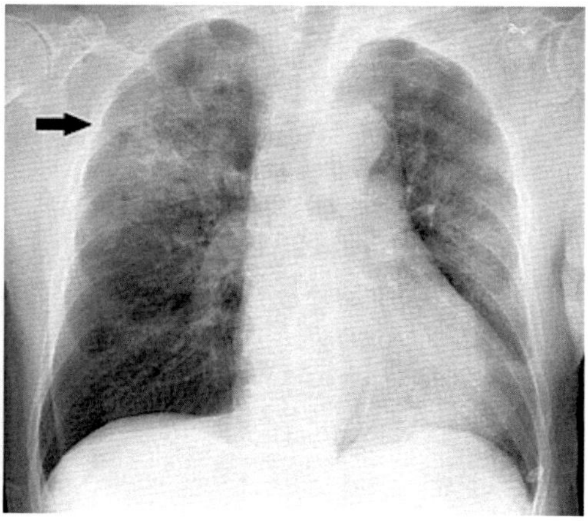

This image is by Mikael Häggström, M.D.- Author info- Reusing imagesMikael HäggströmConsent note: Written informed consent was obtained from the individual, including online publication. - Own work, CC0, https://commons.wikimedia.org/w/index.php?curid=76593347. https://en.wikipedia.org/wiki/Pneumonia#/media/File:Chest_radiograph_in_influensa_and_H_influenzae,_posteroanterior,_annotated.jpg. This file is made available under the Creative Commons CC0 1.0 Universal Public Domain Dedication. Consent note: Written informed consent was obtained from the individual, including online publication. No changes were made to this image.

Exacerbation of chemotherapy-induced neutropenia

HERCEPTIN HYLECTA may exacerbate chemotherapy-induced neutropenia. In randomized, controlled clinical trials with intravenous trastuzumab, the per-patient incidences of NCI-CTC Grade 3–4 neutropenia *(Grade 3: ≥500– < 1,000/mm³; Grade 4: <500/mm³) (Figure 73)* and of febrile neutropenia were higher in patients receiving trastuzumab in combination with myelosuppressive chemotherapy as compared to those who received chemotherapy alone. The incidence of septic death was similar among patients who received trastuzumab and those who did not.

Figure 73. A peripheral blood film with a striking absence of neutrophils, leaving only red blood cells and platelets.

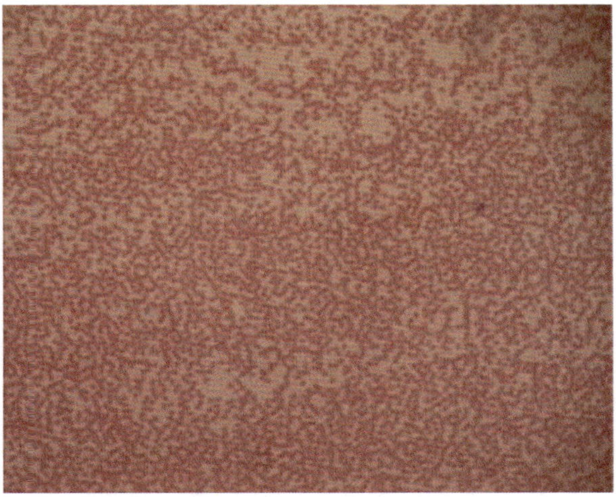

This image is Roberto J. Galindo - Own Work: Foto tomada por Roberto J. Galindo, CC BY-SA 3.0, https://commons.wikimedia.org/w/index.php?curid=2176642. https://en.wikipedia.org/wiki/Neutropenia#/media/File:Neutropenia.JPG. This file is licensed under the Creative Commons Attribution-Share Alike 3.0 Unported license. No changeshave been made to this image.

Hypersensitivity and administration-related reactions

Severe administration-related reactions (ARRs), including hypersensitivity and anaphylaxis, have been reported with HERCEPTIN HYLECTA. Patients experiencing dyspnea at rest due to complications of advanced malignancy and comorbidities may be at increased risk of a severe or of a fatal ARR.

In the HannaH and SafeHER trials, 9% and 4.2% of patients experienced Grade 1-4 hypersensitivity and anaphylaxis, respectively. Grade 3-4 hypersensitivity and anaphylactic reactions occurred in 1% and <1% of the patients treated with HERCEPTIN HYLECTA, respectively. In the SafeHER trial, 2 patients required permanent treatment discontinuation with HERCEPTIN HYLECTA (1 patient due to a hypersensitivity reaction and 1 patient due to anaphylaxis).

Serious and fatal reactions have been reported after treatment with intravenous trastuzumab products.

Closely monitor patients for systemic hypersensitivity reactions, especially during the first administration. Permanently discontinue HERCEPTIN HYLECTA in patients who experience anaphylaxis or severe hypersensitivity reactions. Medications to treat such reactions, as well as emergency equipment, should be available for immediate use. For patients experiencing reversible Grade 1 or 2 hypersensitivity reactions, consider pre-medication with an analgesic, antipyretic, or an antihistamine prior to readministration of HERCEPTIN HYLECTA.

Immunogenicity

As with all therapeutic proteins, there is potential for immunogenicity. The detection of antibody formation is highly dependent on the sensitivity and specificity of the assay. Additionally, the observed incidence of antibody (including neutralizing antibody) positivity in an assay may be influenced by several factors including assay methodology, sample handling, timing of sample collection, concomitant medications, and underlying disease. For these reasons, comparison of the incidence of antibodies to HERCEPTIN HYLECTA and intravenous trastuzumab in the study described below with the incidence of antibodies in other studies or to other products may be misleading. In the HannaH study, at a median follow-up exceeding 60 months, the incidence of treatment-induced/enhanced anti-trastuzumab antibodies was 10% (30/296) in patients treated with intravenous trastuzumab and 16% (47/295) in patients receiving HERCEPTIN HYLECTA. Neutralizing anti-trastuzumab antibodies were detected in postbaseline samples in 2/30 patients in the intravenous trastuzumab arm and 3/47 patients in the HERCEPTIN HYLECTA arm. The incidence of treatment-induced/enhanced anti-recombinant human hyaluronidase antibodies was 21% (62/295) in the HERCEPTIN HYLECTA arm. None of the patients who tested positive for antirecombinant human hyaluronidase antibodies tested positive for neutralizing antibodies. The clinical relevance of the development of anti-trastuzumab or anti-recombinant human hyaluronidase antibodies after treatment with HERCEPTIN HYLECTA is not known.

Postmarketing experience

The following adverse reactions have been identified during post-approval use of trastuzumab. Because these reactions are reported voluntarily from a population of uncertain size, it is not always possible to reliably estimate their frequency or establish a causal relationship to drug exposure.

- Administration-related reaction
- Oligohydramnios or oligohydramnios sequence, including pulmonary hypoplasia, skeletal abnormalities, and neonatal death
- Glomerulopathy
- Immune thrombocytopenia
- Tumor lysis syndrome (TLS)

Cases of possible TLS have been reported in patients treated with trastuzumab. Patients with significant tumor burden (e.g., bulky metastases) may be at a higher risk. Patients could present with hyperuricemia, hyperphosphatemia, and acute renal failure which may represent possible TLS. Providers should consider additional monitoring and/or treatment as clinically indicated.

DRUG INTERACTIONS

Anthracyclines

Patients who receive anthracycline after stopping HERCEPTIN HYLECTA may be at increased risk of cardiac dysfunction because of HERCEPTIN HYLECTA's estimated long washout period. If possible, avoid anthracycline-based therapy for up to 7 months after stopping HERCEPTIN HYLECTA. If anthracyclines are used, carefully monitor the patient's cardiac function.

USE IN SPECIFIC POPULATIONS

Pregnancy

Pregnancy Pharmacovigilance Program

There is a pregnancy pharmacovigilance program for HERCEPTIN HYLECTA. If HERCEPTIN HYLECTA is administered during pregnancy, or if a patient becomes pregnant while receiving HERCEPTIN HYLECTA or within 7 months following the last dose of HERCEPTIN HYLECTA, health care providers and patients should immediately report HERCEPTIN HYLECTA exposure to Genentech at 1-888-835-2555.

Risk summary

HERCEPTIN HYLECTA can cause fetal harm when administered to a pregnant woman. In post-marketing reports, use of trastuzumab during pregnancy resulted in cases of oligohydramnios and of oligohydramnios sequence, manifesting as pulmonary hypoplasia, skeletal abnormalities, and neonatal death. Apprise the patient of the potential risks to a fetus. There are clinical considerations if HERCEPTIN HYLECTA is used in a pregnant woman or if a patient becomes pregnant within 7 months following the last dose of HERCEPTIN HYLECTA. The estimated background risk of major birth defects and miscarriage for the indicated population is unknown. In the U.S. general population, the estimated background risk of major birth defects and miscarriage in clinically recognized pregnancies is 2 to 4% and 15 to 20%, respectively.

Clinical considerations fetal/neonatal adverse reactions

Monitor women who received HERCEPTIN HYLECTA during pregnancy or within 7 months prior to conception for oligohydramnios. If oligohydramnios occurs, perform fetal testing that is appropriate for gestational age and consistent with community standards of care.

Data

Human data

In post-marketing reports, use of trastuzumab during pregnancy resulted in cases of oligohydramnios and of oligohydramnios sequence, manifesting in the fetus as pulmonary hypoplasia, skeletal abnormalities, and neonatal death. These case reports described oligohydramnios in pregnant women who received trastuzumab either alone or in combination with chemotherapy. In some case reports, amniotic fluid index increased after use of trastuzumab was stopped. In one case, therapy with trastuzumab resumed after amniotic index improved and oligohydramnios recurred.

Animal data

HERCEPTIN HYLECTA for subcutaneous injection contains trastuzumab and hyaluronidase.

Trastuzumab: in studies where intravenous trastuzumab was administered to pregnant cynomolgus monkeys during the period of organogenesis at doses up to 25 mg/kg given twice weekly (up to 25 times the recommended weekly human dose of 2 mg/kg), trastuzumab crossed the placental barrier during the early (Gestation Days 20 to 50) and late (Gestation Days 120 to 150) phases of gestation. The resulting concentrations of trastuzumab in fetal serum and amniotic fluid were approximately 33% and 25%, respectively, of those present in the maternal serum but were not associated with adverse developmental effects.

Hyaluronidase: in an embryo-fetal study, mice have been dosed daily by subcutaneous injection during the period of organogenesis with hyaluronidase (recombinant human) at dose levels up to 2,200,000 U/kg, which is >7,200 times higher than the human dose. The study found no evidence of teratogenicity.

Reduced fetal weight and increased numbers of fetal resorptions were observed, with no effects found at a daily dose of 360,000 U/kg, which is >1,200 times higher than the human dose. In a peri-and post-natal reproduction study, mice have been dosed daily by subcutaneous injection, with hyaluronidase (recombinant human) from implantation through lactation and weaning at dose levels up to 1,100,000 U/kg, which is >3,600 times higher than the human dose. The study found no adverse effects on sexual maturation, learning and memory or fertility of the offspring.

Lactation risk summary

There is no information regarding the presence of trastuzumab or hyaluronidase in human milk, the effects on the breastfed infant, or the effects on milk production. Published data suggest human IgG is present in human milk but does not enter the neonatal and infant circulation in substantial amounts. Trastuzumab was present in the milk of lactating cynomolgus monkeys but not associated with neonatal toxicity. Consider the developmental and health benefits of breastfeeding along with the mother's clinical need for HERCEPTIN HYLECTA treatment and any potential adverse effects on the breastfed child from HERCEPTIN HYLECTA or from the underlying maternal condition. This consideration should also take into account the trastuzumab wash out period of 7 months.

Data

In lactating cynomolgus monkeys, trastuzumab was present in breast milk at about 0.3% of maternal serum concentrations after pre- (beginning Gestation Day 120) and post-partum (through Post-partum Day 28) doses of 25 mg/kg administered twice weekly (25 times the recommended weekly human dose of 2 mg/kg of intravenous trastuzumab). Infant monkeys with detectable serum levels of trastuzumab did not exhibit any adverse effects on growth or development from birth to 1 month of age.

Females and males of reproductive potential

Pregnancy Testing

Verify the pregnancy status of females of reproductive potential prior to the initiation of HERCEPTIN HYLECTA.

Contraception

Females

HERCEPTIN HYLECTA can cause embryo-fetal harm when administered during pregnancy. Advise females of reproductive potential to use effective contraception during treatment with HERCEPTIN HYLECTA and for 7 months following the last dose of HERCEPTIN HYLECTA

Pediatric use

The safety and effectiveness of HERCEPTIN HYLECTA in pediatric patients have not been established.

Geriatric use

Of the total number of patients in the HannaH and SafeHER studies treated with HERCEPTIN HYLECTA, 19% were 65 and over, while 4.7% were 75 and over. In patients receiving intravenous trastuzumab, the risk of cardiac dysfunction was increased in geriatric patients as compared to younger patients, in both those receiving treatment for adjuvant therapy or metastatic disease. Other differences in safety or effectiveness were not observed between elderly patients and younger patients.

Efficacy of HERCEPTIN HYLECTA in the treatment of breast cancer

HannaH (NCT00950300) and PrefHer (NCT01401166) studies validated the subcutaneous (H-s.c.) formulation of trastuzumab as effective and safe as intravenous (H-i.v.) and highly preferred by patients in early breast cancer. The present randomised MetaspHer trial (NCT01810393) is the first study assessing patient's preference in metastatic setting.

Pivot, X. et al. European Journal of Cancer 82: 230-236, 2017

9.9. PEMBROLIZUMAB (KEYTRUDA)

Pembrolizumab is a humanized monoclonal IgG4 kappa antibody with an approximate molecular weight of 149 kDa. Pembrolizumab is produced in recombinant Chinese hamster ovary (CHO) cells. It is FDA-approved for therapeutic use in some 15 different malignant disease settings, including triple-negative breast cancer (ie, breast cancers which do not display the estrogen receptor, the progesterone receptor or HER2 on their surface and which are associated with a poorer prognosis that those breast cancers that do display them. Pembrolizumab is one of a class of agents known as checkpoint inhibitors because of their activity in allowing T cell immunity to occur by blocking the PD-1 and CTLA-4 pathways that normally inhibit T cell activity, specifically the CTLA-4 inhibitor: ipilimumab, the PD-1 inhibitors nivolumab and pembrolizumab, and the PD-L1 inhibitors: atezolizumab, avelumab, and durvalumab.

KEYTRUDA® (pembrolizumab) injection, for intravenous use. Initial U.S. Approval: 2014.

MECHANISM OF ACTION

KEYTRUDA is a programmed death receptor-1 (PD-1)-blocking antibody: binding of the PD-1 ligands, PD-L1 and PD-L2, to the PD-1 receptor found on T cells, inhibits T cell proliferation and cytokine production. Upregulation of PD-1 ligands occurs in some tumors and signalling through this pathway can contribute to inhibition of active T-cell immune surveillance of tumors. Pembrolizumab is a monoclonal antibody that binds to the PD-1 receptor and blocks its interaction with PD-L1 and PD-L2, releasing PD-1 pathway-mediated inhibition of the immune response, including the anti-tumor immune response. In syngeneic mouse tumor models, blocking PD-1 activity resulted in decreased tumor growth.

KEYTRUDA is a programmed death receptor-1 (PD-1)-blocking antibody indicated for 15 different malignant disease settings but only the indication in breast cancer is included in this book:

Triple-Negative Breast Cancer (TNBC)

• in combination with chemotherapy, for the treatment of patients with locally recurrent unresectable or metastatic TNBC whose tumors express PD-L1 [Combined Positive Score (CPS) ≥10] as determined by an FDA approved test. This indication is approved under accelerated approval based on tumor response rate and durability of response. Continued approval for this indication may be contingent upon verification and description of clinical benefit in the confirmatory trials. This indication is approved under accelerated approval based on progression-free survival. Continued approval for this indication may be contingent upon verification and description of clinical benefit in the confirmatory trials. This indication is approved under accelerated approval based on pharmacokinetic data, the relationship of exposure to efficacy, and the relationship of exposure to safety. Continued approval for this dosing may be contingent upon verification and description of clinical benefit in the confirmatory trials.

CONTRAINDICATIONS: None.

WARNINGS AND PRECAUTIONS

• Immune-mediated adverse reactions

o Immune-mediated adverse reactions, which may be severe or fatal, can occur in any organ system or tissue, including the following: immune-mediated pneumonitis, immune-mediated colitis, immune-mediated hepatitis, immune-mediated endocrinopathies,immune-mediated nephritis with renal dysfunction, immune-mediated dermatologic adverse reactions, and solid organ transplant rejection.

o Monitor for early identification and management. Evaluate liver enzymes, creatinine, and thyroid function at baseline and periodically during treatment.

o Withhold or permanently discontinue based on severity and type of reaction.

• Infusion-related reactions: interrupt, slow the rate of infusion, or permanently discontinue KEYTRUDA based on the severity of reaction.

• Complications of allogeneic hematopoietic stem cell transplantation (HSCT): fatal and other serious complications can occur in patients who receive allogeneic HSCT before or after being treated with a PD-1/PD-L1 blocking antibody.

• Embryo-fetal toxicity: can cause fetal harm. Advise females of reproductive potential of the potential risk to a fetus and to use effective method of contraception.

More detailed information on WARNINGS AND PRECAUTIONS

Severe and fatal immune-mediated adverse reactions

KEYTRUDA is a monoclonal antibody that belongs to a class of drugs that bind to either the programmed death-receptor 1 (PD-1) or the PD-ligand 1 (PD-L1), blocking the PD-1/PD-L1 pathway, thereby removing inhibition of the immune response, potentially breaking peripheral tolerance and inducing immune-mediated adverse reactions. Immune-mediated adverse reactions, which may be severe or fatal, can occur in any organ system or tissue and can affect more than one body system simultaneously. Immune-mediated adverse reactions can occur at any time after starting treatment with a PD-1/PD-L1 blocking antibody. While immune-mediated adverse reactions usually manifest during treatment with PD-1/PD-L1 blocking antibodies, immune-mediated adverse reactions can also manifest after discontinuation of PD-1/PD-L1 blocking antibodies. Early identification and management of immune-mediated adverse reactions are essential to ensure safe use of PD-1/PD-L1 blocking antibodies. Monitor patients closely for symptoms and signs that may be clinical manifestations of underlying immune-mediated adverse reactions. Evaluate liver enzymes, creatinine, and thyroid function at baseline and periodically during treatment. In cases of suspected immune-mediated adverse reactions, initiate appropriate workup to exclude alternative etiologies, including infection. Institute medical management promptly, including specialty consultation as appropriate. Withhold or permanently discontinue KEYTRUDA depending on severity. In general, if KEYTRUDA requires interruption or discontinuation, administer systemic corticosteroid therapy (1 to 2 mg/kg/day prednisone or equivalent) until improvement to Grade 1 or less. Upon improvement to Grade 1 or less, initiate corticosteroid taper and continue to taper over at least 1 month. Consider administration of other systemic immunosuppressants in patients whose immune-mediated adverse reactions are not controlled with corticosteroid therapy. Toxicity management guidelines for adverse reactions that do not necessarily require systemic steroids (e.g., endocrinopathies and dermatologic reactions) are discussed below.

Immune-mediated pneumonitis

KEYTRUDA can cause immune-mediated pneumonitis. The incidence of pneumonitis is higher in patients who have received prior thoracic radiation. Immune-mediated pneumonitis occurred in 3.4% (94/2799) of patients receiving KEYTRUDA, including fatal (0.1%), Grade 4 (0.3%), Grade 3 (0.9%), and Grade 2 (1.3%) adverse reactions. Systemic corticosteroids were required in 67% (63/94) of patients with pneumonitis. Pneumonitis led to permanent discontinuation of KEYTRUDA in 1.3% (36) of patients and withholding of KEYTRUDA in 0.9% (26) of patients. All patients who were withheld reinitiated KEYTRUDA after symptom improvement; of these,

23% had recurrence of pneumonitis. Pneumonitis resolved in 59% of the 94 patients. In clinical studies enrolling 389 adult patients with classical Hodgkin Lymhoma (cHL) who received KEYTRUDA as a single agent, pneumonitis occurred in 31 (8%) patients, including Grades 3-4 pneumonitis in 2.3% of patients. Patients received high-dose corticosteroids for a median duration of 10 days (range: 2 days to 53 months). Pneumonitis rates were similar in patients with and without prior thoracic radiation. Pneumonitis led to discontinuation of KEYTRUDA in 21 (5.4%) patients. Of the patients who developed pneumonitis, 42% interrupted KEYTRUDA, 68% discontinued KEYTRUDA, and 77% had resolution.

Immune-mediated colitis

KEYTRUDA can cause immune-mediated colitis, which may present with diarrhoea (Figure 74). Cytomegalovirus (CMV) infection/reactivation has been reported in patients with corticosteroid-refractory immune-mediated colitis. In cases of corticosteroid-refractory colitis, consider repeating infectious workup to exclude alternative etiologies. Immune-mediated colitis occurred in 1.7% (48/2799) of patients receiving KEYTRUDA, including Grade 4 (<0.1%), Grade 3 (1.1%), and Grade 2 (0.4%) adverse reactions. Systemic corticosteroids were required in 69% (33/48) of patients with colitis. Additional immunosuppressant therapy was required in 4.2% of patients. Colitis led to permanent discontinuation of KEYTRUDA in 0.5% (15) of patients and withholding of KEYTRUDA in 0.5% (13) of patients.

Figure 74. A high magnification micrograph of the histopathology of collagenous colitis. H&E stain.

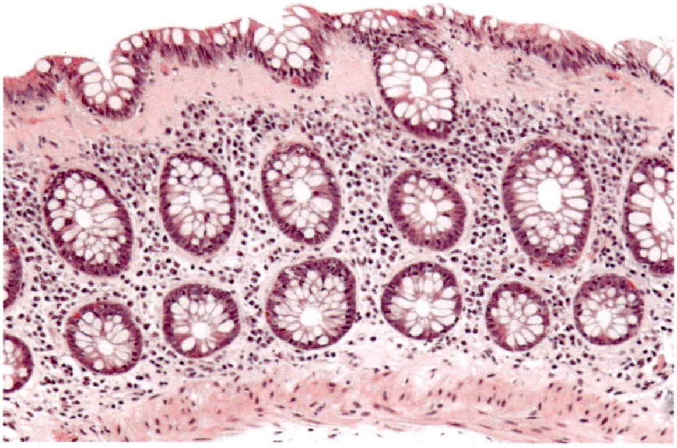

Collagenous colitis is an inflammatory disease of the colon with similarities to immune-mediated colitis. This image is by By Nephron - Own work, CC BY-SA 3.0, https://commons.wikimedia.org/w/index.php?curid=11975287. Collagenous colitis - Wikipedia. This file is licensed under the Creative Commons Attribution-Share Alike 3.0 Unported license. No changes were made to this image.

All patients who were withheld reinitiated KEYTRUDA after symptom improvement; of these, 23% had recurrence of colitis. Colitis resolved in 85% of the 48 patients.

Hepatotoxicity and immune-mediated hepatitis

KEYTRUDA as a Single Agent

KEYTRUDA can cause immune-mediated hepatitis. Immune-mediated hepatitis occurred in 0.7% (19/2799) of patients receiving KEYTRUDA, including Grade 4 (<0.1%), Grade 3 (0.4%), and Grade 2 (0.1%) adverse reactions. Systemic corticosteroids were required in 68% (13/19) of patients with hepatitis. Eleven percent of these patients required additional immunosuppressant therapy. Hepatitis led to permanent discontinuation of KEYTRUDA in 0.2% (6) of patients and withholding of KEYTRUDA in 0.3% (9) of patients. All patients who were withheld reinitiated KEYTRUDA after symptom improvement; of these, none had recurrence of hepatitis. Hepatitis resolved in 79% of the 19 patients.

KEYTRUDA with axitinib

KEYTRUDA in combination with axitinib can cause hepatic toxicity with higher than expected frequencies of Grades 3 and 4 ALT and AST elevations compared to KEYTRUDA alone. Monitor liver enzymes before initiation of and periodically throughout treatment. Consider more frequent monitoring of liver enzymes as compared to when the drugs are administered as single agents. For elevated liver enzymes, interrupt KEYTRUDA and axitinib, and consider administering corticosteroids as needed. With the combination of KEYTRUDA and axitinib, Grades 3 and 4 increased ALT (20%) and increased AST (13%) were seen. Fifty-nine percent of the patients with increased ALT received systemic corticosteroids. In patients with ALT ≥3 times ULN (Grades 2-4, n=116), ALT resolved to Grades 0-1 in 94%. Among the 92 patients who were rechallenged with either KEYTRUDA (n=3) or axitinib (n=34) administered as a single agent or with both (n=55), recurrence of ALT ≥3 times ULN was observed in 1 patient receiving KEYTRUDA, 16 patients receiving axitinib, and 24 patients receiving both KEYTRUDA and axitinib. All patients with a recurrence of ALT ≥3 ULN subsequently recovered from the event.

Immune-mediated endocrinopathies

Adrenal Insufficiency

KEYTRUDA can cause primary or secondary adrenal insufficiency *(Figures 75 and 76).*

For Grade 2 or higher adrenal insufficiency, initiate symptomatic treatment, including hormone replacement as clinically indicated. Withhold KEYTRUDA depending on severity. Adrenal insufficiency occurred in 0.8% (22/2799) of patients receiving KEYTRUDA, including Grade 4 (<0.1%), Grade 3 (0.3%), and Grade 2 (0.3%) adverse reactions. Systemic corticosteroids were required in 77% (17/22) of patients with adrenal insufficiency; of these, the majority remained on systemic corticosteroids.

Figure 75. Pigmentation of the lower legs in a Caucasian woman with Addison's disease (adrenal insufficiency).

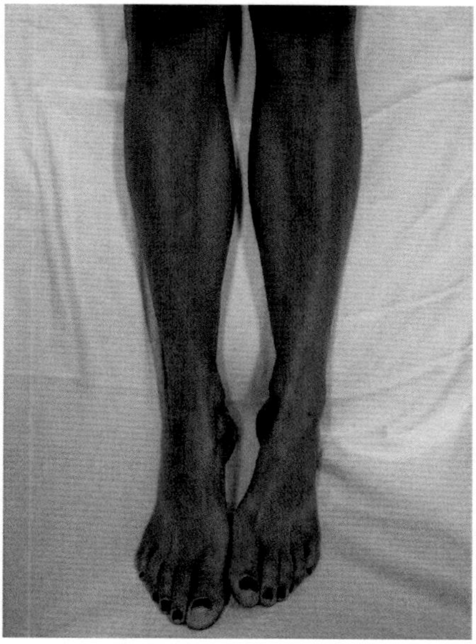

This image is By James Heilman, MD - Own work, CC BY-SA 4.0, https://commons.wikimedia.org/w/index.php?curid=73507970. https://en.wikipedia.org/wiki/Addison%27s_disease#/media/File:Addison'sLegs.jpg. This file is licensed under the Creative Commons Attribution-Share Alike 4.0 International license. No changes have been made to this image.

Figure 76. Darkening of the gums due to increased pigment as seen in Addison's disease (adrenal insufficiency)

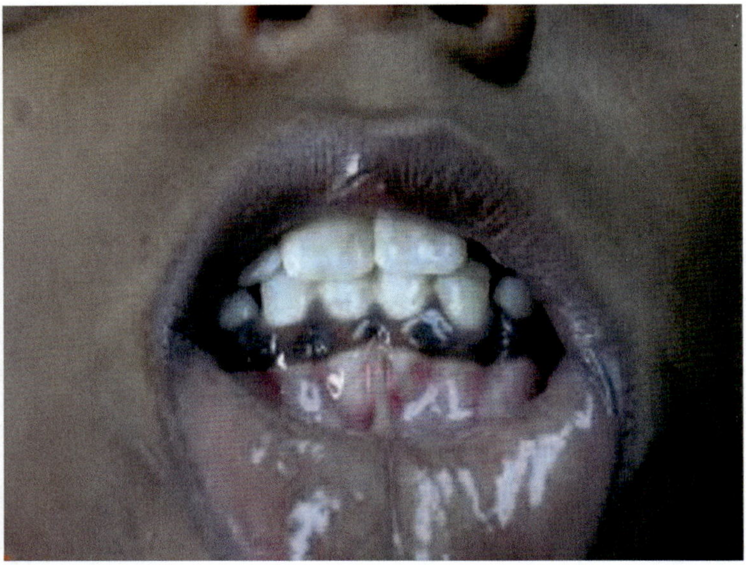

This image is By FlatOut - Dermatology Online Journal http://dermatology.cdlib.org/, CC0, https://commons.wikimedia.org/w/index.php?curid=25847348. https://en.wikipedia.org/wiki/Addison%27s_disease#/media/File:Addisons_hyperpigmentation.jpg. This file is made available under the Creative Commons CC0 1.0 Universal Public Domain Dedication. No changes have been made to this image.

Adrenal insufficiency led to permanent discontinuation of KEYTRUDA in <0.1%, (1) of patients and withholding of KEYTRUDA in 0.3% (8) of patients. All patients who were withheld reinitiated KEYTRUDA after symptom improvement.

Hypophysitis

KEYTRUDA can cause immune-mediated hypophysitis. *Hypophysitis is inflammation of the pituitary gland (Figure 77)* and can present with acute symptoms associated with mass effect such as headache, photophobia, or visual field defects.

Figure 77. Anatomy of the ***pituitary gland***

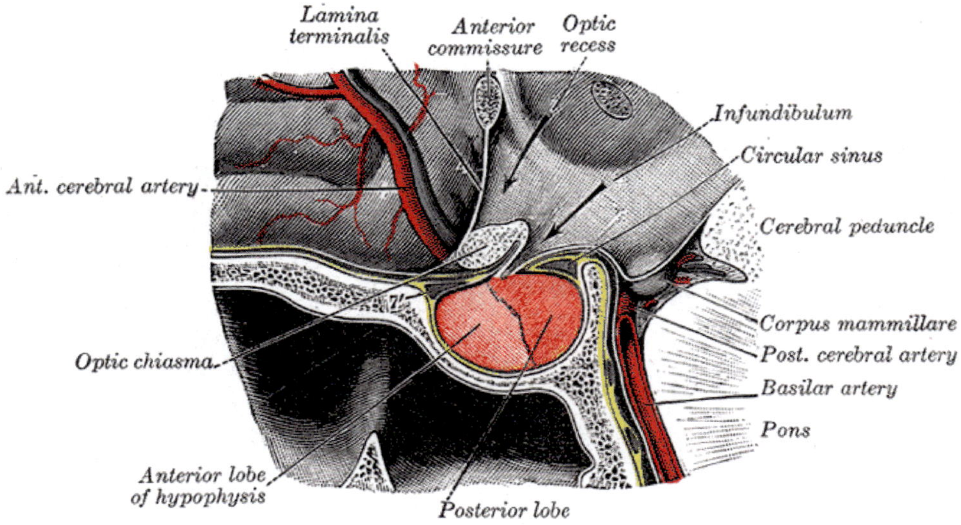

This image is By Henry Vandyke Carter - Henry Gray (1918) Anatomy of the Human Body (See "Book" section below)Bartleby.com: Gray's Anatomy, Plate 1180, Public Domain, https://commons.wikimedia.org/w/index.php?curid=567162. https://en.wikipedia.org/wiki/Hypophysitis#/media/File:Gray1180.png. This work is in the public domain in its country of origin and other countries and areas where the copyright term is the author's life plus 100 years or fewer. This work is in the public domain in the United States because it was published (or registered with the U.S. Copyright Office) before January 1, 1926 (PD 1925).

Hypophysitis can cause hypopituitarism. Initiate hormone replacement as indicated. Withhold or permanently discontinue KEYTRUDA depending on severity. Hypophysitis occurred in 0.6% (17/2799) of patients receiving KEYTRUDA, including Grade 4 (<0.1%), Grade 3 (0.3%), and Grade 2 (0.2%) adverse reactions. Systemic corticosteroids were required in 94% (16/17) of patients with hypophysitis; of these, the majority remained on systemic corticosteroids. Hypophysitis led to permanent discontinuation of KEYTRUDA in 0.1% (4) of patients and withholding of KEYTRUDA in 0.3% (7) of patients. All patients who were withheld reinitiated KEYTRUDA after symptom improvement.

Thyroid disorders *(Figure 78)*

KEYTRUDA can cause immune-mediated thyroid disorders. Thyroiditis can present with or without endocrinopathy. Hypothyroidism can follow hyperthyroidism. Initiate hormone replacement for hypothyroidism or institute medical management of hyperthyroidism as clinically indicated. Withhold or permanently discontinue KEYTRUDA depending on severity. Thyroiditis occurred in 0.6% (16/2799) of patients receiving KEYTRUDA, including Grade 2 (0.3%). No patients discontinued KEYTRUDA due to thyroiditis. KEYTRUDA was withheld in <0.1%), (2) of patients and withholding of KEYTRUDA in 0.3% (7) of patients. All patients who were withheld reinitiated KEYTRUDA after symptom improvement. Hypothyroidism occurred in 8% (237/2799) of patients receiving KEYTRUDA, including Grade 3 (0.1%) and Grade 2 (6.2%). Hypothyroidism led to permanent discontinuation of KEYTRUDA in <0.1%, (1) of patients and withholding of KEYTRUDA in 0.5% (14) of patients. All patients who were withheld reinitiated KEYTRUDA after symptom improvement. The majority of patients with hypothyroidism required long-term thyroid hormone replacement. The incidence of new or worsening hypothyroidism was higher in 1185 patients with HNSCC, occurring in 16% of patients receiving KEYTRUDA as a single agent or in combination with platinum and FU, including Grade 3 (0.3%) hypothyroidism. The incidence of new or worsening hypothyroidism was higher in 389 patients with cHL (17%) receiving KEYTRUDA as a single agent, including Grade 1 (6.2%) and Grade 2 (10.8%) hypothyroidism.

Figure 78. The thyroid system: Diagram of the hypothalamic–pituitary–thyroid axis. The hypothalamus secretes TRH (green), which stimulates the production of TSH (red) by the pituitary gland. This, in turn, stimulates the production of thyroxine by the thyroid (blue). Thyroxine levels decrease TRH and TSH production by a negative feedback process.

The following image is By Mikael Häggström - All used images are in public domain. Public Domain, https://commons.wikimedia.org/w/index.php?curid=8567011. https://en.wikipedia.org/wiki/Hypothyroidism#/media/File:Thyroid_system.svg. The copyrightholder of this work has released the work into the public domain.

Figure 78. The thyroid system.

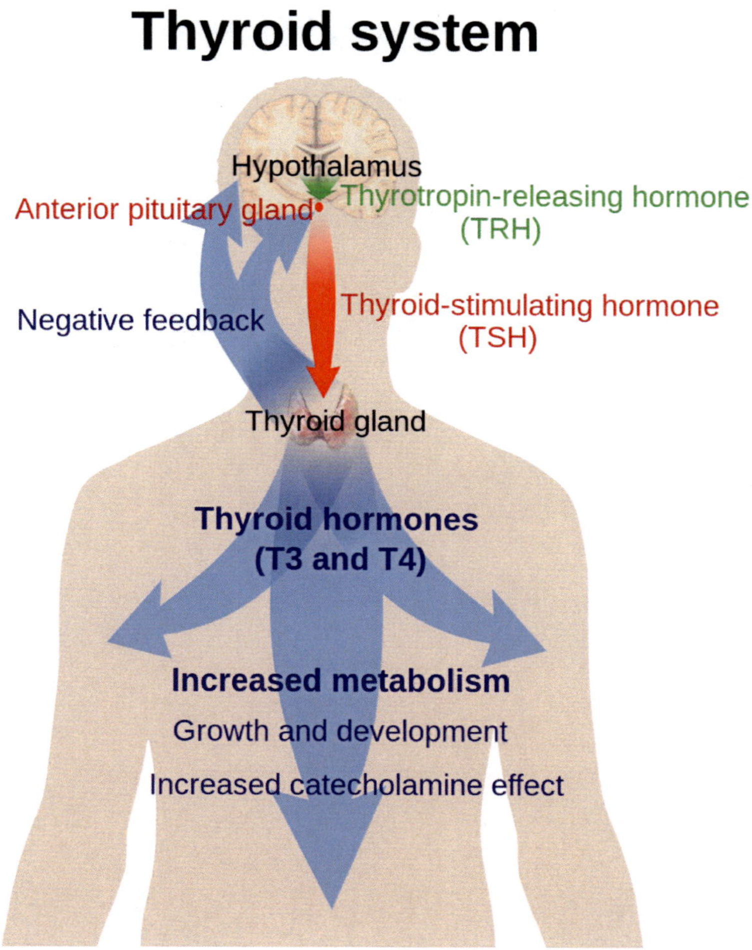

Figure 79. A man with myxedema (severe hypothyroidism) showing an expressionless face, puffiness around the eyes and pallor.

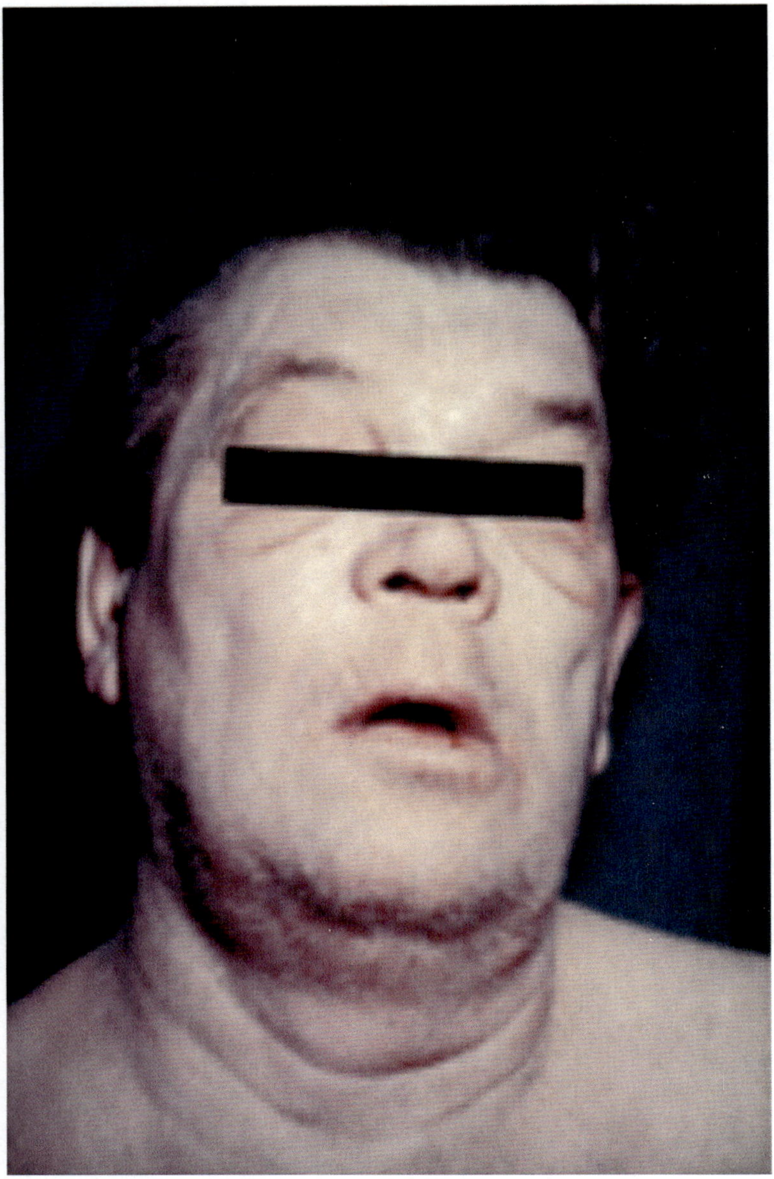

https://en.wikipedia.org/wiki/Hypothyroidism#/media/File:Myxedema_face.png.

Type 1 Diabetes mellitus, which can present with diabetic ketoacidosis

Monitor patients for hyperglycemia or other signs and symptoms of diabetes. Initiate treatment with insulin as clinically indicated. Withhold KEYTRUDA depending on severity. Type 1 diabetes mellitus occurred in 0.2% (6/2799) of patients receiving KEYTRUDA. Type 1 diabetes mellitus led to permanent discontinuation in <0.1%, (1) of patients and withholding of KEYTRUDA in <0.1%, Grade 3 (0.1%), and Grade 2 (0.1%) adverse reactions. Systemic corticosteroids were required in 89% (8/9) of patients with nephritis. Nephritis led to permanent discontinuation of KEYTRUDA in 0.1% (3) of patients and withholding of KEYTRUDA in 0.1% (3) of patients. All patients who were withheld reinitiated KEYTRUDA after symptom improvement; of these, none had recurrence of nephritis. Nephritis resolved in 56% of the 9 patients.

Immune-mediated dermatologic adverse reactions

KEYTRUDA can cause immune-mediated rash or dermatitis. Exfoliative dermatitis, including Stevens Johnson Syndrome *(Figures 80 and 81),* DRESS, and toxic epidermal necrolysis (TEN) *(Figure 82),* has occurred with PD-1/PD-L1 blocking antibodies. Topical emollients and/or topical corticosteroids may be adequate to treat mild to moderate non-exfoliative rashes. Withhold or permanently discontinue KEYTRUDA depending on severity. Immune-mediated dermatologic adverse reactions occurred in 1.4% (38/2799) of patients receiving KEYTRUDA, including Grade 3 (1%) and Grade 2 (0.1%) adverse reactions. Systemic corticosteroids were required in 40% (15/38) of patients with immune-mediated dermatologic adverse reactions. Immune-mediated dermatologic adverse reactions led to permanent discontinuation of KEYTRUDA in 0.1% (2) of patients and withholding of KEYTRUDA in 0.6% (16) of patients. All patients who were withheld reinitiated KEYTRUDA after symptom improvement; of these, 6% had recurrence of immune-mediated dermatologic adverse reactions. Immune-mediated dermatologic adverse reactions resolved in 79% of the 38 patients.

DRESS, drug reaction with eosinophilia and systemic symptoms. DRESS syndrome is classified as one form of severe cutaneous adverse reactions (SCARs). In addition to DRESS, SCARs includes four other drug-induced skin reactions, the Stevens–Johnson syndrome (SJS); Toxic epidermal necrolysis (TEN), Stevens–Johnson/toxic epidermal necrolysis overlap syndrome (SJS/TEN)

Figure 80. Stevens-Johnson syndrome.

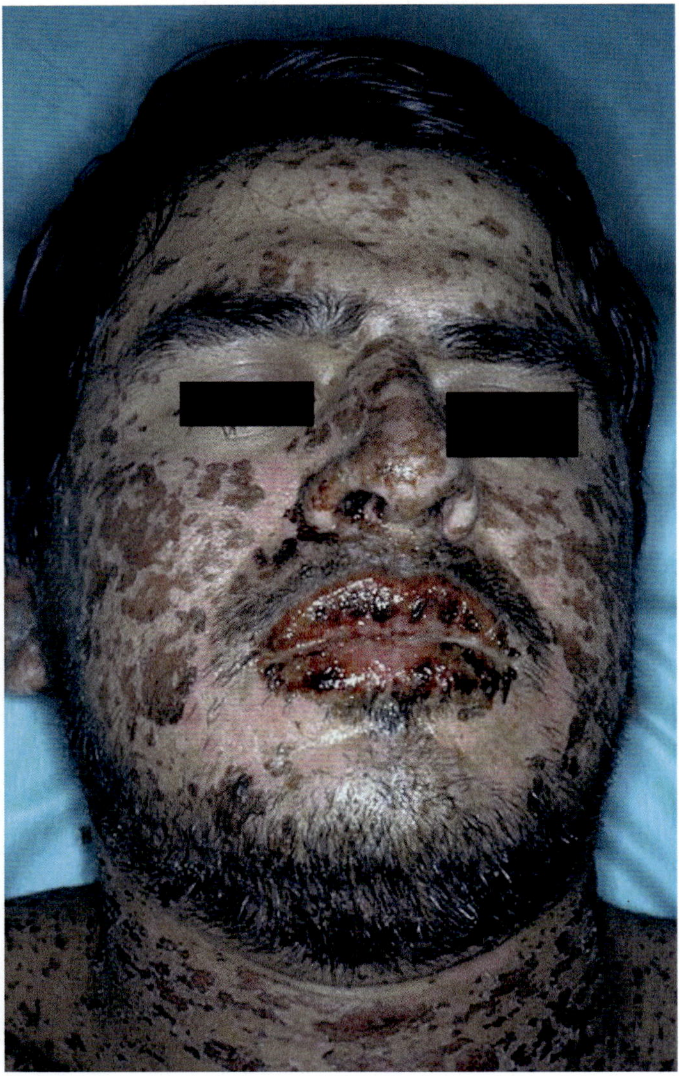

https://commons.wikimedia.org/w/index.php?curid=9699327. https://en.wikipedia.org/wiki/Stevens%E2%80%93Johnson_syndrome#/media/File:Stevens-johnson-syndrome.jpg. This file is licensed under the Creative Commons Attribution-Share Alike 3.0 Unported license. No changes were made to this image.

Figure 81. Stevens-Johnson syndrome showing the characteristic skin loss.

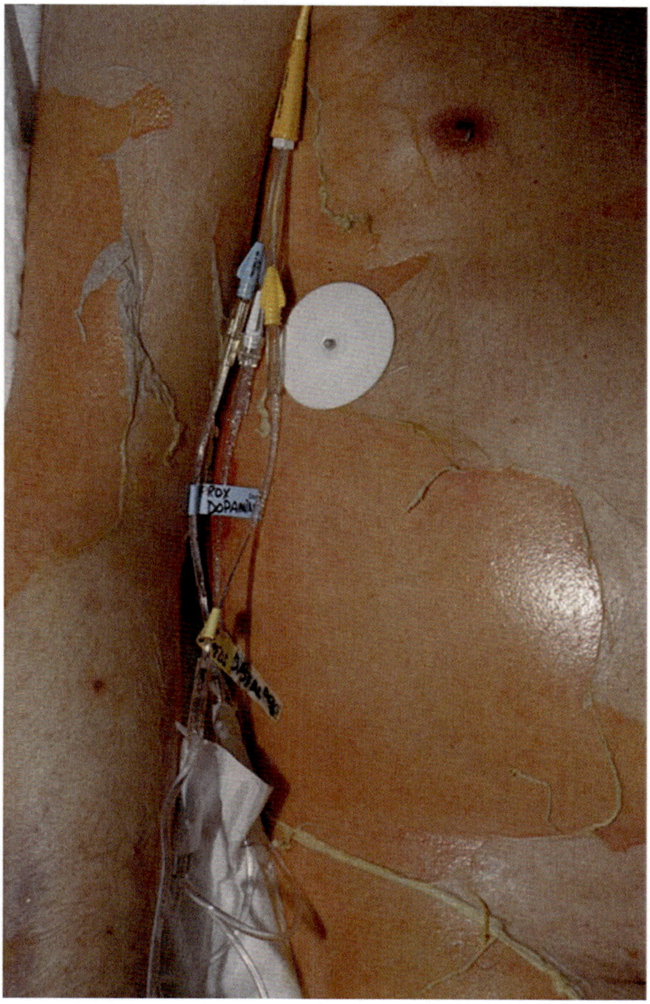

This image is By Madhero88 - http://www.dermnet.com/Toxic-Epidermal-Necrolysis/picture/14991, CC BY-SA 3.0, https://commons.wikimedia.org/w/index.php?curid=9699513. https://en.wikipedia.org/wiki/Toxic_epidermal_necrolysis#/media/File:Toxic-

epidermal-necrolysis.jpg. This file is licensed under the Creative Commons Attribution-Share Alike 3.0 Unported license. No changes have been made to the image.

Figure 82. The back of a toxic epidermal necrolysis (TEN) patient on day 10, at the peak of the condition.

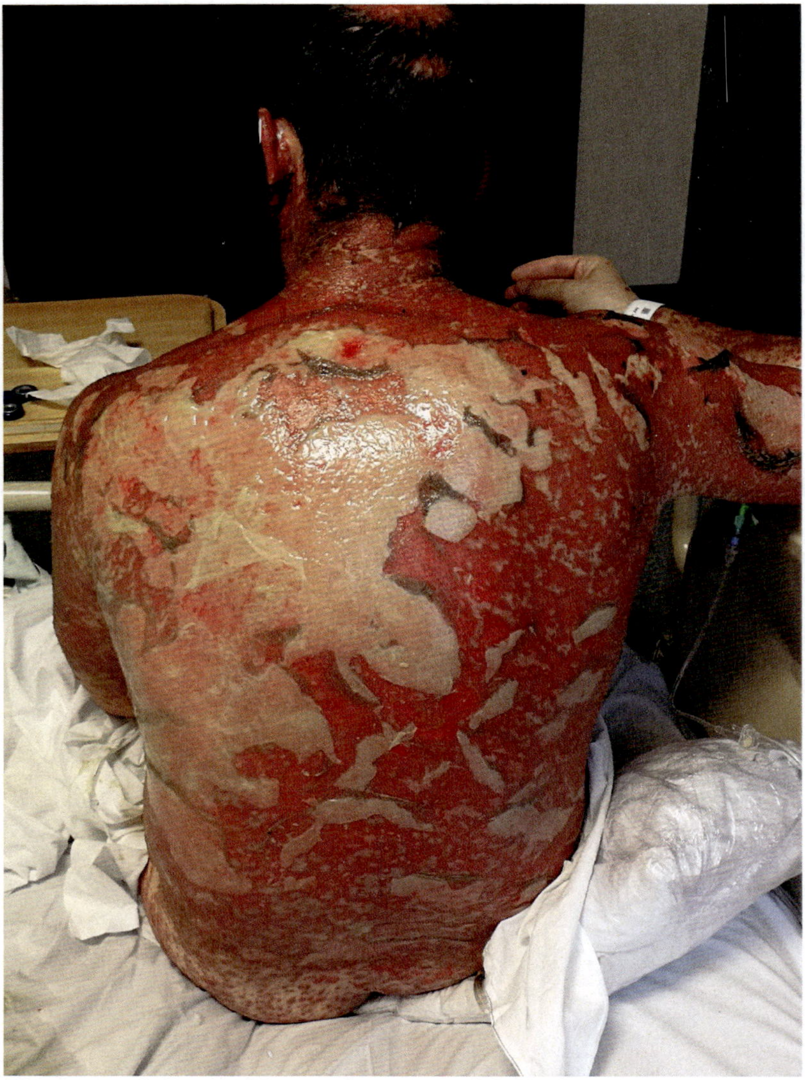

*This image is By Jay2Base - Own work, CC BY-SA 4.0, https://commons.wikimedia.org/w/index.php?curid=67491133. https://en.wikipedia.org/wiki/Toxic_epidermal_necrolysis#/media/File:TENS_patient_*

on_day_10.jpg. This file is licensed under the Creative Commons Attribution-Share Alike 4.0 International license. No changes have been made to this image

Other immune-mediated adverse reactions

The following clinically significant immune-mediated adverse reactions occurred at an incidence of <0.1%, (unless otherwise noted) in patients who received KEYTRUDA or were reported with the use of other PD1/PD-L1 blocking antibodies. Severe or fatal cases have been reported for some of these adverse reactions.

Cardiac/vascular

Myocarditis, pericarditis, vasculitis *(Figure 33)*

Figure 83. *Petechia / purpura on the low limb due to medication-induced vasculitis.*

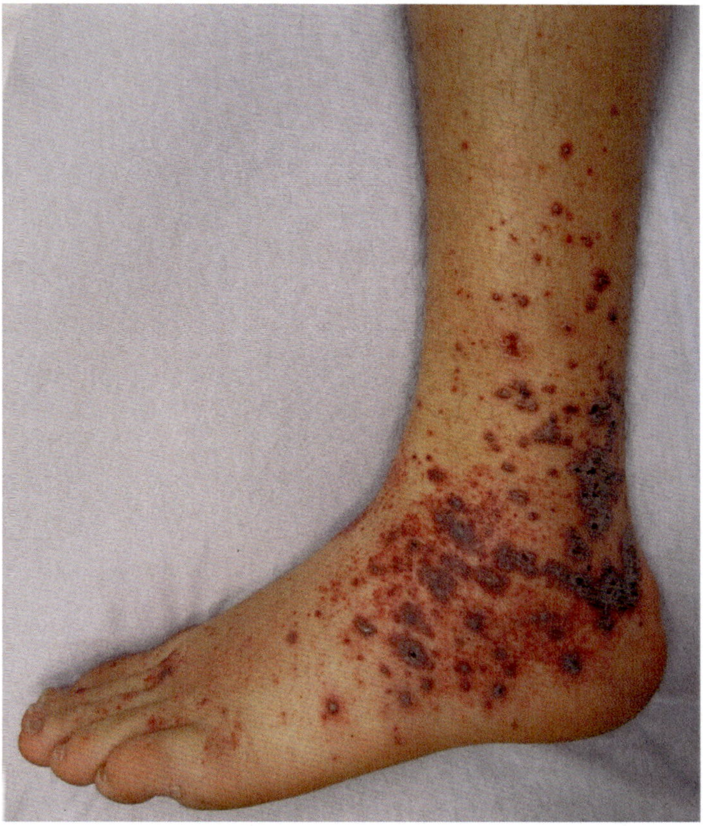

This image is by James Heilman, MD - Own work, CC BY-SA 3.0, https://commons.wikimedia.org/w/index.php?curid=11857197.

https://en.wikipedia.org/wiki/Vasculitis#/media/File:Vasculitis.JPG. This file is licensed under the Creative Commons Attribution-Share Alike 3.0 Unported license. No changes have been made to this image.

Nervous system

Meningitis, encephalitis, myelitis and demyelination, myasthenic syndrome/myasthenia gravis (including exacerbation) *(Figure 84),* Guillain-Barré syndrome, nerve paresis, autoimmune neuropathy

Figure 84. Eye deviation and a drooping eyelid in a person with myasthenia gravis trying to open her eyes.

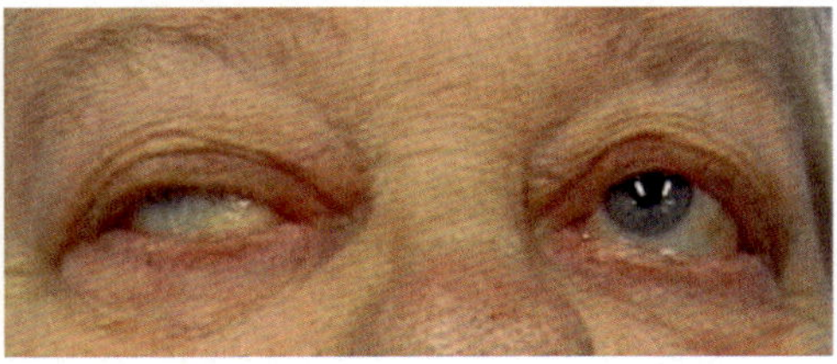

This image is by James Heilman, MD - Own work, CC BY-SA 3.0, https://commons.wikimedia.org/w/index.php?curid=17978809. https://en.wikipedia.org/wiki/Myasthenia_gravis#/media/File:DiplopiaMG1.jpg. This file is licensed under the Creative Commons Attribution-Share Alike 3.0 Unported license. No changes have been made to this image

Ocular

Uveitis, iritis, and other ocular inflammatory toxicities can occur. Some cases can be associated with retinal detachment. Various grades of visual impairment, including blindness, can occur. If uveitis occurs in combination with other immune-mediated adverse reactions, consider a Vogt-Koyanagi-Harada-like syndrome, as this may require treatment with systemic steroids to reduce the risk of permanent vision loss.

Figure 85 shows hypopyon in anterior uveitis, seen as yellowish exudation in lower part of anterior chamber of eye.

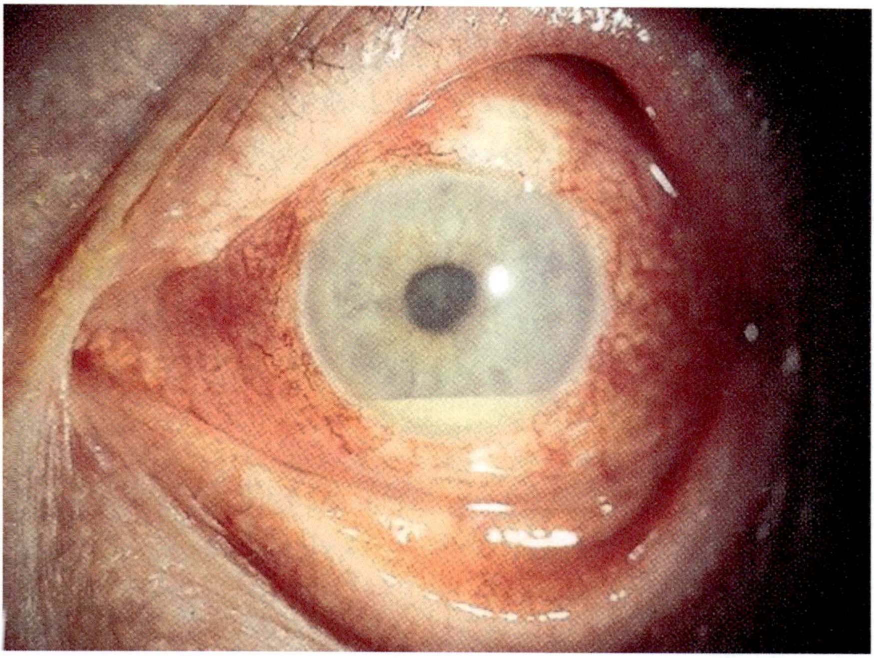

This image is by EyeMD (Rakesh Ahuja, M.D.). - Own work. CC BY-SA 2.5, https://commons.wikimedia.org/w/index.php?curid=1229578. https://en.wikipedia.org/wiki/Uveitis#/media/File:Hypopyon.jpg. This file is licensed under the Creative Commons Attribution-Share Alike 2.5 Generic license. No changes have been made to this image.

Figure 86. Keratic precipitate due to Vogt-Koyanagi-Harada Disease

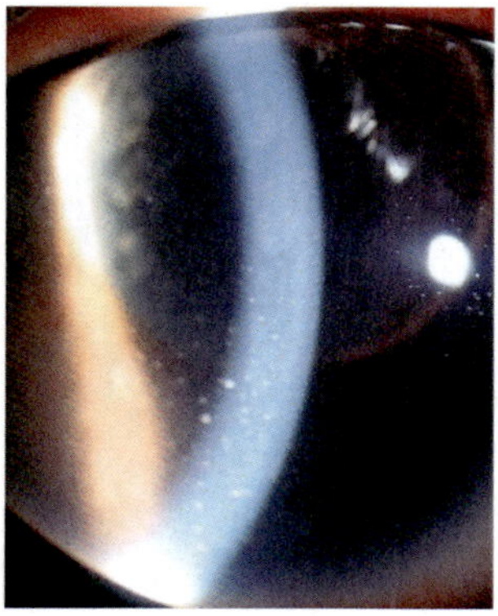

Gastrointestinal

Pancreatitis, to include increases in serum amylase and lipase levels, gastritis, duodenitis

Musculoskeletal and connective tissue

Myositis/polymyositis, rhabdomyolysis (and associated sequelae, including renal failure), arthritis (1.5%), and polymyalgia rheumatic *(Figure 87).*

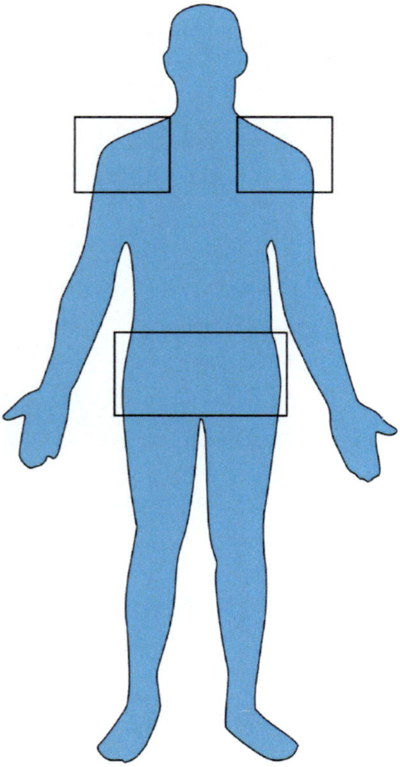

Figure 87. In polmyalgia rheumatica, pain is usually located in the shoulders and hips.

https://en.wikipedia.org/wiki/Polymyalgia_rheumatica#/media/File:Polymyalgia_rheumatica_man.svg. The copyright holder of this work has released it into the public domain. No changes have been made to this image.

Other endocrine

Hypoparathyroidism

Hematologic/immune systems

Hemolytic anemia, aplastic anemia, hemophagocytic lymphohistiocytosis[1], systemic inflammatory response syndrome[2], histiocytic necrotizing lymphadenitis[3] (Kikuchi lymphadenitis), sarcoidosis[4], immune thrombocytopenic purpura, solid organ transplant rejection.

[1]Hemophagocytic lymphohistiocytosis (HLH), also known as haemophagocytic lymphohistiocytosis (British spelling), and hemophagocytic or haemophagocytic syndrome, is an uncommon hematologic disorder seen more often in children than in adults. It is a life-threatening disease of severe hyperinflammation caused by uncontrolled proliferation of activated lymphocytes and macrophages, characterised by proliferation of morphologically benign lymphocytes and macrophages that secrete high amounts of inflammatory cytokines. It is classified as one of the cytokine storm syndromes.

Figure 89. Light microscopic image of bone marrow showing stromal macrophages containing numerous red blood cells in their cytoplasm.

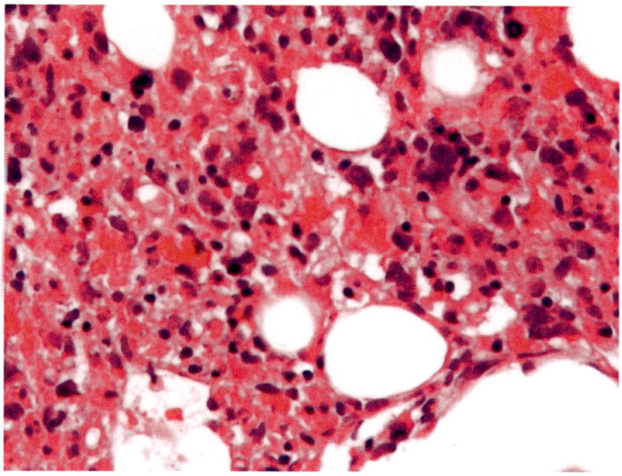

This image is by Jon salisbury at English Wikipedia - Transferred from en.wikipedia to Commons, Public Domain, https://commons.wikimedia.org/w/index.php?curid=11557969. https://en.wikipedia.org/wiki/Hemophagocytic_lymphohistiocytosis#/media/File:Haemophagocytic_lymphohistiocytosis_Bone_marrow.JPG.
This work has been released into the public domain by its author, Jon salisbury at English Wikipedia. No changes to this image have been made.

[2]Systemic inflammatory response syndrome (SIRS), is an inflammatory state affecting the whole body. It is the body's response to an infectious or noninfectious insult. Although the definition of SIRS refers to it as an "inflammatory" response, it actually has pro- and anti-inflammatory components.

[3]Histiocytic necrotizing lymphadenitis (aka Kikuchi disease) was described in 1972 in Japan. It is also known as histiocytic necrotizing lymphadenitis, Kikuchi necrotizing lymphadenitis, phagocytic necrotizing lymphadenitis, subacute necrotizing lymphadenitis, and necrotizing lymphadenitis. Kikuchi disease occurs sporadically in people with no family history of the condition. The signs and symptoms of Kikuchi disease are fever, enlargement of the lymph nodes (lymphadenopathy), skin rashes, and headache. Rarely, enlargement of the liver and spleen and nervous system involvement resembling meningitis are seen. It is diagnosed by lymph node excision biopsy. Kikuchi disease is a self-limiting illness which has symptoms which may overlap with Hodgkin's lymphoma leading to misdiagnosis in some patients.

Figure 90. Histopathology of a lymph node in histiocytic necrotizing lymphadenitis showing the characteristic features of abundant histiocytes, necrosis without neutrophils. H&E stain.

This image is by Nephron - Own work, CC BY-SA 3.0, https://commons.wikimedia.org/w/index.php?curid=11102211. https://en.wikipedia.org/wiki/Kikuchi_disease#/media/File:Histiocytic_necrotizing_lymphadenitis_-_intermed_mag.jpg. This file is licensed under the Creative Commons Attribution-Share Alike 3.0 Unported license. No changes have been made to this image.

Figure 90. Lypmph node histpathology in histiocytic necrotizing lymphadenitis.

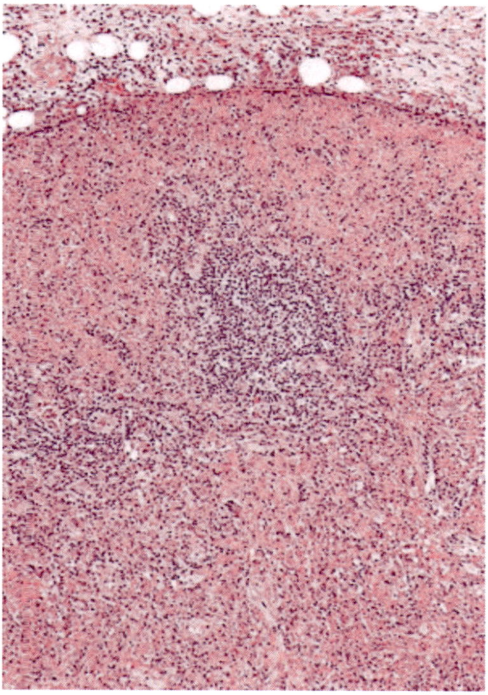

[4]Sarcoid or sarcoidosis

Sarcoidosis (also known as Besnier-Boeck-Schaumann disease) is a disease involving abnormal collections of inflammatory cells that form lumps known as granulomata. The disease usually begins in the lungs, skin, or lymph nodes. Less commonly affected are the eyes, liver, heart, and brain. Any organ, however, can be affected. The signs and symptoms depend on the organ involved. Often, no, or only mild, symptoms are seen. When it affects the lungs, wheezing, coughing, shortness of breath, or chest pain may occur. Some may have Löfgren syndrome with fever, large lymph nodes, arthritis, and a rash known as erythema nodosum. The cause of sarcoidosis is unknown. Treatments for sarcoidosis vary greatly depending on the patient. At least half of patients require no systemic therapy. Most people (>75%) only require symptomatic treatment with nonsteroidal anti-inflammatory drugs (NSAIDs) like ibuprofen or aspirin. For those presenting with lung symptoms, unless the respiratory impairment is devastating, active pulmonary sarcoidosis is observed usually without therapy for two to three months; if the inflammation does not subside spontaneously, therapy is instituted. Major categories of drug interventions include glucocorticoids, antimetabolites, biologic agents especially monoclonal anti-tumor necrosis factor antibodies. Corticosteroids, most commonly prednisone or prednisolone, have been the standard treatment for many years. In some people, this treatment can slow or reverse the course of the disease, but other people do not respond to steroid therapy. The use of corticosteroids in mild disease is controversial because in many cases the disease remits spontaneously.

Figure 91. The symptoms and signs of sarcoid

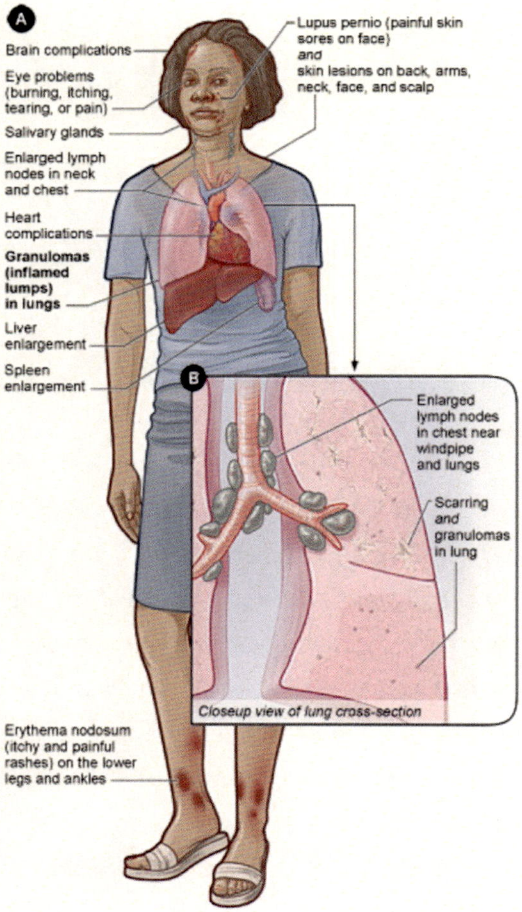

This image is by NHLBI authors. Minor editing by Mikael Häggström - National Heart, Lung, and Blood Institute: DCI Home: Lung Diseases: Sarcoidosis: Signs &

Symptoms Retrieved on May 9, 2009. Public Domain, https://commons.wikimedia.org/w/index.php?curid=6738077. https://en.wikipedia.org/wiki/Sarcoidosis#/media/File:Sarcoidosis_signs_and_symptoms.png. This work is in the public domain in the United States because it is a work prepared by an officer or employee of the United States Government as part of that person's official duties under the terms of Title 17, Chapter 1, Section 105 of the US Code.

Figure 92. Chest x-ray showing the typical nodularity of sarcoidosis, predominantly in the bases of the lungs.

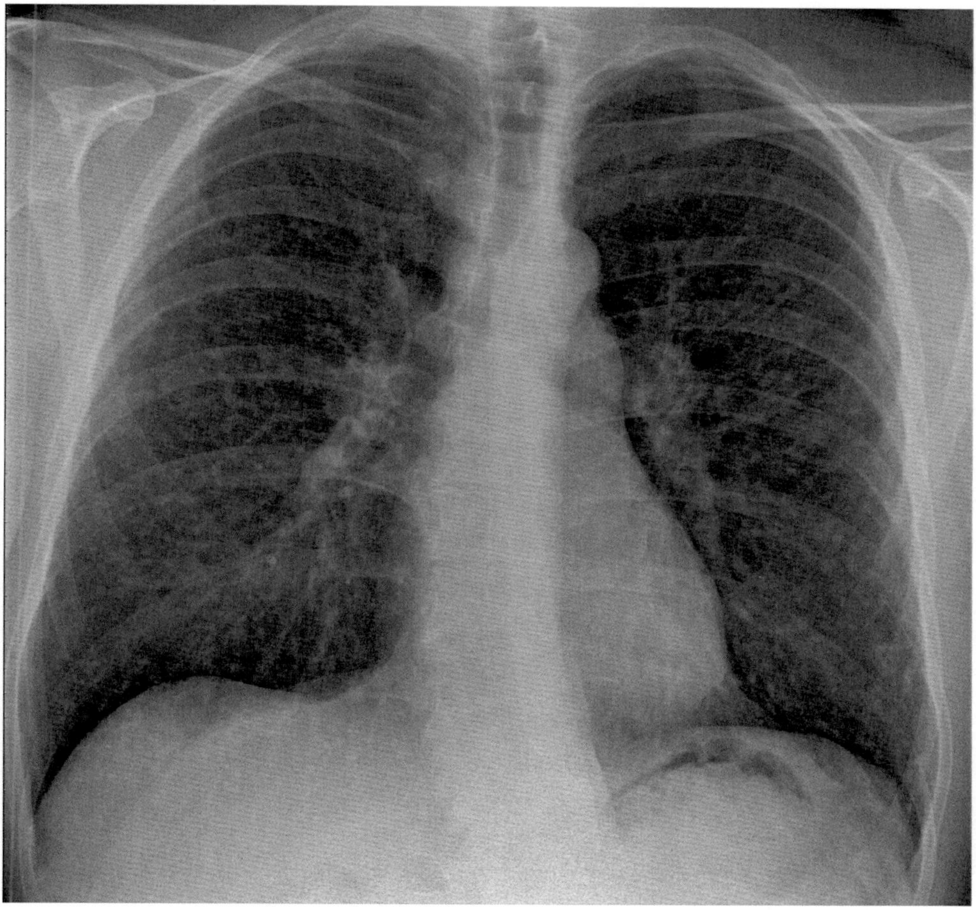

By Mikael Häggström - Own work, CC0, https://commons.wikimedia.org/w/index.php?curid=12149898. https://en.wikipedia.org/wiki/Sarcoidosis#/media/File:Chest_X-

ray_of_sarcoidosis_nodules.png. This file is made available under the Creative Commons CC0 1.0 Universal Public Domain Dedication. No changes were made to this image.

Infusion-related reactions

KEYTRUDA can cause severe or life-threatening infusion-related reactions, including hypersensitivity and anaphylaxis, which have been reported in 0.2% of 2799 patients receiving KEYTRUDA. Monitor patients for signs and symptoms of infusion-related reactions including rigors, chills, wheezing, pruritus, flushing, rash, hypotension, hypoxemia, and fever. Interrupt or slow the rate of infusion for mild (Grade 1) or moderate (Grade 2) infusion-related reactions. For severe (Grade 3) or life-threatening (Grade 4) infusion-related reactions, stop infusion and permanently discontinue KEYTRUDA.

Complications of allogeneic HSCT

Fatal and other serious complications can occur in patients who receive allogeneic hematopoietic stem cell transplantation (HSCT) before or after being treated with a PD-1/PD-L1 blocking antibody. Transplant-related complications include hyperacute graft-versus-host-disease (GVHD), acute GVHD, chronic GVHD, hepatic veno-occlusive disease (VOD, aka hepatic sinusoidal obstructive syndrome) after reduced intensity conditioning, and steroid-requiring febrile syndrome (without an identified infectious cause). These complications may occur despite intervening therapy between PD-1/PD-L1 blockade and allogeneic HSCT. Follow patients closely for evidence of transplant-related complications and intervene promptly. Consider the benefit versus risks of treatment with a PD-1/PD-L1 blocking antibody prior to or after an allogeneic HSCT.

ADVERSE REACTIONS

Most common adverse reactions (reported in ≥20% of patients) were:

• KEYTRUDA as a single agent

Fatigue, musculoskeletal pain, decreased appetite, pruritus, diarrhoea, nausea, rash, pyrexia, cough, dyspnea, constipation, pain, and abdominal pain.

• KEYTRUDA in combination with chemotherapy

Fatigue/asthenia, nausea, constipation, diarrhoea, decreased appetite, rash, vomiting, cough, dyspnoea, pyrexia, alopecia, peripheral neuropathy, mucosal inflammation, stomatitis *(Figure 93),* headache, and weight loss.

Figure 93. Apthous stomatitis of the oral mucosa

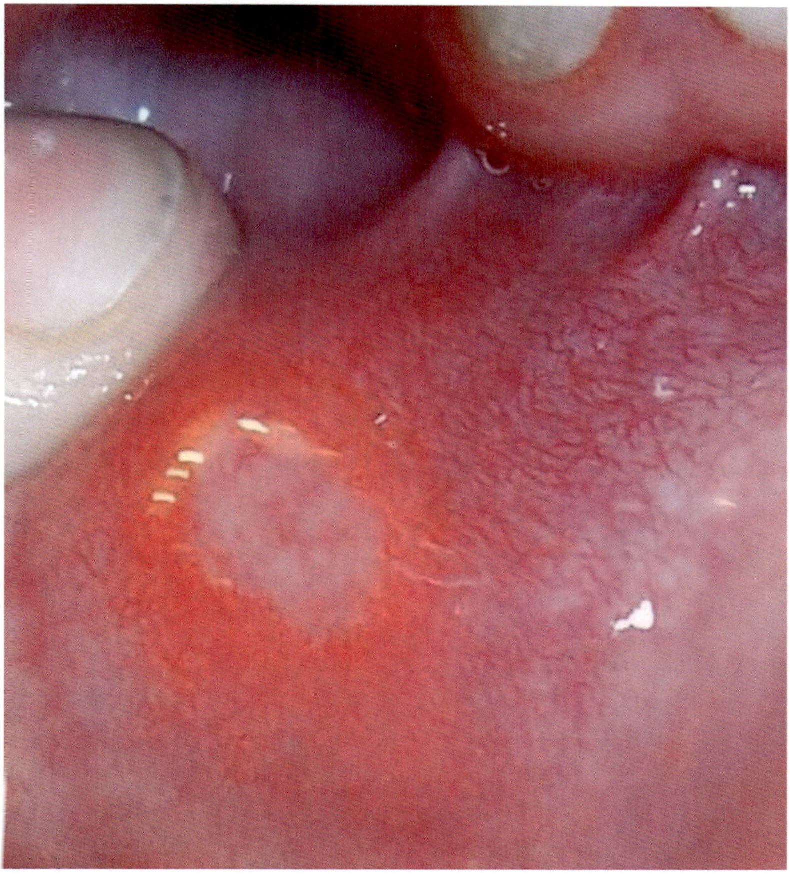

KEYTRUDA in combination with axitinib

Diarrhoea, fatigue/asthenia, hypertension, hepatotoxicity, hypothyroidism, decreased appetite, palmar-plantar erythrodysesthesia, nausea, stomatitis/mucosal inflammation, dysphonia, rash, cough, and constipation.

• KEYTRUDA in combination with lenvatinib

Fatigue, hypertension, musculoskeletal pain, diarrhoea, decreased appetite, hypothyroidism, nausea, stomatitis, vomiting, weight loss, abdominal pain, headache, constipation, urinary tract infection, dysphonia, hemorrhagic events, hypomagnesemia, palmar-plantar erythrodysesthesia,, dyspnea, cough, and rash.

Dose modifications

No dose reduction for KEYTRUDA is recommended. In general, withhold KEYTRUDA for severe (Grade 3) immune-mediated adverse reactions. Permanently discontinue KEYTRUDA for Life-threatening (Grade 4) immune-mediated adverse reactions, recurrent severe (Grade 3) immune-mediated reactions that require systemic immunosuppressive treatment, or an inability to reduce corticosteroid dose to 10 mg or less of prednisone or equivalent per day within 12 weeks of initiating steroids.

USE IN SPECIFIC POPULATIONS

Lactation risk summary

There are no data on the presence of pembrolizumab in either animal or human milk or its effects on the breastfed child or on milk production. Because of the potential for serious adverse reactions in breastfed children, advise women not to breastfeed during treatment with KEYTRUDA and for 4 months after the final dose.

Pregnancy testing

Verify pregnancy status in females of reproductive potential prior to initiating KEYTRUDA. Contraception KEYTRUDA can cause fetal harm when administered to a pregnant woman. Advise females of reproductive potential to use effective contraception during treatment with KEYTRUDA and for at least 4 months following the final dose.

Embryo-fetal toxicity

Based on its mechanism of action, KEYTRUDA can cause fetal harm when administered to a pregnant woman. Animal models link the PD-1/PD-L1 signalling pathway with maintenance of pregnancy through induction of maternal immune tolerance to fetal tissue. Advise women of the potential risk to a fetus. Advise females of reproductive potential to use effective contraception during treatment with KEYTRUDA and for 4 months after the last dose.

Pediatric use

The safety and effectiveness of KEYTRUDA as a single agent have been established in pediatric patients with classical Hodgkin lymphoma (cHL), primary mediastinal B cell lymphoma (PMBCL), Merkel cell carcinoma (MCC), microsatellite instability – high (MSI-H) cancer, and tumor mutational burden – high (TMB-H) cancer. Use of KEYTRUDA in pediatric patients for these indications is supported by evidence from adequate and well-controlled studies in adults with additional pharmacokinetic and safety data in pediatric patients. In KEYNOTE-051, 161 pediatric patients (62 pediatric patients aged 6 months to younger than 12 years and 99 pediatric patients aged 12 to 17 years) with advanced melanoma, lymphoma, or PD-L1 positive solid tumors received KEYTRUDA 2 mg/kg every 3 weeks. The median duration of exposure was 2.1 months (range: 1 day to 24 months). Adverse reactions that occurred at a ≥10% higher rate in pediatric patients when compared to adults included pyrexia (33%), vomiting (30%), upper respiratory tract infection (29%), and headache (25%). Laboratory abnormalities that occurred at a ≥10% higher rate in pediatric patients when compared to adults were leukopenia (30%), neutropenia (26%), and Grade 3 anemia (17%). The safety and effectiveness of KEYTRUDA in pediatric patients have not been established in the other approved indications.

Geriatric use

Of 3781 patients with melanoma, NSCLC, HNSCC, or urothelial carcinoma who were treated with KEYTRUDA in clinical studies, 48% were 65 years and over and 17% were 75 years and over. No overall differences in safety or effectiveness were observed between elderly patients and younger patients. Of 389 adult patients with cHL who were treated with KEYTRUDA in clinical studies, 46 (12%) were 65 years and over. Patients aged 65 years and over had a higher incidence of serious adverse reactions (50%) than patients aged younger than 65 years (24%). Clinical studies of KEYTRUDA in cHL did not include sufficient numbers of patients aged 65 years and over to determine whether effectiveness differs from that in younger patients. Of 596 adult patients with TNBC who were treated with KEYTRUDA in combination with paclitaxel, paclitaxel protein-bound, or gemcitabine and carboplatin in KEYNOTE-355, 137 (23%) were 65 years and over. No overall differences in safety or effectiveness were observed between elderly patients and younger patients.

Therapeutic efficacy of prembolizumab in the management of breast cancer

Pembrolizumab plus standard neoadjuvant therapy for high-risk breast cancer (BC): Results from I-SPY 2. In one trial reported in 2017, pebrolizumab added to standard therapy (AC) improved pCR rates in all HER2- BCs that met I-SPY 2 trial eligibility, especially in TNBC. Immune-mediated AEs were observed (one case of hypophysitis and 4 of adrenal insufficiency.

Nanda, R et al., Journal of Clinical Oncology 2017 35:15_suppl, 506-506

9.10 PALBOCICLIB (IBRANCE)

IBRANCE® (palbociclib) capsules, for oral use. Initial U.S. Approval: 2015

RECENT MAJOR CHANGES

INDICATIONS AND USAGE

IBRANCE is a kinase inhibitor indicated for the treatment of adult patients with hormone receptor (HR)-positive, human epidermal growth factor receptor 2 (HER2)-negative advanced or metastatic breast cancer in combination with:

• an aromatase inhibitor as initial endocrine-based therapy in postmenopausal women or in men; or

• fulvestrant in patients with disease progression following endocrine therapy.

MECHANISM OF ACTION

Palbociclib is an inhibitor of cyclin-dependent kinases (CDK) 4 and 6. Cyclin D1 and CDK4/6 are downstream of signaling pathways which lead to cellular proliferation. In vitro, palbociclib reduced cellular proliferation of estrogen receptor (ER)-positive breast cancer cell lines by blocking progression of the cell from G1 into S phase of the cell cycle. Treatment of breast cancer cell lines with the combination of palbociclib and antiestrogens leads to decreased retinoblastoma (Rb) protein phosphorylation resulting in reduced E2F expression and signaling, and increased growth arrest compared to treatment with each drug alone. In vitro treatment of ER-positive breast cancer cell lines with the combination of palbociclib and antiestrogens led to increased cell senescence compared to each drug alone, which was sustained for up to 6 days following palbociclib removal and was greater if antiestrogen treatment was continued. In vivo studies using a patient-derived ER-positive breast cancer xenograft model demonstrated that the combination of palbociclib and letrozole increased the inhibition of Rb phosphorylation, downstream signaling, and tumor growth compared to each drug alone. Human bone marrow mononuclear cells treated with palbociclib in the presence or absence of an anti-estrogen in vitro did not become senescent and resumed proliferation following palbociclib withdrawal.

DESCRIPTION

IBRANCE capsules for oral administration contain 125 mg, 100 mg, or 75 mg of palbociclib, a kinase inhibitor. The molecular formula for palbociclib is C24H29N7O2. The molecular weight is 447.54 daltons. The chemical name is 6-acetyl-8-cyclopentyl-5-methyl-2-{[5-(piperazin-1-yl)pyridin-2-yl]amino}pyrido[2,3-d]pyrimidin7(8H)-one, and its structural formula is: MMe e MMe e N N HHN N N N N N OO O O N N N N NN H H.

Palbociclib is a yellow to orange powder with pKa of 7.4 (the secondary piperazine nitrogen) and 3.9 (the pyridine nitrogen). At or below pH 4, palbociclib behaves as a high-solubility compound. Above pH 4, the solubility of the drug substance reduces significantly. Inactive ingredients: Microcrystalline cellulose, lactose monohydrate, sodium starch glycolate, colloidal silicon dioxide, magnesium stearate, and hard gelatin capsule shells. The light orange, light orange/caramel, and caramel opaque capsule shells contain gelatin, red iron oxide, yellow iron oxide, and titanium dioxide;

the printing ink contains shellac, titanium dioxide, ammonium hydroxide, propylene glycol, and simethicone.

PHARMACODYNAMICS

Cardiac

Electrophysiology The effect of palbociclib on the QT interval corrected for heart rate (QTc) was evaluated using time-matched electrocardiograms (ECGs) evaluating the change from baseline and corresponding pharmacokinetic data in 77 patients with breast cancer. Palbociclib had no large effect on QTc (i.e., >20 ms) at 125 mg once daily for 21 consecutive days followed by 7 days off treatment to comprise a complete cycle of 28 days.

PHARMACOKINETICS

The pharmacokinetics (PK) of palbociclib were characterized in patients with solid tumors including advanced breast cancer and in healthy subjects.

Absorption

The mean maximum observed concentration (Cmax) of palbociclib is generally observed between 6 to 12 hours (time to reach maximum concentration, Tmax) following oral administration. The mean absolute bioavailability of IBRANCE after an oral 125 mg dose is 46%. In the dosing range of 25 mg to 225 mg, the AUC and Cmax increased proportionally with dose in general. Steady state was achieved within 8 days following repeated once daily dosing. With repeated once daily administration, palbociclib accumulated with a median accumulation ratio of 2.4 (range 1.5 to 4.2).

Food effect

Palbociclib absorption and exposure were very low in approximately 13% of the population under the fasted condition. Food intake increased the palbociclib exposure in this small subset of the population but did not alter palbociclib exposure in the rest of the population to a clinically relevant extent. Therefore, food intake reduced the intersubject variability of palbociclib exposure, which supports administration of IBRANCE with food. Compared to IBRANCE given under overnight fasted conditions, the population average area under the concentration-time curve from zero to infinity (AUCINF) and Cmax of palbociclib increased by 21% and 38%, respectively, when given with high-fat, high-calorie food (approximately 800 to 1000 calories with 150, 250, and 500 to 600 calories from protein, carbohydrate, and fat, respectively), by 12% and 27%, respectively, when given with low-fat, low-calorie food (approximately 400 to 500 calories with 120, 250, and 28 to 35 calories from protein, carbohydrate, and fat, respectively), and by 13% and 24%, respectively, when moderate-fat, standard calorie food (approximately 500 to 700 calories with 75 to 105, 250 to 350 and 175 to 245 calories from protein, carbohydrate, and fat, respectively) was given 1 hour before and 2 hours after IBRANCE dosing.

Distribution

Binding of palbociclib to human plasma proteins in vitro was approximately 85%, with no concentration dependence over the concentration range of 500 ng/mL to 5000 ng/mL. The mean fraction unbound (fu) of palbociclib in human plasma in vivo increased incrementally with worsening hepatic function. There was no obvious trend in the mean palbociclib fu in human plasma in vivo with worsening renal function. The geometric mean apparent volume of distribution (Vz/F) was 2583 L with a coefficient of variation (CV) of 26%.

Metabolism

In vitro and in vivo studies indicated that palbociclib undergoes hepatic metabolism in humans. Following oral administration of a single 125 mg dose of [14C] palbociclib to humans, the primary metabolic pathways for palbociclib involved oxidation and sulfonation, with acylation and glucuronidation contributing as minor pathways. Palbociclib was the major circulating drug-derived entity in plasma (23%). The major circulating metabolite was a glucuronide conjugate of palbociclib, although it only represented 1.5% of the administered dose in the excreta. Palbociclib was extensively metabolized with unchanged drug accounting for 2.3% and 6.9% of radioactivity in feces and urine, respectively. In feces, the sulfamic acid conjugate of palbociclib was the major drug-related component, accounting for 26% of the administered dose. In vitro studies with human hepatocytes, liver cytosolic and S9 fractions, and recombinant SULT enzymes indicated that CYP3A and SULT2A1 are mainly involved in the metabolism of palbociclib.

Elimination

The geometric mean apparent oral clearance (CL/F) of palbociclib was 63.1 L/hr (29% CV), and the mean (± standard deviation) plasma elimination half-life was 29 (±5) hours in patients with advanced breast cancer. In 6 healthy male subjects given a single oral dose of [14C]palbociclib, a median of 91.6% of the total administered radioactive dose was recovered in 15 days; feces (74.1% of dose) was the major route of excretion, with 17.5% of the dose recovered in urine. The majority of the material was excreted as metabolites.

Age, gender, and body eight

Based on a population pharmacokinetic analysis in 183 patients with cancer (50 male and 133 female patients, age range from 22 to 89 years, and body weight range from 37.9 to 123 kg), gender had no effect on the exposure of palbociclib, and age and body weight had no clinically important effect on the exposure of palbociclib.
Pediatric population

Pharmacokinetics of IBRANCE have not been evaluated in patients ULN, or total bilirubin >1.0 to 1.5 × ULN and any AST), mild hepatic impairment had no effect on the exposure of palbociclib, further supporting the findings from the dedicated hepatic impairment study.

Renal Impairment

Data from a pharmacokinetic trial in subjects with varying degrees of renal impairment indicate that palbociclib AUCINF increased by 39%, 42%, and 31% with mild (60 mL/min ≤ CrCl < 90 mL/min), moderate (30 mL/min ≤ CrCl

FULL PRESCRIBING INFORMATION

INDICATIONS AND USAGE

IBRANCE is indicated for the treatment of adult patients with hormone receptor (HR)-positive, human epidermal growth factor receptor 2 (HER2)-negative advanced or metastatic breast cancer in combination with:

• an aromatase inhibitor as initial endocrine-based therapy in postmenopausal women or in men; or

• fulvestrant in patients with disease progression following endocrine therapy.

DOSAGE AND ADMINISTRATION

Recommended dose and schedule

The recommended dose of IBRANCE is a 125 mg capsule taken orally once daily for 21 consecutive days followed by 7 days off treatment to comprise a complete cycle of 28 days. IBRANCE should be taken with food. Administer the recommended dose of an aromatase inhibitor when given with IBRANCE. When given with IBRANCE, the recommended dose of fulvestrant is 500 mg administered on Days 1, 15, 29, and once monthly thereafter. Patients should be encouraged to take their dose of IBRANCE at approximately the same time each day. If the patient vomits or misses a dose, an additional dose should not be taken. The next prescribed dose should be taken at the usual time. IBRANCE capsules should be swallowed whole (do not chew, crush, or open them prior to swallowing). Capsules should not be ingested if they are broken, cracked, or otherwise not intact. Pre/perimenopausal women treated with the combination IBRANCE plus fulvestrant therapy should also be treated with luteinizing hormone-releasing hormone (LHRH) agonists according to current clinical practice standards. For men treated with combination IBRANCE plus aromatase inhibitor therapy, consider treatment with an LHRH agonist according to current clinical practice standards.

Dose modification

Dose

Recommended starting dose 125 mg/day First dose reduction 100 mg/day Second dose reduction 75 mg/day. If further dose reduction below 75 mg/day is required, discontinue.

Dose modification and management – hematologic toxicities[a]

Monitor complete blood counts prior to the start of IBRANCE therapy and at the beginning of each cycle, as well as on Day 15 of the first 2 cycles, and as clinically indicated. For patients who experience a maximum of Grade 1 or 2 neutropenia in the first 6 cycles, monitor complete blood counts for subsequent cycles every 3 months, prior to the beginning of a cycle and as clinically indicated.

CTCAE grade dose modifications

Grade 1 or 2: No dose adjustment is required.

Grade 3 Day 1 of cycle: Withhold IBRANCE, repeat complete blood count monitoring within 1 week. When recovered to Grade ≤2, start the next cycle at the *same dose.*

Day 15 of first 2 cycles: If Grade 3 on Day 15, continue IBRANCE at current dose to complete cycle and repeat complete blood count on Day 22.

If Grade 4 on Day 22, see Grade 4 dose modification guidelines below.

Consider dose reduction in cases of prolonged (>1 week) recovery from Grade 3 neutropenia or recurrent Grade 3 neutropenia on Day 1 of subsequent cycles.

Grade 3 neutropenia[b] with fever ≥38.5 °C and/or infection at any time: Withhold IBRANCE until recovery to Grade ≤2. Resume at the *next lower dose*.

Grade 4 At any time: Withhold IBRANCE until recovery to Grade ≤2. Resume at the *next lower dose.*

Grading according to CTCAE 4.0. *(*CTCAE = Common Terminology Criteria for Adverse Events*)*

LLN = lower limit of normal.

[a]Table applies to all hematologic adverse reactions except lymphopenia (unless associated with clinical events, e.g., opportunistic infections).

[b]Absolute neutrophil count (ANC): Grade 1: ANC < LLN - 1500/mm^3; Grade 2: ANC 1000 – <1500/mm^3; Grade 4: ANC <500/mm^3.

Dose modification and management – non-hematologic toxicities

CTCAE Grade Dose Modifications

Grade 1 or 2: No dose adjustment is required.

Grade ≥3 non-hematologic toxicity (if persisting despite optimal medical treatment): withhold until symptoms resolve to:

- Grade ≤1;
- Grade ≤2 (if not considered a safety risk for the patient).

Resume at the *next lower* dose. Permanently discontinue IBRANCE in patients with severe interstitial lung disease (ILD)/pneumonitis.

DRUG INTERACTIONS

Palbociclib is primarily metabolized by CYP3A and sulfotransferase (SULT) enzyme SULT2A1. In vivo, palbociclib is a time-dependent inhibitor of CYP3A.

Agents that may increase palbociclib plasma concentrations

Effect of CYP3A Inhibitors

Coadministration of a strong CYP3A inhibitor (*eg,* itraconazole) increased the plasma exposure of palbociclib in healthy subjects by 87%. Avoid concomitant use of strong CYP3A inhibitors (e.g., clarithromycin, indinavir, itraconazole, ketoconazole, lopinavir/ritonavir, nefazodone, nelfinavir, posaconazole, ritonavir, saquinavir, telaprevir, telithromycin, and voriconazole).

Avoid grapefruit or grapefruit juice during IBRANCE treatment.

If coadministration of IBRANCE with a strong CYP3A inhibitor cannot be avoided, reduce the dose of IBRANCE

Agents that may decrease palbociclib plasma concentrations

Effect of CYP3A Inducers

Coadministration of a strong CYP3A inducer (*eg,* rifampin) decreased the plasma exposure of palbociclib in healthy subjects by 85%. Avoid concomitant use of strong CYP3A inducers (e.g., phenytoin, rifampin, carbamazepine, enzalutamide, and St John's Wort

Drugs that may have their plasma concentrations altered by palbociclib

Coadministration of midazolam with multiple doses of IBRANCE increased the midazolam plasma exposure by 61%, in healthy subjects, compared to administration of midazolam alone. The dose of the sensitive CYP3A substrate with a narrow therapeutic index (e.g., alfentanil, cyclosporine, dihydroergotamine, ergotamine, everolimus, fentanyl, pimozide, quinidine, sirolimus, and tacrolimus) may need to be reduced, as IBRANCE may increase its exposure

USE IN SPECIFIC POPULATIONS

Pregnancy risk summary

Based on findings from animal studies and its mechanism of action, IBRANCE can cause fetal harm when administered to a pregnant woman. There are no available data in pregnant women to inform the drug-associated risk. In animal reproduction studies, administration of palbociclib to pregnant rats and rabbits during organogenesis resulted in Embryo-fetal toxicity at maternal exposures that were ≥4 times the human clinical exposure based on AUC. Advise pregnant women of the potential risk to a fetus. The estimated background risk of major birth defects and miscarriage for the indicated population is unknown. In the U.S. general population, the estimated background risk of major birth defects and miscarriage in clinically recognized pregnancies is 2%-4% and 15%-20%, respectively.

Data

Animal data

In a fertility and early embryonic development study in female rats, palbociclib was administered orally for 15 days before mating through to Day 7 of pregnancy, which did not cause embryo toxicity at doses up to 300 mg/kg/day with maternal systemic exposures approximately 4 times the human exposure (AUC) at the recommended dose. In embryo-fetal development studies in rats and rabbits, pregnant animals received oral doses of palbociclib up to 300 mg/kg/day and 20 mg/kg/day, respectively, during the period of organogenesis. The maternally toxic dose of 300 mg/kg/day was fetotoxic in rats, resulting in reduced fetal body weights. At doses ≥100 mg/kg/day in rats, there was an increased incidence of a skeletal variation (increased incidence of a rib present at the seventh cervical vertebra). At the maternally toxic dose of 20 mg/kg/day in rabbits, there was an increased incidence of skeletal variations, including small phalanges in the forelimb. At 300 mg/kg/day in rats and 20 mg/kg/day in rabbits, the maternal systemic exposures were approximately 4 and 9 times the human exposure (AUC) at the recommended dose, respectively. CDK4/6 double knockout mice have been reported to die in late stages of fetal development (gestation Day 14.5 until birth) due to severe anemia. However, knockout mouse data may not be predictive of effects in humans due to differences in degree of target inhibition.

Lactation risk summary

There is no information regarding the presence of palbociclib in human milk, its effects on milk production, or the breastfed infant. Because of the potential for serious adverse reactions in breastfed infants from IBRANCE, advise a lactating woman not to breastfeed during treatment with IBRANCE and for 3 weeks after the last dose.

Females and males of reproductive potential

Pregnancy testing

Based on animal studies, IBRANCE can cause fetal harm when administered to a pregnant woman. Females of reproductive potential should have a pregnancy test prior to starting treatment with IBRANCE.

Contraception

Females

IBRANCE can cause fetal harm when administered to a pregnant woman Advise females of reproductive potential to use effective contraception during treatment with IBRANCE and for at least 3 weeks after the last dose.

Males

Because of the potential for genotoxicity, advise male patients with female partners of reproductive potential to use effective contraception during treatment with IBRANCE and for 3 months after the last dose

Infertility

Males

Based on animal studies, IBRANCE may impair fertility in males of reproductive potential.

Pediatric use

The safety and efficacy of IBRANCE in pediatric patients have not been studied. Altered glucose metabolism (glycosuria, hyperglycemia, decreased insulin) associated with changes in the pancreas (islet cell vacuolation), eye (cataracts, lens degeneration), kidney (tubule vacuolation, chronic progressive nephropathy) and adipose tissue (atrophy) were identified in a 27 week repeat-dose toxicology study in rats that were immature at the beginning of the studies and were most prevalent in males at oral palbociclib doses ≥30 mg/kg/day (approximately 11 times the adult human exposure [AUC] at the recommended dose). Some of these findings (glycosuria/hyperglycemia, pancreatic islet cell vacuolation, and kidney tubule vacuolation) were present with lower incidence and severity in a 15-week repeat-dose toxicology study in immature rats. Altered glucose metabolism or associated changes in the pancreas, eye, kidney and adipose tissue were not identified in a 27-week repeat-dose toxicology study in rats that were mature at the beginning of the study and in dogs in repeat-dose toxicology studies up to 39 weeks duration.

Toxicities in teeth independent of altered glucose metabolism were observed in rats. Administration of 100 mg/kg palbociclib for 27 weeks (approximately 15 times the adult human exposure [AUC] at the recommended dose) resulted in abnormalities in growing incisor teeth (discolored, ameloblast degeneration/necrosis, mononuclear cell infiltrate). Other toxicities of potential concern to pediatric patients have not been evaluated in juvenile animals.

Geriatric use

Of 444 patients who received IBRANCE in Study 1, 181 patients (41%) were ≥65 years of age and 48 patients (11%) were ≥75 years of age. Of 347 patients who received IBRANCE in Study 2, 86 patients (25%) were ≥65 years of age and 27 patients (8%) were ≥75 years of age. No overall differences in safety or effectiveness of IBRANCE were observed between these patients and younger patients.

Hepatic impairment

No dose adjustment is required in patients with mild or moderate hepatic impairment (Child-Pugh classes A and B). For patients with severe hepatic impairment (Child-Pugh class C), the recommended dose of IBRANCE is 75 mg once daily for 21 consecutive days followed by 7 days off treatment to comprise a complete cycle of 28 days Based on a pharmacokinetic trial in subjects with varying degrees of hepatic function, the palbociclib unbound exposure (unbound AUCINF) decreased by 17% in subjects with mild hepatic impairment (Child-Pugh class A), and increased by 34% and 77% in subjects with moderate (Child-Pugh class B) and severe (Child-Pugh class C) hepatic impairment, respectively, relative to subjects with normal hepatic function. Peak palbociclib unbound exposure (unbound Cmax) increased by 7%, 38% and 72% for mild, moderate and severe hepatic impairment, respectively, relative to subjects with normal hepatic function.

Review the full prescribing information for the aromatase inhibitor or fulvestrant for dose modifications related to hepatic impairment.

Renal impairment

No dose adjustment is required in patients with mild, moderate, or severe renal impairment (CrCl >15 mL/min). Based on a pharmacokinetic trial in subjects with varying degrees of renal function, the total palbociclib exposure (AUCINF) increased by 39%, 42%, and 31% with mild (60 mL/min ≤ CrCl

The efficacy of palbociclib in the treatment of breast cancer

i). The available clinical data from both controlled clinical trials and real-life experiences concerning palbociclib-based combinations in patients with hormone receptor-positive (HR+)/human epidermal growth factor receptor 2-negative (HER2−) metastatic disease, including patient-reported outcomes and subgroup analyses, have been reviewed and discussed. Palbociclib significantly improved progression-free survival and clinical benefit rates when added to letrozole in postmenopausal women as initial endocrine-based therapy, and it prolonged progression-free survival and overall survival when added to fulvestrant in women who progressed on previous endocrine therapy in randomized clinical trials. Tolerability profile was manageable, with neutropenia occurring most commonly, without detrimental impact on quality of life. Available data from real-life experiences confirm the good performance of palbociclib in unselected, heavily pretreated populations. Palbociclib in combination with endocrine therapy is a valuable emerging option for patients with HR+/HER2− advanced or metastatic breast cancer. Further investigation is needed to provide solutions for palbociclib resistance and to identify the best sequence to use for the best patient benefit with a minimal toxicity.

Serra F, et al. Palbociclib in metastatic breast cancer: current evidence and real-life data. Drugs Context. 2019;8: 212579. Published 2019 Jul 16. doi:10.7573/dic.212579.

ii). In this first real-world assessment of clinical outcomes in US patients with HR+/HER- ABC/MBC, treatment with palbociclib in combination with AI or fulvestrant demonstrated favorable effectiveness in terms of progression-free and survival rates. Ongoing studies are needed to deliver mature clinical outcome data beyond 12/24 months in the real-world setting.

Taylor-Stokes G, et al. Treatment patterns and clinical outcomes among patients receiving palbociclib in combination with an aromatase inhibitor or fulvestrant for HR+/HER2-negative advanced/metastatic breast cancer in real-world settings in the US: Results from the IRIS study. Breast. 2019 Feb; 43:22-27. doi: 10.1016/j.breast.2018.10.009. Epub 2018 Oct 20. PMID: 30391832.

9.11. RIBOCICLIB (KISKALI)

KISQALI® (ribociclib) tablets, for oral use. Initial U.S. Approval: 2017.

INDICATIONS AND USAGE

KISQALI is a kinase inhibitor indicated in combination with an aromatase inhibitor as initial endocrine-based therapy for the treatment of postmenopausal women with hormone receptor (HR)-positive, human epidermal growth factor receptor 2 (HER2)-negative advanced or metastatic breast cancer.

MECHANISM OF ACTION

Ribociclib is an inhibitor of cyclin-dependent kinase (CDK) 4 and 6. These kinases are activated upon binding to D cyclins and play a crucial role in signaling pathways which lead to cell cycle progression and cellular proliferation. The cyclin D-CDK4/6 complex regulates cell cycle progression through phosphorylation of the retinoblastoma protein (pRb). In vitro, ribociclib decreased pRb phosphorylation leading to arrest in the G1 phase of the cell cycle and reduced cell proliferation in breast cancer cell lines. In vivo, treatment with single agent ribociclib in a rat xenograft model with human tumor cells led to decreased tumor volumes, which correlated with inhibition of pRb phosphorylation. In studies using patient-derived estrogen receptor positive breast cancer xenograft models, combination of ribociclib and antiestrogen (e.g., letrozole) resulted in increased tumor growth inhibition compared to each drug alone.

DESCRIPTION

KISQALI (ribociclib) is a kinase inhibitor. The chemical name of ribociclib succinate is: Butanedioic acid—7-cyclopentyl-N,N-dimethyl-2-{[5-(piperazin-1-yl) pyridin-2-yl]amino}-7H-pyrrolo[2,3-d]pyrimidine-6-carboxamide (1/1). Ribociclib succinate is a light yellow to yellowish brown crystalline powder. The molecular formula for ribociclib succinate is $C23H30N8O \cdot C4H6O4$ and the molecular weight is 552.64 g/mol (Free base: 434.55 g/mol). The chemical structure of ribociclib is shown below: KISQALI film-coated tablets are supplied for oral use and contain 200 mg of ribociclib free base (equivalent to 254.40 mg ribociclib succinate). The tablets also contain colloidal silicon dioxide, crospovidone, hydroxypropylcellulose, magnesium stearate and microcrystalline cellulose. The film-coating contains iron oxide black, iron oxide red, lecithin (soya), polyvinyl alcohol (partially hydrolysed), talc, titanium dioxide, and xanthan gum as inactive ingredients.

DOSAGE AND ADMINISTRATION

KISQALI tablets are taken orally with or without food in combination with letrozole.

- Recommended starting dose: 600 mg orally (three 200 mg tablets) taken once daily with or without food for 21 consecutive days followed by 7 days off treatment.

- Dose interruption, reduction, and/or discontinuation may be required based on individual safety and tolerability.

DOSAGE FORMS AND STRENGTHS

- Tablets: 200 mg

CONTRAINDICATIONS: None.

WARNINGS AND PRECAUTIONS

- QT interval prolongation: monitor electrocardiograms (ECGs) and electrolytes prior to initiation of treatment with KISQALI. Repeat ECGs at approximately Day 14 of the first cycle and at the beginning of the second cycle, and as clinically indicated. Monitor electrolytes at the beginning of each cycle for 6 cycles, and as clinically indicated.

(The QT interval [Figure 94] is a measurement made on an electrocardiogram used to assess some of the electrical properties of the heart. It is calculated as the time from the start of the Q wave to the end of the T wave, and approximates to the time taken from when the cardiac ventricles start to contract to when they finish relaxing. An abnormally long or abnormally short QT interval is associated with an increased risk of developing abnormal heart rhythms and sudden cardiac death. Abnormalities in the QT interval can be caused by genetic conditions such as long QT syndrome, by certain medications such as sotalol or pitolisant, by disturbances in the concentrations of certain salts within the blood such as hypokalaemia, or by hormonal imbalances such as hypothyroidism).

Figure 94. Cartoon showing measurement of the QT interval.

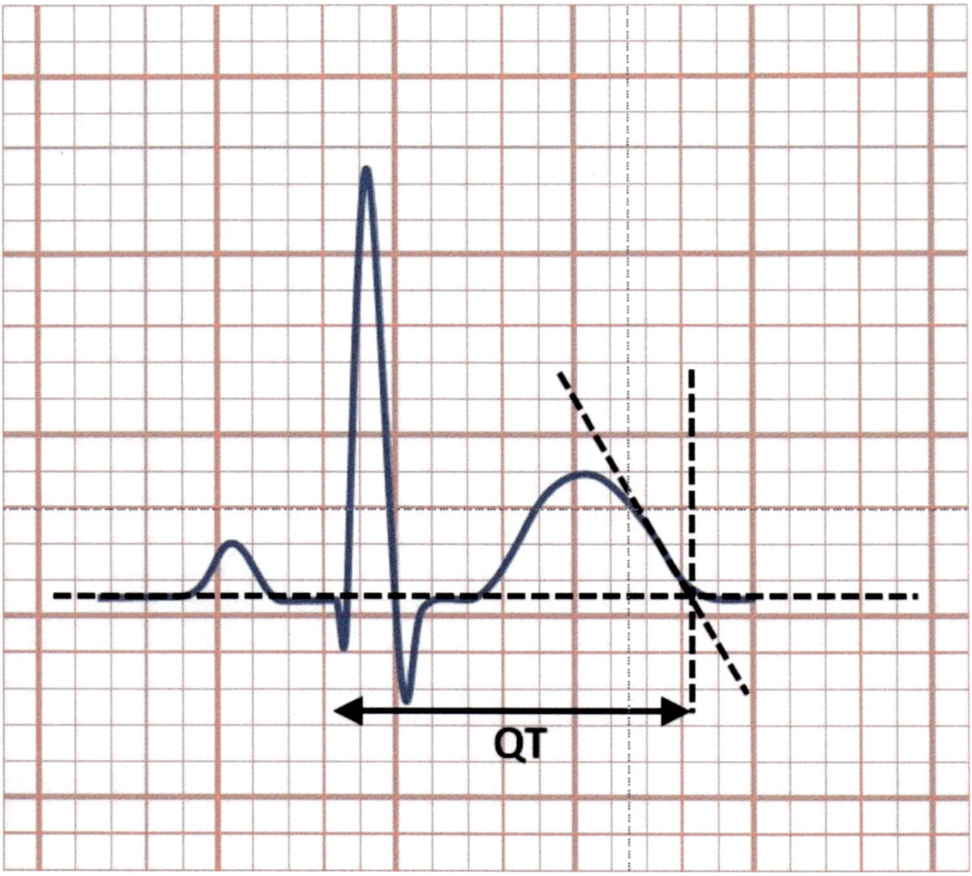

This image is by PeaBrainC - Own work, CC BY-SA 4.0, https://commons.wikimedia.org/w/index.php?curid=74185800. https://en.wikipedia.org/wiki/QT_interval#/media/File:QT_interval.jpg. This file is licensed under the Creative Commons Attribution-Share Alike 4.0 International license. No changeshave been made to this image.

A prolonged QT interval can lead to the Long QT syndrome (LQTS), a condition in which repolarization of the heart after a heartbeat is affected It results in an increased risk of an irregular heartbeat which can result in fainting, drowning, seizures, or sudden death. A prolonged QT interval is defined as being longer than 480 milliseconds (Figure 95).

Figure 95. An ECG demonstrating typical LQT1 pattern, annotated to demonstrate measurement of QT interval and cutoff for diagnosis of Long QT syndrome.

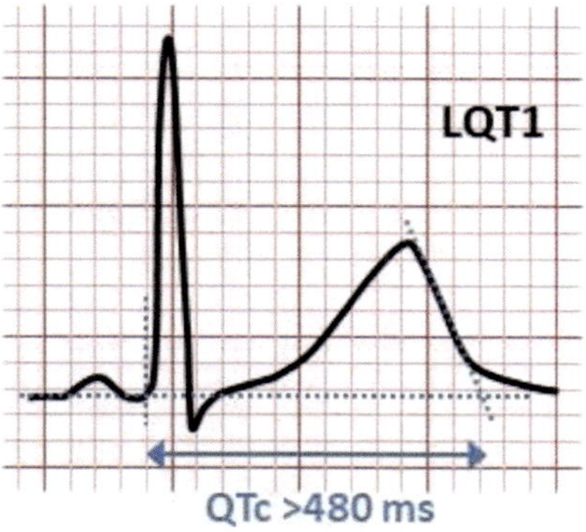

This image is by By PeaBrainC - Own work, CC BY-SA 4.0, https://commons.wikimedia.org/w/index.php?curid=89699845. https://en.wikipedia.org/wiki/Long_QT_syndrome#/media/File:Long_QT_syndrome_type_1.jpg. This file is licensed under the Creative Commons Attribution-Share Alike 4.0 International license. No changeshave been made to this image.

• Hepatobiliary toxicity: increases in serum transaminase levels have been observed. Perform Liver Function Tests (LFTs) before initiating treatment with KISQALI. Monitor LFTs every 2 weeks for the first 2 cycles, at the beginning of each subsequent 4 cycles, and as clinically indicated. Figure 96 shows yellowing of the skin and sclera due to marked hyperbilirubinemia (jaundice).

Figure 96. A person with jaundice, due in this case to pancreatic cancer obstructing outflow from the biliary tract.

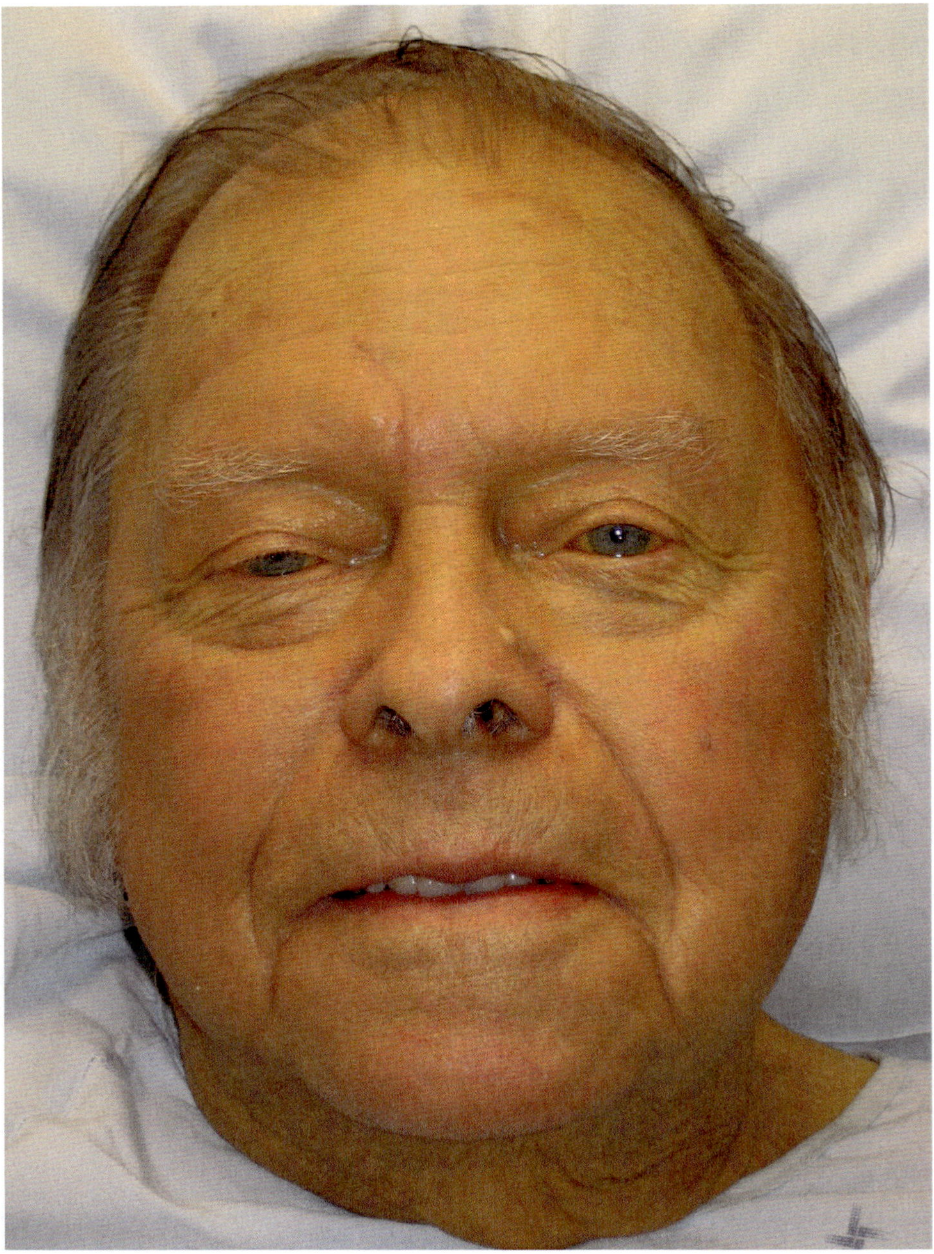

This image is by By James Heilman, MD - Own work, CC BY 3.0, https://commons.wikimedia.org/w/index.php?curid=9389660. https://en.wikipedia.org/wiki/Jaundice#/media/File:Jaundice08.jpg. This file is licensed under the Creative Commons Attribution 3.0 Unported license. No changeshave ben made to this image. ***Important note from the creator of this image****: the uploader of this image asserts the following regarding consent of identifiable persons: I personally created this media. All identifiable persons shown specifically consented to publication of this photograph or video.*

• Neutropenia: perform Complete Blood Count (CBC) before initiating therapy with KISQALI. Monitor CBC every 2 weeks for the first 2 cycles, at the beginning of each subsequent 4 cycles, and as clinically indicated.

• Embryo-fetal toxicity: can cause fetal harm. Advise patients of potential risk to a fetus and to use effective contraception during therapy.

ADVERSE REACTIONS

The most common adverse reactions (incidence ≥ 20%) are neutropenia, nausea, fatigue, diarrhea, leukopenia, alopecia, vomiting, constipation, headache and back pain. To report SUSPECTED ADVERSE REACTIONS, contact Novartis Pharmaceuticals Corporation at 1-888-669-6682 or FDA at 1-800-FDA1088 or www.fda.gov/medwatch.

DRUG INTERACTIONS

• CYP3A4 Inhibitors: avoid concomitant use of KISQALI with strong CYP3A inhibitors. If strong inhibitors cannot be avoided, reduce KISQALI dose.

• CYP3A4 Inducers: avoid concomitant use of KISQALI with strong CYP3A inducers.

• CYP3A substrates: the dose of sensitive CYP3A substrates with narrow therapeutic indices may need to be reduced when given concurrently with KISQALI.

• Drugs known to prolong QT interval: avoid concomitant use of drugs known to prolong QT interval such as anti-arrhythmic medicines.

FULL PRESCRIBING INFORMATION

INDICATIONS AND USAGE

KISQALI® is indicated in combination with an aromatase inhibitor as initial endocrine-based therapy for the treatment of postmenopausal women with hormone receptor (HR)-positive, human epidermal growth factor receptor 2 (HER2)- negative advanced or metastatic breast cancer.

DOSAGE AND ADMINISTRATION

Dosing and Administration

The recommended dose of KISQALI is 600 mg (three 200 mg film-coated tablets) taken orally, once daily for 21 consecutive days followed by 7 days off treatment resulting in a complete cycle of 28 days. KISQALI can be taken with or without food. Coadminister KISQALI with letrozole 2.5 mg taken once daily throughout the 28-day cycle. Refer to the full prescribing information of letrozole. For dosing and administration with other aromatase inhibitors refer to the applicable full prescribing information. Patients should take their dose of KISQALI and letrozole at approximately the same time each day, preferably in the morning. If the patient vomits after taking the dose, or misses a dose, no additional dose should be taken that day. The next prescribed dose should be taken at the usual time. KISQALI tablets should be swallowed whole (tablets should not be chewed, crushed or split prior to swallowing). No tablet should be ingested if it is broken, cracked, or otherwise not intact.

Dose modifications dose modifications for adverse reactions

Level	KISQALI DOSE	KISQALI NUMBER OF TABLETS
Starting dose	600 mg/day	Three 200 mg tablets
First dose reduction	400 mg/day	Two 200 mg tablets
Second dose reduction	200 mg/day□	One 200 mg tablet

*If further dose reduction below 200 mg/day is required, discontinue the treatment.

Dose modification and management for neutropenia

Grade 1 or 2: ANC 1000/m^3 – lower limit of normal	Grade 3: ANC 500-1000/m^3	Grade 3 with febrile neutropenia	Grade 4: ANC <500/m^3
No dose adjustment is required.	Dose interruption until recovery to Grade 2. Resume KISQALI at same dose level. If toxicity recurs at Grade 3, dose interruption until recovery, then resume KISQALI at the next lower dose level.	Grade 3 ANC with febrile neutropenia□: dose interruption until recovery of ANC to Grade 2. Resume KISQALI at next lower dose level.	Dose interruption until recovery to Grade ≤ 2. Resume KISQALI at the next lower dose level

□ Grade 3 neutropenia with single episode of fever >38°C (or) above 38°C for more than one hour and/or concurrent infection.

Perform complete blood count (CBC) before initiating treatment with KISQALI. Monltor CBC every 2 weeks for the first 2 cycles, at the beginning of each subsequent 4 cycles and as clinically indicated.

Modification and management for hepatobiliary dose toxicity

AST and/or ALT elevations from baseline*, WITHOUT increase in total bilirubin above 2 x ULN	Grade 1 (> ULN – 3 x ULN) No dose adjustment is required.	Grade 2 (>3 to 5 x ULN) Baseline* at < Grade 2: Dose interruption until recovery to ≤ baseline grade, then resume KISQALI at same dose level. If Grade 2 recurs, resume KISQALI at next lower dose level. Baseline* at Grade 2: No dose interruption	Grade 3 (>5 to 20 x ULN) Dose interruption until recovery to ≤ baseline* grade, then resume at next lower dose level. If Grade 3 recurs, discontinue KISQALI	Grade 4 (>20 x ULN) Discontinue KISQALI
Combined elevations in AST and/or ALT	If patients develop ALT and/or AST > 3	If patients develop ALT and/or AST > 3	If patients develop ALT and/or AST > 3	If patients develop ALT and/or AST > 3

of baseline grade, WITH total bilirubin increase, in the absence of cholestasis	x ULN along with total bilirubin > 2 x ULN irrespective of baseline grade, discontinue KISQALI	x ULN along with total bilirubin > 2 x ULN irrespective of baseline grade, discontinue KISQALI	x ULN along with total bilirubin > 2 x ULN irrespective of baseline grade, discontinue KISQALI	x ULN along with total bilirubin > 2 x ULN irrespective of baseline grade, discontinue KISQALI

Perform liver function tests (LFTs) before initiating treatment with KISQALI. Monitor LFTs every 2 weeks for the first 2 cycles, at the beginning of each subsequent 4 cycles, and as clinically indicated. If Grade ≥2 abnormalities are noted, more frequent monitoring is recommended.

*Baseline = prior to treatment initiation.

Grading according to CTCAE Version 4.03. ULN = upper limit of normal AST = aspartate aminotransferase; ALT = alanine aminotransferase

Dose modification and management for QT prolongation

ECGs with QTcF > 480 msec

1. Interrupt KISQALI Treatment

2. If QTcF prolongation resolves to < 481 msec, resume treatment at the same dose level

3. If QTcF ≥ 481 msec recurs, interrupt dose until QTcF resolves to < 481 msec; then resume KISQALI at next lower dose level.

ECGs with QTcF > 500

1. Interrupt KISQALI treatment if QTcF greater than 500 msec on at least 2 separate ECGs msec (within the same visit).

2. If QTcF prolongation resolves to < 481 msec, resume treatment at the next lower dose level. Permanently discontinue KISQALI if QTcF interval prolongation is either greater than 500 msec or greater than 60 msec change from baseline AND associated with any of the following:

Torsades de Pointes (Figure 97)

Polymorphic ventricular tachycardia

Unexplained syncope

Signs/symptoms of serious arrhythmia.

Electrocardiograms should be assessed prior to initiation of treatment. Repeat ECGs at approximately Day 14 of the first cycle and at the beginning of the second cycle, and as clinically indicated. In case of (QTcF) prolongation at any given time during treatment, more frequent ECG monitoring is recommended.

Figure 97. Prolonged QT interval; Torsades de Pointes (TdP).

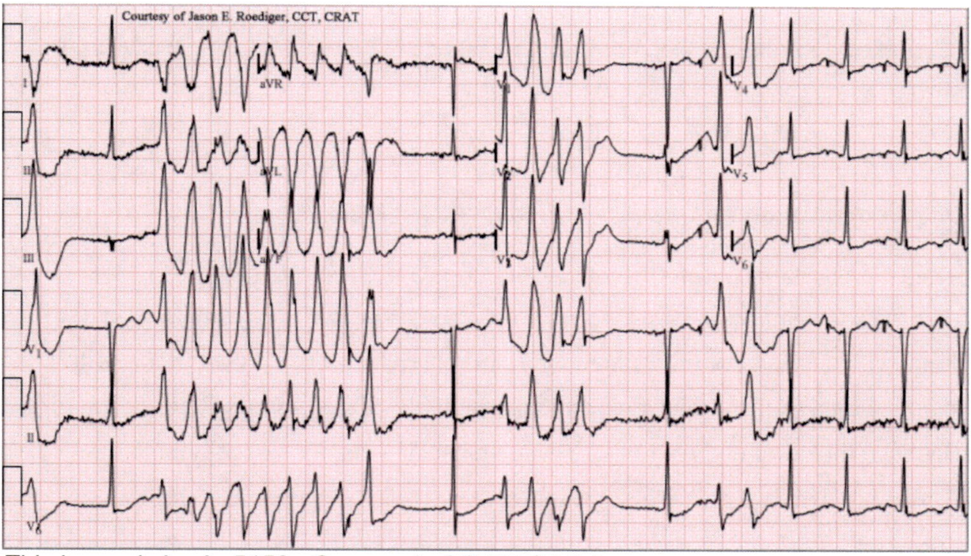

This image is by Jer5150 - Own work, CC BY-SA 3.0, https://commons.wikimedia.org/w/index.php?curid=19738256. https://en.wikipedia.org/wiki/Torsades_de_pointes#/media/File:Torsades_de_Pointes_TdP.png. This file is licensed under the Creative Commons Attribution-Share Alike 3.0 Unported license. No changeshave been made to this image.

Torsades de pointes (TdP), translated from French as "twisting of peaks", is a specific type of abnormal heart rhythm that can lead to sudden cardiac death. It is a polymorphic ventricular tachycardia that exhibits distinct characteristics on the electrocardiogram. It was described by French physician François Dessertenne in 1966. Prolongation of the QT interval can increase a person's risk of developing this abnormal heart rhythm, occurring in between 1% and 10% of patients who receive QT-prolonging antiarrhythmic drugs.

Dose modification and management for other toxicities*

Grade 1 or 2	Grade 3	Grade 4
No dose adjustment is required. Initiate appropriate medical therapy and monitor as clinically indicated.	Dose interruption until recovery to Grade ≤1 then resume KISQALI at same dose level. If Grade 3 recurs, Discontinue KISQALI. resume KISQALI at the next lower dose level	Discontinue KISQALI.

*Excluding neutropenia, hepatobiliary toxicity and QT interval prolongation. Grading according to CTCAE Version 4.03.

Dose modification for use with strong CYP3A inhibitors

Avoid concomitant use of KISQALI with strong CYP3A inhibitors and consider an alternative concomitant medication with less potential for CYP3A inhibition. If a strong CYP3A inhibitor must be coadministered, reduce the KISQALI dose to 400 mg once daily. If the strong inhibitor is discontinued, change the KISQALI dose (after at least 5 half-lives of the strong CYP3A inhibitor) to the dose used prior to the initiation of the strong CYP3A inhibitor Dose

Modification for hepatic impairment

No dose adjustment is necessary in patients with mild hepatic impairment (Child-Pugh class A). The recommended starting dose is 400 mg KISQALI once daily for patients with moderate (Child-Pugh class B) and severe hepatic impairment (Child-Pugh class C)

CONTRAINDICATIONS: None.

Further information on **WARNINGS AND PRECAUTIONS**

QT Interval prolongation

KISQALI has been shown to prolong the QT interval in a concentration-dependent manner, with estimated mean increase in QTc interval exceeding 20 ms (22.9 ms (90% CI: 21.6, 24.1)) at the mean steady-state Cmax following administration at 600 mg once daily dose In Study 1 (MONALEESA-2), one patient (0.3%) had >500 msec post-baseline QTcF value (average of triplicate), and nine patients out of 329 patients (3%) had a >60 msec increase from baseline in QTcF intervals (average of triplicate). These ECG changes occurred within the first four weeks of treatment and were reversible with dose interruption. There were no reported cases of Torsades de Pointes. Syncope occurred in 9 patients (2.7%) in the KISQALI plus letrozole arm versus 3 (0.9%) in placebo plus letrozole arm. On the KISQALI plus letrozole treatment arm, there was one (0.3%) sudden death in a patient with Grade 3 hypokalemia and Grade 2 QT prolongation. Assess ECG prior to initiation of treatment. Initiate treatment with KISQALI only in patients with QTcF values less than 450 msec. Repeat ECG at approximately Day 14 of the first cycle and the beginning of the second cycle, and as clinically indicated. Monitor serum electrolytes (including potassium, calcium, phosphorous and magnesium) prior to the initiation of treatment, at the beginning of the first 6 cycles, and as clinically indicated. Correct any abnormality before starting KISQALI therapy.

Avoid the use of KISQALI in patients who already have or who are at significant risk of developing QTc prolongation, including patients with:

- long QT syndrome
- uncontrolled or significant cardiac disease including recent myocardial infarction, congestive heart failure, unstable angina and bradyarrhythmias
- electrolyte abnormalities

Avoid using KISQALI with drugs known to prolong QTc interval and/or strong CYP3A inhibitors as this may lead to prolongation of the QTcF interval. Based on the observed QT prolongation during treatment, KISQALI may require dose interruption, reduction or discontinuation as described.

Hepatobiliary toxicity

In Study 1, increases in transaminases were observed. Grade 3 or 4 increases in ALT (10% versus 1%) and AST (7% versus 2%) were reported in the KISQALI and placebo arms, respectively. Among the patients who had Grade ≥ 3 ALT/AST elevation, the median time-to-onset was 57 days for the KISQALI plus letrozole treatment group. The median time to resolution to Grade ≤ 2 was 24 days in the

KISQALI plus letrozole treatment group. Concurrent elevations in ALT or AST greater than three times the ULN and total bilirubin greater than two times the ULN, with normal alkaline phosphatase, in the absence of cholestasis occurred in 4 (1%) patients in Study 1 and all patients recovered after discontinuation of KISQALI.

Perform LFTs before initiating therapy with KISQALI.

Monitor LFTs every 2 weeks for first 2 cycles, at the beginning of each subsequent 4 cycles, and as clinically indicated. Based on the severity of the transaminase elevations, KISQALI may require dose interruption, reduction, or discontinuation as described (Dose Modification and Management for Hepatobiliary Toxicity) Recommendations for patients who have elevated AST/ALT Grade ≥ 3 at baseline have not been established.

Neutropenia

In Study 1, neutropenia was the most frequently reported adverse reaction (75%) and a Grade 3/4 decrease in neutrophil count (based on laboratory findings) was reported in 60% of patients receiving KISQALI plus letrozole. Among the patients who had Grade 2, 3, or 4 neutropenia, the median time to Grade > 2 neutropenia was 16 days. The median time to resolution of Grade ≥ 3 (to normalization or Grade < 3) was 15 days in the KISQALI plus letrozole treatment group.

Febrile neutropenia was reported in 1.5% of patients receiving KISQALI and letrozole. Treatment discontinuation due to neutropenia was 0.9%. Perform CBC before initiating therapy with KISQALI.

Monitor CBC every 2 weeks for the first 2 cycles, at the beginning of each subsequent 4 cycles, and as clinically indicated.

Based on the severity of the neutropenia, KISQALI may require dose interruption, reduction or discontinuation as described in above.

Embryo-fetal toxicity

Based on findings from animal studies and the mechanism of action, KISQALI can cause fetal harm when administered to a pregnant woman. In animal reproduction studies, administration of ribociclib to pregnant rats and rabbits during organogenesis caused embryo-fetal toxicities at maternal exposures that were 0.6

and 1.5 times the human clinical exposure, respectively, based on area under the curve (AUC). Advise pregnant women of the potential risk to a fetus. Advise women of reproductive potential to use effective contraception during therapy with KISQALI and for at least 3 weeks after the last dose.

ADVERSE REACTIONS

The following adverse reactions are discussed in greater detail in other sections of the labeling:

- QT interval prolongation
- Hepatobiliary toxicity
- Neutropenia

DRUG INTERACTIONS

Drugs that may increase ribociclib plasma concentrations

CYP3A4 inhibitors

Coadministration of a strong CYP3A4 inhibitor (*eg,* ritonavir) increased ribociclib exposure in healthy subjects by 3.2-fold. Avoid concomitant use of strong CYP3A inhibitors (e.g., boceprevir, clarithromycin, conivaptan, grapefruit juice, indinavir, itraconazole, ketoconazole, lopinavir/ritonavir, nefazodone, nelfinavir, posaconazole, ritonavir, saquinavir, and voriconazole) and consider alternative concomitant medications with less potential for CYP3A inhibition. If coadministration of KISQALI with a strong CYP3A inhibitor cannot be avoided, reduce the dose of KISQALI to 400 mg once daily. Instruct patients to avoid pomegranates or pomegranate juice, grapefruit, all of which are known to inhibit cytochrome CYP3A enzymes and may increase the exposure to ribociclib.

Drugs that may decrease ribociclib plasma concentrations

CYP3A4 Inducers

Coadministration of a strong CYP3A4 inducer (eg, rifampin) decreased the plasma exposure of ribociclib in healthy subjects by 89%. Avoid concomitant use of strong CYP3A inducers and consider an alternate concomitant medication with no or minimal potential to induce CYP3A (e.g., phenytoin, rifampin, carbamazepine and St John's Wort (Hypericum perforatum)).

Effect of KISQALI on other drugs

CYP3A substrates with narrow therapeutic index

Coadministration of midazolam (a sensitive CYP3A4 substrate) with multiple doses of KISQALI (400 mg) increased the midazolam exposure by 3.8-fold in healthy subjects, compared with administration of midazolam alone. KISQALI given at the clinically relevant dose of 600 mg is predicted to increase the midazolam AUC by 5.2-fold. Therefore, caution is recommended when KISQALI is administered with CYP3A substrates with a narrow therapeutic index. The dose of a sensitive CYP3A substrate with a narrow therapeutic index, including but not limited to alfentanil, cyclosporine, dihydroergotamine, ergotamine, everolimus, fentanyl, pimozide, quinidine, sirolimus and tacrolimus, may need to be reduced as ribociclib can increase their exposure.

Drugs that prolong the QT interval

Avoid coadministration of KISQALI with medicinal products with a known potential to prolong QT such as antiarrhythmic medicines (including, but not limited to amiodarone, disopyramide, procainamide, quinidine and sotalol), and other drugs that are known to prolong the QT interval (including, but not limited to, chloroquine, halofantrine, clarithromycin, haloperidol, methadone, moxifloxacin, bepridil, pimozide and ondansetron (i.v)).

USE IN SPECIFIC POPULATIONS

Pregnancy risk summary

Based on findings from animal studies and the mechanism of action, KISQALI can cause fetal harm when administered to a pregnant woman. There are no available human data informing the drug-associated risk. In animal reproduction studies, administration of ribociclib to pregnant animals during organogenesis resulted in increased incidences of postimplantation loss and reduced fetal weights in rats and increased incidences of fetal abnormalities in rabbits at exposures 0.6 or 1.5 times the exposure in humans, respectively, at the highest recommended dose of 600 mg/day based on AUC [see Data]. Advise pregnant women of the potential risk to a fetus. The background risk of major birth defects and miscarriage for the indicated population is unknown. However, the background risk of major birth defects is 2-4% and of miscarriage is 15-20% of clinically recognized pregnancies in the U.S. general population.

Data

Animal data

In embryo-fetal development studies in rats and rabbits, pregnant animals received oral doses of ribociclib up to 1000 mg/kg/day and 60 mg/kg/day, respectively, during the period of organogenesis. In rats, 300 mg/kg/day resulted in reduced maternal body weight gain and reduced fetal weights accompanied by skeletal changes related to the lower fetal weights. There were no significant effects on embryo-fetal viability or fetal morphology at 50 or 300 mg/kg/day. In rabbits at doses ≥ 30 mg/kg/day, there were adverse effects on embryo-fetal development including increased incidences of fetal abnormalities (malformations and external, visceral and skeletal variants) and fetal growth (lower fetal weights). These findings included reduced/small lung lobes, additional vessel on the descending aorta, additional vessel on the aortic arch, small eyes, diaphragmatic hernia, absent accessory lobe or (partly) fused lung lobes, reduced/small accessory lung lobe, extra/rudimentary 13th ribs, misshapen hyoid bone, bent hyoid bone alae, and reduced number of phalanges in the pollex. There was no evidence of increased incidence of embryo-fetal mortality. There was no maternal toxicity observed at 30 mg/kg/day. At 300 mg/kg/day in rats and 30 mg/kg/day in rabbits, the maternal systemic exposures (AUC) were approximately 0.6 and 1.5 times, respectively, the exposure in patients at the highest recommended dose of 600 mg/day.

Lactation risk summary

It is not known if ribociclib is present in human milk. There are no data on the effects of ribociclib on the breastfed infant or on milk production. Ribociclib and its metabolites readily passed into the milk of lactating rats. Because of the potential for serious adverse reactions in breastfed infants from KISQALI, advise lactating women not to breastfeed while taking KISQALI and for at least 3 weeks after the last dose.

Data In lactating rats administered a single dose of 50 mg/kg, exposure to ribociclib was 3.56-fold higher in milk compared to maternal plasma.

Females and males of reproductive potential

Pregnancy testing

Based on animal studies, KISQALI can cause fetal harm when administered to a pregnant woman Females of reproductive potential should have a pregnancy test prior to starting treatment with KISQALI.

Contraception

Females

Based on animal studies, KISQALI can cause fetal harm when administered to a pregnant woman. Advise females of reproductive potential to use effective contraception (methods that result in less than 1% pregnancy rates) during treatment with KISQALI and for at least 3 weeks after the last dose.

Infertility

Males

Based on animal studies, KISQALI may impair fertility in males of reproductive potential.

Pediatric use

The safety and efficacy of KISQALI in pediatric patients has not been established.
Geriatric use

Of 334 patients who received KISQALI in Study 1, 150 patients (45%) were ≥65 years of age and 35 patients (11%) were ≥75 years of age. No overall differences in safety or effectiveness of KISQALI were observed between these patients and younger patients.

Hepatic impairment

No dose adjustment is necessary in patients with mild hepatic impairment (Child-Pugh A). A reduced starting dose of 400 mg is recommended in patients with moderate (Child-Pugh B) and severe hepatic impairment (Child-Pugh C). Based on a pharmacokinetic trial in patients with hepatic impairment, mild hepatic impairment had no effect on the exposure of ribociclib. The mean exposure for ribociclib was increased less than 2-fold in patients with moderate (geometric mean ratio [GMR]: 1.50 for Cmax; 1.32 for AUCinf) and severe (GMR: 1.34 for Cmax; 1.29 for AUCinf) hepatic impairment.

OVERDOSAGE

There are no known cases of overdose with KISQALI. General symptomatic and supportive measures should be initiated in all cases of overdose where necessary.

DESCRIPTION

KISQALI (ribociclib) is a kinase inhibitor. The chemical name of ribociclib succinate is: Butanedioic acid—7-cyclopentyl-N,N-dimethyl-2-{[5-(piperazin-1-yl) pyridin-2-yl]amino}-7H-pyrrolo[2,3-d]pyrimidine-6-carboxamide (1/1). Ribociclib succinate is a light yellow to yellowish brown crystalline powder. The molecular formula for ribociclib succinate is $C_{23}H_{30}N_8O \cdot C_4H_6O_4$ and the molecular weight is 552.64 g/mol (Free base: 434.55 g/mol). The chemical structure of ribociclib is shown below: KISQALI film-coated tablets are supplied for oral use and contain 200 mg of ribociclib free base (equivalent to 254.40 mg ribociclib succinate). The tablets also contain colloidal silicon dioxide, crospovidone, hydroxypropylcellulose, magnesium stearate and microcrystalline cellulose. The film-coating contains iron oxide black, iron oxide red, lecithin (soya), polyvinyl alcohol (partially hydrolysed), talc, titanium dioxide, and xanthan gum as inactive ingredients.

CLINICAL PHARMACOLOGY

Pharmacodynamics

Cardiac electrophysiology

Serial, triplicate ECGs were collected following a single dose and at steady-state to evaluate the effect of ribociclib on the QTc interval in patients with advanced cancer. A pharmacokinetic-pharmacodynamic analysis included a total of 267 patients treated with ribociclib at doses ranging from 50 to 1200 mg, including 193 patients treated with ribociclib 600 mg. The analysis suggested that ribociclib causes concentration-dependent increases in the QTc interval. The estimated mean change from baseline in QTcF was 22.9 ms (90% CI: 21.6, 24.1) at the mean observed Cmax at steady state following administration at the recommended 600 mg dose.

Pharmacokinetics

Ribociclib exhibited over-proportional increases in exposure (peak plasma concentrations (Cmax) and area under the time concentration curve (AUC)) across the dose range of 50 mg to 1200 mg following both single dose and repeated doses. Following repeated 600 mg once daily administration, steady state was generally achieved after 8 days and ribociclib accumulated with a geometric mean accumulation ratio of 2.51 (range: 0.972 to 6.40).

Absorption

The time to reach Cmax (Tmax) following ribociclib administration was between 1 and 4 hours.

Food Effect

Compared to the fasted state, oral administration of a single 600 mg dose of KISQALI film-coated tablet with a high-fat, high-calorie meal (approximately 800 to 1000 calories with ~50% calories from fat, ~35% calories from carbohydrates, and ~15% calories from protein) had no effect on the rate and extent of absorption of ribociclib (Cmax GMR: 1.00; 90% CI: 0.898, 1.11; AUCinf GMR: 1.06; 90% CI: 1.01, 1.12).

Distribution

Binding of ribociclib to human plasma proteins in vitro was approximately 70% and independent of concentration (10 to 10,000 ng/mL). Ribociclib was equally distributed between red blood cells and plasma with a mean in vivo blood-toplasma ratio of 1.04. The apparent volume of distribution at steady state (Vss/F) was 1090 L based on population PK analysis.

Metabolism

In vitro and in vivo studies indicated ribociclib undergoes extensive hepatic metabolism mainly via CYP3A4 in humans. Following oral administration of a single 600 mg dose of radio-labeled ribociclib to humans, the primary metabolic pathways for ribociclib involved oxidation (dealkylation, C and/or N-oxygenation, oxidation (-

2H)) and combinations thereof. Phase II conjugates of ribociclib Phase I metabolites involved N-acetylation, sulfation, cysteine conjugation, glycosylation and glucuronidation. Ribociclib was the major circulating drug-derived entity in plasma (44%). The major circulating metabolites included metabolite M13 (CCI284, N-hydroxylation), M4 (LEQ803, N-demethylation), and M1 (secondary glucuronide), each representing an estimated 9%, 9%, and 8% of total radioactivity, and 22%, 20%, and 18% of ribociclib exposure.

Clinical activity (pharmacological and safety) of ribociclib

This was due primarily to parent drug, with negligible contribution from circulating metabolites. Ribociclib was extensively metabolized with unchanged drug accounting for 17% and 12% in feces and urine, respectively. Metabolite LEQ803 was a significant metabolite in excreta and represented approximately 14% and 4% of the administered dose in feces and urine, respectively. Numerous other metabolites were detected in both feces and urine in minor amounts (≤ 3% of the administered dose).

Elimination

The geometric mean plasma effective half-life (based on accumulation ratio) was 32.0 hours (63% CV) and the geometric mean apparent oral clearance (CL/F) was 25.5 L/hr (66% CV) at steady-state at 600 mg in patients with advanced cancer. The geometric mean apparent plasma terminal half-life (T1/2) of ribociclib ranged from 29.7 to 54.7 hours and geometric mean CL/F of ribociclib ranged from 39.9 to 77.5 L/hr at 600 mg across studies in healthy subjects. Ribociclib is eliminated mainly via feces, with a small contribution of the renal route. In 6 healthy male subjects, following a single oral dose of radio-labeled ribociclib, 92% of the total administered radioactive dose was recovered within 22 days; feces was the major route of excretion (69%), with 23% of the dose recovered in urine.

Specific populations

Patients with hepatic impairment

Based on a pharmacokinetic trial in patients with hepatic impairment, mild (Child-Pugh class A) hepatic impairment had no effect on the exposure of ribociclib. The mean exposure for ribociclib was increased less than 2-fold in patients with moderate (Child-Pugh class B; geometric mean ratio [GMR]: 1.50 for Cmax; 1.32 for AUCinf) and severe (Child-Pugh class C; GMR: 1.34 for Cmax; 1.29 for AUCinf) hepatic impairment. Based on a population pharmacokinetic analysis that included 160 patients with normal hepatic function and 47 patients with mild hepatic impairment, mild hepatic impairment had no effect on the exposure of ribociclib, further supporting the findings from the dedicated hepatic impairment study.

Patients with renal impairment

The pharmacokinetics of ribociclib in patients with severe renal impairment (eGFR < 30 mL/min/1.73m^2) is unknown. Mild (60 mL/min/1.73m^2 ≤ eGFR < 90 mL/min/1.73m^2) and moderate (30 mL/min/1.73m^2 ≤ eGFR < 60 mL/min/1.73m^2) renal impairment had no effect on the exposure of ribociclib based on a population pharmacokinetic analysis (PK) analysis.

Effect of age, weight, gender, and race

Population PK analysis showed that there are no clinically relevant effects of age, body weight, gender, or race on the systemic exposure of ribociclib.

Drug interaction studies

Drugs that affect ribociclib plasma concentrations

CYP3A inhibitors

A drug interaction trial in healthy subjects was conducted with ritonavir (a strong CYP3A inhibitor). Compared to ribociclib alone, ritonavir (100 mg twice a day for 14 days) increased ribociclib Cmax and AUCinf by 1.7-fold and 3.2-fold, respectively, following a single 400 mg ribociclib dose. Cmax and AUC for LEQ803 (a prominent metabolite of LEE011, accounting for less than 10% of parent exposure) decreased by 96% and 98%, respectively. A moderate CYP3A4 inhibitor (erythromycin) is predicted to increase ribociclib Cmax and AUC by 1.3-fold and 1.9-fold, respectively.

CYP3A inducers

A drug interaction trial in healthy subjects was conducted with rifampicin (a strong CYP3A4 inducer). Compared to ribociclib alone, rifampicin (600 mg daily for 14 days) decreased ribociclib Cmax and AUCinf by 81% and 89%, respectively, following a single 600 mg ribociclib dose. Cmax increased 1.7-fold and AUCinf decreased by 27%, respectively. A moderate CYP3A inducer (efavirenz) is predicted to decrease ribociclib Cmax and AUC by 37% and 60%, respectively.

Drugs that are affected by KISQALI

CYP3A4 and CYP1A2 substrates

A drug interaction trial in healthy subjects was conducted as a cocktail study with midazolam (sensitive CYP3A4 substrate) and caffeine (sensitive CYP1A2 substrate). Compared to midazolam and caffeine alone, multiple doses of ribociclib (400 mg once daily for 8 days) increased midazolam Cmax and AUCinf by 2.1- fold and 3.8-fold, respectively. Administration of ribociclib at 600 mg once daily is predicted to increase midazolam Cmax and AUC by 2.4-fold and 5.2-fold, respectively. The effect of multiple doses of 400 mg ribociclib on caffeine was minimal, with Cmax decreased by 10% and AUCinf increased slightly by 20%. Only weak inhibitory effects on CYP1A2 substrates are predicted at 600 mg ribociclib once daily dose.

Gastric pH-elevating agents

Coadministration of ribociclib with drugs that elevate the gastric pH was not evaluated in a clinical trial; however, altered ribociclib absorption was not identified in a population PK analysis and was not predicted using physiology-based PK models.

Letrozole

Data from a clinical trial in patients with breast cancer and population PK analysis indicated no drug interaction between ribociclib and letrozole following coadministration of the drugs.

Anastrozole

Data from a clinical trial in patients with breast cancer indicated no clinically relevant drug interaction between ribociclib and anastrozole following coadministration of the drugs.

Exemestane

Data from a clinical trial in patients with breast cancer indicated no clinically relevant drug interaction between ribociclib and exemestane following coadministration of the drugs.

Effect of ribociclib on CYP enzymes

In vitro, ribociclib was a reversible inhibitor of CYP1A2, CYP2E1 and CYP3A4/5 and a time-dependent inhibitor of CYP3A4/5, at clinically relevant concentrations. In vitro evaluations indicated that KISQALI has no potential to inhibit the activities of CYP2A6, CYP2B6, CYP2C8, CYP2C9, CYP2C19, and CYP2D6 at clinically relevant concentrations. It has no potential for time-dependent inhibition of CYP1A2, CYP2C9, and CYP2D6, and no induction of CYP1A2, CYP2B6, CYP2C9 and CYP3A4 at clinically relevant concentrations.

Effect of ribociclib on transporters

In vitro evaluations indicated that KISQALI has a low potential to inhibit the activities of drug transporters P-gp, OATP1B1/B3, OCT1, MATEK2 at clinically relevant concentrations. KISQALI may inhibit BCRP, OCT2, MATE1, and human BSEP at clinically relevant concentrations.

Effect of transporters on ribociclib

Based on in vitro data, P-gp and BCRP mediated transport are unlikely to affect the extent of oral absorption of ribociclib at therapeutic doses.

Therapeutic efficacy in the management of breast cancer

i). Ribociclib, when added to endocrine therapy, significantly improves PFS and has manageable toxicity in premenopausal/perimenopausal and postmenopausal women with HR+/HER2− advanced breast cancer.

Rascon K, et al. Ribociclib in HR+/HER2− Advanced or Metastatic Breast Cancer Patients. Annals of Pharmacotherapy. 2019; 53(5):501-509. doi:10.1177/1060028018817904

ii). Novartis press release, 2017

Novartis Kisqali® (ribociclib) receives EU approval as first-line treatment for HR+/HER2- locally advanced or metastatic breast cancer in combination with any aromatase inhibitor.

- *Approval is based on pivotal MONALEESA-2 trial, which showed Kisqali plus letrozole reduced risk of disease progression or death by 43% versus letrozole alone*
- *Kisqali plus letrozole demonstrated a median progression-free survival (PFS) of 25.3 months versus 16.0 months of patients who received letrozole alone*
- *Kisqali plus letrozole demonstrated rapid clinical improvement in patients with measurable disease, with 76% seeing a reduction in tumor size after only eight weeks versus 67% with letrozole alone*
- *Up to one-third of patients with early-stage breast cancer will subsequently develop advanced disease3; globally an estimated 250,000 women are diagnosed with advanced breast cancer each year*

9.12. LAPATINIB (TYKERB®)

TYKERB® (lapatinib) tablets, for oral use. Initial U.S. Approval: 2007.

WARNING: HEPATOTOXICITY See full prescribing information for complete boxed warning. Hepatotoxicity has been observed in clinical trials and postmarketing experience. The hepatotoxicity may be severe and deaths have been reported. Causality of the deaths is uncertain

RECENT MAJOR CHANGES

Warnings and Precautions, QT Prolongation 09/2018

Warnings and Precautions, Embryo-fetal toxicity 09/2018

MECHANISM OF ACTION

Lapatinib is a 4-anilinoquinazoline kinase inhibitor of the intracellular tyrosine kinase domains of both Epidermal Growth Factor Receptor (EGFR [ErbB1]) and of Human Epidermal Receptor Type 2 (HER2 [ErbB2]) receptors (estimated Ki app values of 3nM and 13nM, respectively) with a dissociation half-life of greater than or equal to 300 minutes. Lapatinib inhibits ErbB-driven tumor cell growth in vitro and in various animal models. An additive effect was demonstrated in an in vitro study when lapatinib and 5-FU (the active metabolite of capecitabine) were used in combination in the 4 tumor cell lines tested. The growth inhibitory effects of lapatinib were evaluated in trastuzumab-conditioned cell lines. Lapatinib retained significant activity against breast cancer cell lines selected for long-term growth in trastuzumab-containing medium in vitro. These in vitro findings suggest non-cross-resistance between these two agents. Hormone receptor-positive breast cancer cells (with ER [Estrogen Receptor] and/or PgR [Progesterone Receptor]) that coexpress the HER2 tend to be resistant to established endocrine therapies. Similarly, hormone receptor-positive breast cancer cells that initially lack EGFR or HER2 upregulate these receptor proteins as the tumor becomes resistant to endocrine therapy.

DESCRIPTION

Lapatinib is a small molecule and a member of the 4-anilinoquinazoline class of kinase inhibitors. It is present as the monohydrate of the ditosylate salt, with chemical name N-(3-chloro-4-{[(3- fluorophenyl)methyl]oxy}phenyl)-6-[5-({[2-(methylsulfonyl)ethyl]amino}methyl)-2-furanyl]-4- quinazolinamine bis(4-methylbenzenesulfonate) monohydrate. It has the molecular formula C29H26ClFN4O4S (C7H8O3S)2 H2O and a molecular weight of 943.5. Lapatinib ditosylate monohydrate has the following chemical structure: Lapatinib is a yellow solid, and its solubility in water is 0.007 mg/mL and in 0.1N HCl is 0.001 mg/mL at 25°C. Each 250 mg tablet of TYKERB contains 405 mg of lapatinib ditosylate monohydrate, equivalent to 398 mg of lapatinib ditosylate or 250 mg lapatinib free base.

INDICATIONS AND USAGE

TYKERB is a kinase inhibitor indicated in combination with:

• capecitabine for the treatment of patients with advanced or metastatic breast cancer whose tumors overexpress human epidermal growth factor receptor 2 (HER2) and who have received prior therapy including an anthracycline, a taxane, and trastuzumab.

Limitations of use

Patients should have disease progression on trastuzumab prior to initiation of treatment with TYKERB in combination with capecitabine.

• letrozole for the treatment of postmenopausal women with hormone receptorpositive metastatic breast cancer that overexpresses the HER2 receptor for whom hormonal therapy is indicated. TYKERB in combination with an aromatase inhibitor has not been compared to a trastuzumab-containing chemotherapy regimen for the treatment of metastatic breast cancer.

DOSAGE AND ADMINISTRATION

The recommended dosage of TYKERB for advanced or metastatic breast cancer is 1,250 mg (5 tablets) given orally once daily on Days 1-21 continuously in combination with capecitabine 2,000 mg/m^2 /day (administered orally in 2 doses approximately 12 hours apart) on Days 1-14 in a repeating 21-day cycle.

The recommended dose of TYKERB for hormone receptor-positive, HER2-positive metastatic breast cancer is 1,500 mg (6 tablets) given orally once daily continuously in combination with letrozole. When TYKERB is coadministered with letrozole, the recommended dose of letrozole is 2.5 mg once daily.

• TYKERB should be taken at least one hour before or one hour after a meal. However, capecitabine should be taken with food or within 30 minutes after food.

• TYKERB should be taken once daily. Do not divide daily doses of TYKERB.

• Modify dose for cardiac and other toxicities, severe hepatic impairment, diarrhea, and CYP3A4 drug interactions.

DOSAGE FORMS AND STRENGTHS

250 mg tablets

CONTRAINDICATIONS

Known severe hypersensitivity (e.g., anaphylaxis) to this product or any of its components.

WARNINGS AND PRECAUTIONS

• Decreases in left ventricular ejection fraction (LVEF) have been reported. Confirm normal LVEF before starting TYKERB and continue evaluations during treatment.

Ejection fraction is commonly measured by echocardiography, although cardiac magnetic resonance imaging (MRI), cardiac computed tomography, ventriculography and nuclear medicine (gated SPECT and radionuclide angiography) scans may also be used. Measurements by different modalities are not interchangeable. Historically, the gold standard for measurement of the ejection fraction was ventriculography but cardiac MRI is now considered the best method. Healthy 8ndividuals typically have ejection fractions between 50% and 65%.

Figure 98. Four chamber view on cardiovascular magnetic resonance imaging using a steady-state free precession imaging technique.

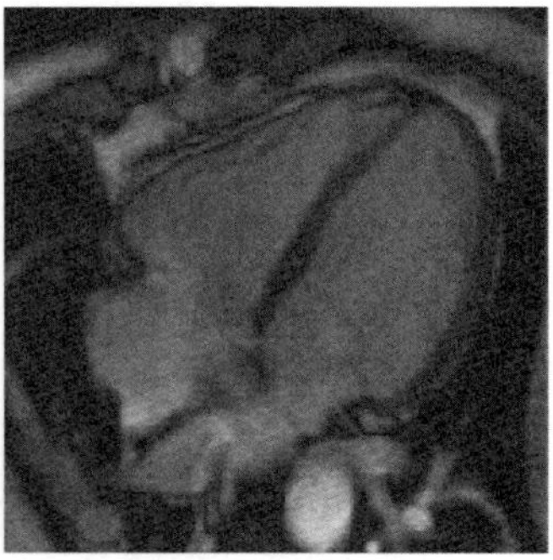

- TYKERB has been associated with hepatotoxicity. Monitor liver function tests before initiation of treatment, every 4 to 6 weeks during treatment, and as clinically indicated. Discontinue and do not restart TYKERB if patients experience severe changes in liver function tests.
- Dose reduction in patients with severe hepatic impairment should be considered.
- Diarrhea, including severe diarrhea, has been reported during treatment. Manage with antidiarrheal agents, and replace fluids and electrolytes if severe.

• TYKERB has been associated with interstitial lung disease and pneumonitis. Discontinue TYKERB if patients experience severe pulmonary symptoms.

• TYKERB may prolong the QT interval in some patients. Consider electrocardiogram (ECG) and electrolyte monitoring.

• Severe cutaneous reactions have been reported. Discontinue TYKERB if life-threatening reactions are suspected.

• TYKERB can cause fetal harm. Advise patients of the potential risk to the fetus and to use effective contraception.

ADVERSE REACTIONS

The most common (greater than 20%) adverse reactions during treatment with TYKERB plus capecitabine were diarrhea, palmar-plantar erythrodysesthesia, nausea, rash, vomiting, and fatigue. The most common (greater than or equal to 20%) adverse reactions during treatment with TYKERB plus letrozole were diarrhea, rash, nausea, and fatigue. To report SUSPECTED ADVERSE REACTIONS, contact Novartis Pharmaceuticals Corporation at 1-888-669-6682 or FDA at 1-800-FDA-1088 or www.fda.gov/medwatch.

USE IN SPECIFIC POPULATIONS

• Lactation

Advise not to breastfeed

• Females and males of reproductive potential

Verify the pregnancy status of females prior to initiation of TYKERB

DRUG INTERACTIONS

• TYKERB is likely to increase exposure to concomitantly administered drugs which are substrates of CYP3A4, CYP2C8, or P-glycoprotein (ABCB1).

• Avoid strong CYP3A4 inhibitors. If unavoidable, consider dose reduction of TYKERB in patients coadministered a strong CYP3A4 inhibitor.

• Avoid strong CYP3A4 inducers. If unavoidable, consider gradual dose increase of TYKERB in patients coadministered a strong CYP3A4 inducer.

FULL PRESCRIBING INFORMATION WARNING: HEPATOTOXICITY

Hepatotoxicity has been observed in clinical trials and postmarketing experience. The hepatotoxicity may be severe, and deaths have been reported. Causality of the deaths is uncertain.

Figure 99. Acute liver failure (with hepatocellular necrosis and sinusoidal bleeding). This case was caused by Marburg virus, a rare cause of acute liver failure.

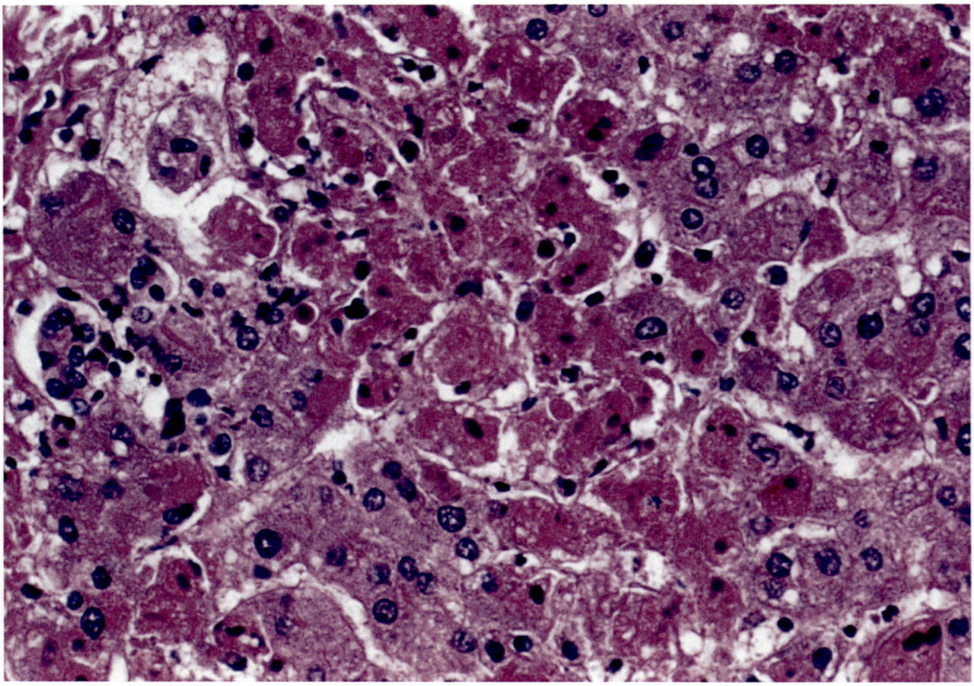

This image is by By Photo Credit:Content Providers(s): CDC/ Dr. J. Lyle Conrad - This media comes from the Centers for Disease Control and Prevention's Public Health Image Library (PHIL), with identification number #6559. Public Domain, https://commons.wikimedia.org/w/index.php?curid=2309971. https://en.wikipedia.org/wiki/Acute_liver_failure#/media/File:Marburg_virus_liver_injury.jpg. This image is a work of the Centers for Disease Control and Prevention, part of the United States Department of Health and Human Services, taken or made as part of an employee's official duties. As a work of the U.S. federal government, the image is in the public domain. No changes have been made to this image.

Figure 100.. A person with massive ascites and caput medusae due to cirrhotic liver failure.(Caput medusae is the appearance of distended and engorged superficial epigastric veins, which are seen radiating from the umbilicus across the abdomen. The name caput medusae (Latin for "head of Medusa") originates from the apparent similarity to Medusa's head, which had venomous snakes in place of hair. It is also a sign of portal hypertension)

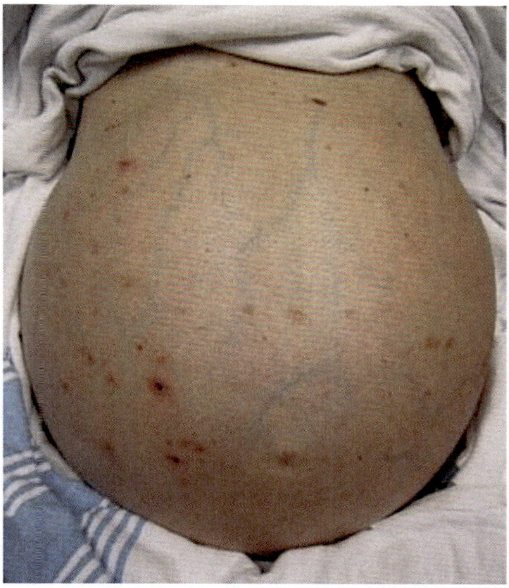

This image is by By James Heilman, MD - Own work, CC BY-SA 3.0, https://commons.wikimedia.org/w/index.php?curid=15335623. https://en.wikipedia.org/wiki/Liver_failure#/media/File:Hepaticfailure.jpg. This file is licensed under the Creative Commons Attribution-Share Alike 3.0 Unported license. No changes have been made to this image.

INDICATIONS AND USAGE

TYKERB® is indicated in combination with:

• capecitabine for the treatment of patients with advanced or metastatic breast cancer whose tumors overexpress human epidermal growth factor receptor 2 (HER2) and who have received prior therapy including an anthracycline, a taxane, and trastuzumab.

Limitations of use

Patients should have disease progression on trastuzumab prior to initiation of treatment with TYKERB in combination with capecitabine.

• letrozole for the treatment of postmenopausal women with hormone receptor-positive metastatic breast cancer that overexpresses the HER2 receptor for whom hormonal therapy is indicated. TYKERB in combination with an aromatase inhibitor has not been compared to a trastuzumab-containing chemotherapy regimen for the treatment of metastatic breast cancer.

DOSAGE AND ADMINISTRATION

Recommended Dosing

HER2-Positive Metastatic Breast Cancer

The recommended dose of TYKERB is 1,250 mg given orally once daily on Days 1-21 continuously in combination with capecitabine 2,000 mg/m^2 /day (administered orally in 2 doses approximately 12 hours apart) on Days 1-14 in a repeating 21-day cycle. TYKERB should be taken at least one hour before or one hour after a meal. The dose of TYKERB should be once daily (5 tablets administered all at once); dividing the daily dose is not recommended. Capecitabine should be taken with food or within 30 minutes after food. If a day's dose is missed, the patient should not double the dose the next day. Treatment should be continued until disease progression or unacceptable toxicity occurs.

Hormone receptor-positive, HER2-positive metastatic breast cancer

The recommended dose of TYKERB is 1,500 mg given orally once daily continuously in combination with letrozole. When coadministered with TYKERB, the recommended dose of letrozole is 2.5 mg once daily. TYKERB should be taken at least one hour before or one hour after a meal. The dose of TYKERB should be once daily (6 tablets administered all at once); dividing the daily dose is not recommended.

Dose modification guidelines

Cardiac events

TYKERB should be discontinued in patients with a decreased left ventricular ejection fraction (LVEF) that is Grade 2 or greater by National Cancer Institute Common

Terminology Criteria for Adverse Events (NCI CTCAE v3.0), and in patients with an LVEF that drops below the institution's lower limit of normal (LLN).

TYKERB in combination with capecitabine may be restarted at a reduced dose (1,000 mg/day) and in combination with letrozole may be restarted at a reduced dose of 1,250 mg/day after a minimum of 2 weeks if the LVEF recovers to normal and the patient is asymptomatic.

Hepatic Impairment

Patients with severe hepatic impairment (Child-Pugh Class C) should have their dose of TYKERB reduced (see below). A dose reduction from 1,250 mg/day to 750 mg/day (HER2-positive metastatic breast cancer indication) or from 1,500 mg/day to 1,000 mg/day (hormone receptor-positive, HER2-positive breast cancer indication) in patients with severe hepatic impairment is predicted to adjust the area under the curve (AUC) to the normal range and should be considered. However, there are no clinical data with this dose adjustment in patients with severe hepatic impairment.

Table 3. The Child-Pugh score for cirrhosis mortality

Bilirubin (Total) <2 mg/dL (<34.2 µmol/L) +1. 2-3 mg/dL (34.2-51.3 µmol/L) +2. ...

Albumin. >3.5 g/dL (>35 g/L) +1. 2.8-3.5 g/dL (28-35 g/L) +2. ...

INR. <1.7. +1. 1.7-2.2. +2. ...

Ascites. Absent. +1. Slight. +2. ...

Encephalopathy. See encephalopathy grades in Evidence > Facts & Figures. No Encephalopathy. +1.

The severity of cirrhosis is as follows: Child-Pugh A: 5 to 6 points. Child-Pugh B: 7 to 9 points. Child-Pugh C: 10 to 15 points.

Diarrhea

TYKERB should be interrupted in patients with diarrhea which is NCI CTCAE Grade 3 or Grade 1 or 2 with complicating features (moderate to severe abdominal cramping, nausea or vomiting greater than or equal to NCI CTCAE Grade 2, decreased performance status, fever, sepsis, neutropenia, frank bleeding, or dehydration). TYKERB may be reintroduced at a lower dose (reduced from 1,250 mg/day to 1,000 mg/day or from 1,500 mg/day to 1,250 mg/day) when diarrhea resolves to Grade 1 or less. TYKERB should be permanently discontinued in patients with diarrhea which is NCI CTCAE Grade 4.

Concomitant strong CYP3A4 inhibitors

The concomitant use of strong CYP3A4 inhibitors should be avoided (e.g., ketoconazole, itraconazole, clarithromycin, atazanavir, indinavir, nefazodone, nelfinavir, ritonavir, saquinavir, telithromycin, voriconazole). Grapefruit may also increase plasma concentrations of lapatinib and should be avoided. If patients must be coadministered a strong CYP3A4 inhibitor, based on pharmacokinetic studies, a dose reduction to 500 mg/day of lapatinib is predicted to adjust the lapatinib AUC to the range observed without inhibitors and should be considered. However, there are no clinical data with this dose adjustment in patients receiving strong CYP3A4 inhibitors. If the strong inhibitor is discontinued, a washout period of approximately 1 week should be allowed before the TYKERB dose is adjusted upward to the indicated dose.

Concomitant strong CYP3A4 inducers

The concomitant use of strong CYP3A4 inducers should be avoided (e.g., dexamethasone, phenytoin, carbamazepine, rifampin, rifabutin, rifapentin, phenobarbital, St. John's wort). If patients must be coadministered a strong CYP3A4 inducer, based on pharmacokinetic studies, the dose of TYKERB should be titrated gradually from 1,250 mg/day up to 4,500 mg/day (HER2-positive metastatic breast cancer indication) or from 1,500 mg/day up to 5,500 mg/day (hormone receptor-positive, HER2-positive breast cancer indication) based on tolerability. This dose of TYKERB is predicted to adjust the lapatinib AUC to the range observed without inducers and should be considered. However, there are no clinical data with this dose adjustment in patients receiving strong CYP3A4 inducers. If the strong inducer is discontinued the TYKERB dose should be reduced to the indicated dose

Other toxicities

Discontinuation or interruption of dosing with TYKERB may be considered when patients develop greater than or equal to Grade 2 NCI CTCAE toxicity, and can be restarted at the standard dose of 1,250 or 1,500 mg/day when the toxicity improves to Grade 1 or less. If the toxicity recurs, then TYKERB in combination with capecitabine should be restarted at a lower dose (1,000 mg/day) and in combination with letrozole should be restarted at a lower dose of 1,250 mg/day.

DOSAGE FORMS AND STRENGTHS: 250 mg tablets

CONTRAINDICATIONS

TYKERB is contraindicated in patients with known severe hypersensitivity (e.g., anaphylaxis) to this product or any of its components.

Further information on **WARNINGS AND PRECAUTIONS**

Decreased left ventricular ejection fraction

TYKERB has been reported to decrease LVEF. In clinical trials, the majority (greater than 57%) of LVEF decreases occurred within the first 12 weeks of treatment; however, data on longterm exposure are limited. Caution should be taken if TYKERB is to be administered to patients with conditions that could impair left ventricular function. LVEF should be evaluated in all patients prior to initiation of treatment with TYKERB to ensure that the patient has a baseline LVEF that is within the institution's normal limits. LVEF should continue to be evaluated during treatment with TYKERB to ensure that LVEF does not decline below the institutions normal.

Hepatotoxicity

Hepatotoxicity [alanine aminotransferase, (ALT) or aspartate aminotransferase], (AST) greater than 3 times the upper limit of normal (ULN) and total bilirubin greater than 2 times the ULN] has been observed in clinical trials (less than 1% of patients) and postmarketing experience. The hepatotoxicity may be severe and deaths have been reported. Causality of the deaths is uncertain. The hepatotoxicity may occur days to several months after initiation of treatment. Liver function tests (transaminases, bilirubin, and alkaline phosphatase) should be monitored before initiation of treatment, every 4 to 6 weeks during treatment, and as clinically indicated. If changes in liver function are severe, therapy with TYKERB should be discontinued and patients should not be retreated with TYKERB.

Patients with severe hepatic impairment

If TYKERB is to be administered to patients with severe preexisting hepatic impairment, dose reduction should be considered. In patients who develop severe hepatotoxicity while on therapy, TYKERB should be discontinued, and patients should not be retreated with TYKERB

Diarrhea

Diarrhea has been reported during treatment with TYKERB. The diarrhea may be severe, and deaths have been reported. Diarrhea generally occurs early during treatment with TYKERB, with almost half of those patients with diarrhea first experiencing it within 6 days. This usually lasts 4 to 5 days. TYKERB-induced diarrhea is usually low-grade, with severe diarrhea of NCI CTCAE Grades 3 and 4 occurring in less than 10% and less than 1% of patients, respectively. Early identification and intervention is critical for the optimal management of diarrhea. Patients should be instructed to report any change in bowel patterns immediately. Prompt treatment of diarrhea with antidiarrheal agents (such as loperamide) after the first unformed stool is recommended. Severe cases of diarrhea may require administration of oral or intravenous electrolytes and fluids, use of antibiotics such as fluoroquinolones (especially if diarrhea is persistent beyond 24 hours, there is fever, or Grade 3 or 4 neutropenia), and interruption or discontinuation of therapy with TYKERB.

Interstitial lung disease/pneumonitis

TYKERB has been associated with interstitial lung disease and pneumonitis in monotherapy or in combination with other chemotherapies. Patients should be monitored for pulmonary symptoms indicative of interstitial lung disease or pneumonitis. TYKERB should be discontinued in patients who experience pulmonary symptoms indicative of interstitial lung disease/pneumonitis which are greater than or equal to Grade 3 (NCI CTCAE v3.0).

QT Prolongation

A concentration-dependent QT prolongation has been associated with TYKERB. Monitor patients who have or may develop prolongation of QTc during treatment with TYKERB. These conditions include patients with hypokalemia or hypomagnesemia, with congenital long QT syndrome, patients taking antiarrhythmic medicines or other medicinal products with known risk for QT prolongation/ Torsades de Pointes (TdP), and cumulative high-dose anthracycline therapy. Correct hypokalemia or hypomagnesemia prior to TYKERB administration.

Severe cutaneous reactions

Severe cutaneous reactions have been reported with TYKERB. If life-threatening reactions such as erythema multiforme *(Figures 101, 102 and 103)*), Stevens-Johnson syndrome, or toxic epidermal necrolysis (e.g., progressive skin rash often with blisters or mucosal lesions) are suspected, discontinue treatment with TYKERB.

Figure 101. A case of erythema nodosum.

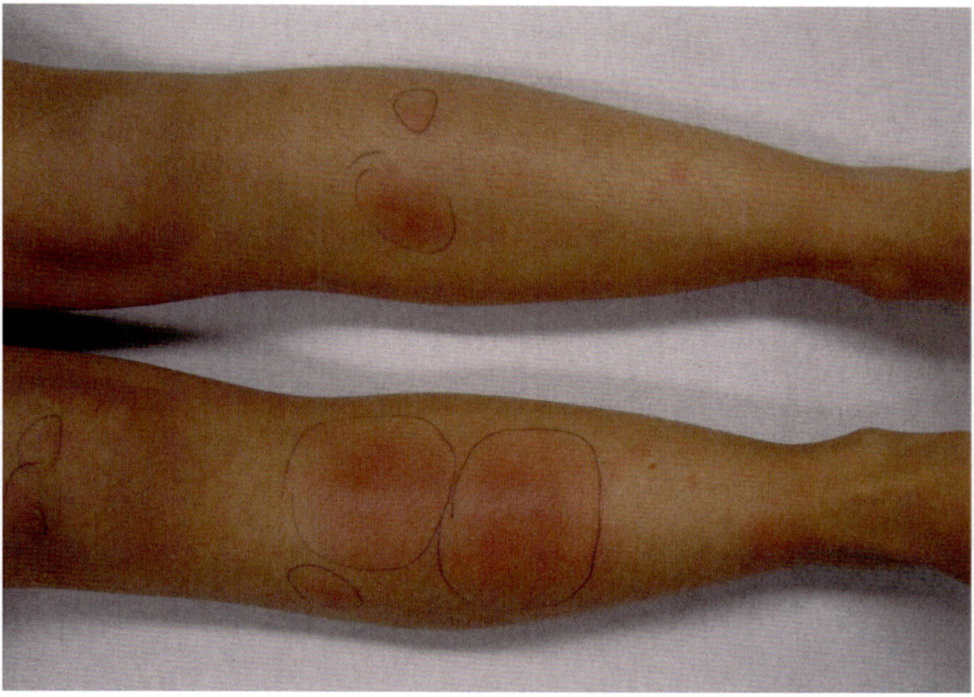

This image is by James Heilman, MD - Own work, CC BY-SA 3.0, https://commons.wikimedia.org/w/index.php?curid=11520780. https://en.wikipedia.org/wiki/Erythema_nodosum#/media/File:ENlegs.JPG. This file is licensed under the Creative Commons Attribution-Share Alike 3.0 Unported license. No changes were made to this image.

Figure 102. A single lesion of erythema nodosum.

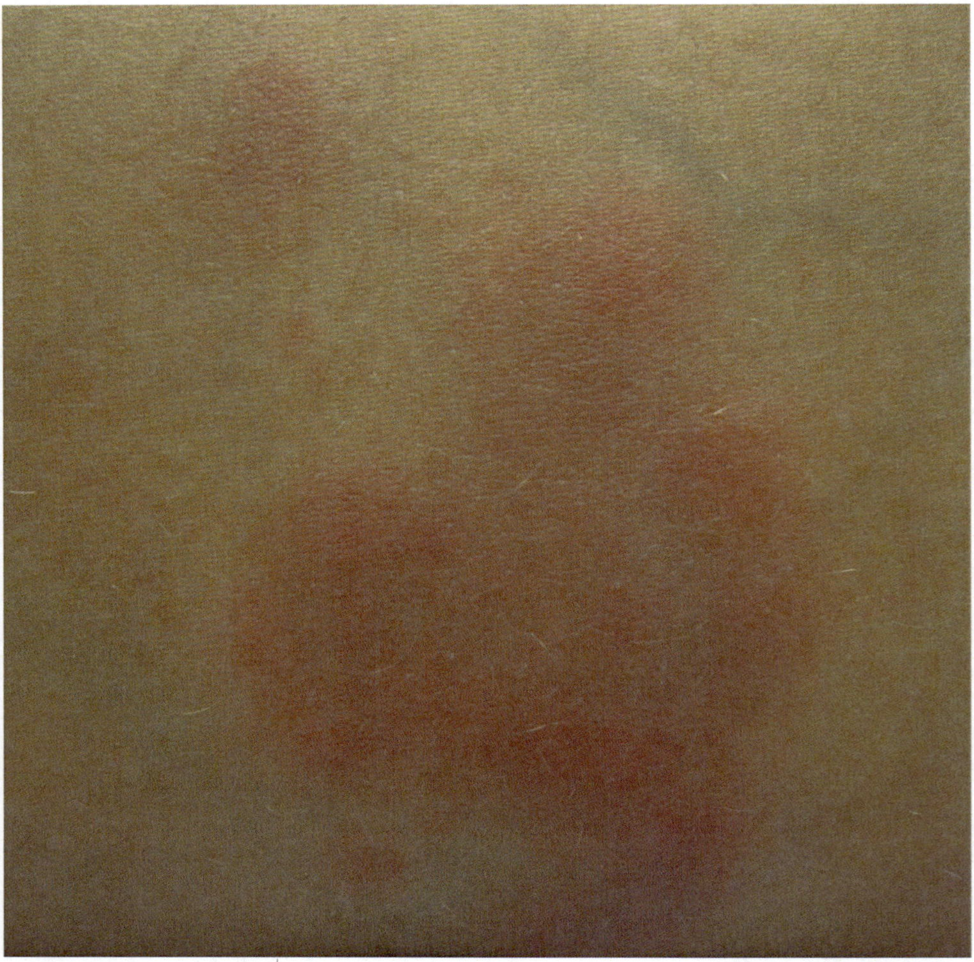

This image is by James Heilman, MD - Own work, CC BY-SA 3.0, https://commons.wikimedia.org/w/index.php?curid=11520795. https://en.wikipedia.org/wiki/Erythema_nodosum#/media/File:A_single_EN.JPG.

Figure 103. Several lesions of erythema nodosum in an individual with dark skin.

This image is by By Medicalpal - Own work, CC BY-SA 4.0, https://commons.wikimedia.org/w/index.php?curid=67154089. https://en.wikipedia.org/wiki/Erythema_nodosum#/media/File:Erythema_Nodosum.jp

g. This file is licensed under the Creative Commons Attribution-Share Alike 4.0 International license. No changeswere made to this image.

Figure 103. Several lesions of erythema nodosum in an individual with dark skin.

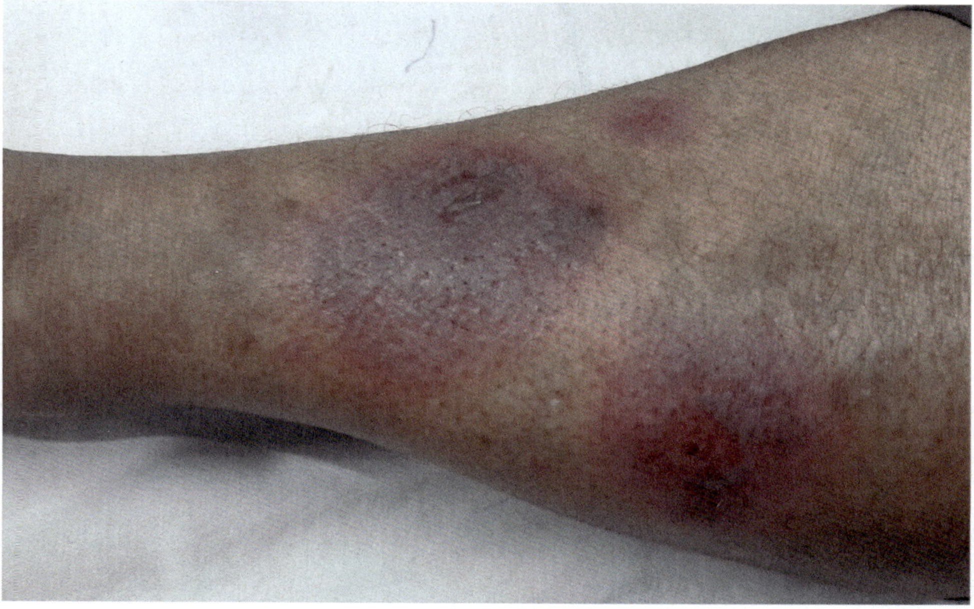

Embryo-fetal toxicity

Based on its mechanism of action and findings in animal studies, TYKERB can cause fetal harm when administered to a pregnant woman. In animal reproductive studies, administration of lapatinib to pregnant rats during the period of organogenesis and through lactation led to death of offspring within the first 4 days after birth at maternal exposures that were ≥ 3.3 times the human clinical exposure based on AUC following 1250 mg dose of lapatinib plus capecitabine. When administered to pregnant animals during the period of organogenesis, lapatinib caused fetal anomalies (rats) or abortions (rabbits) at maternally toxic doses (with maternal exposures approximately 6.4 and 0.2 times, respectively, the human clinical exposure based on AUC following 1250 mg dose of lapatinib plus capecitabine). Advise pregnant women and females of reproductive potential of the potential risk to the fetus. Verify the pregnancy status of females of reproductive potential prior to initiation of TYKERB. Advise females of reproductive potential to use effective contraception during treatment with TYKERB and for 1 week after the last dose. Advise male patients with female partners of reproductive potential to use effective contraception during treatment with TYKERB and for 1 week after the last dose

HER2-positive metastatic breast cancer

The safety of TYKERB has been evaluated in more than 12,000 patients in clinical trials. The efficacy and safety of TYKERB in combination with capecitabine in breast cancer was evaluated in 198 patients in a randomized, Phase 3 trial. The most common adverse reactions (greater than 20%) during therapy with TYKERB plus capecitabine were gastrointestinal (diarrhea, nausea, and vomiting), dermatologic (palmar-plantar erythrodysesthesia *(Figure 104)* and rash), and fatigue.

Figure 104. Capecitabine-induced acral erythema of the foot

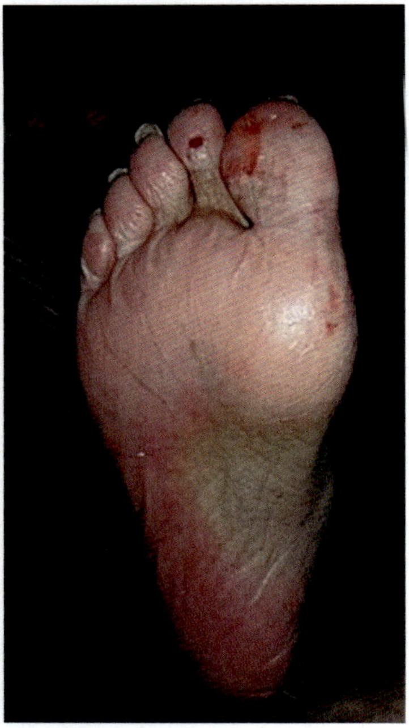

This image is by Maria Sieglinda von Nudeldorf - Own work, CC BY-SA 4.0, https://commons.wikimedia.org/w/index.php?curid=61228494. https://en.wikipedia.org/wiki/Chemotherapy-induced_acral_erythema#/media/File:Foot_on_capecitabine_Natasa_R.jpg. This file

Diarrhea was the most common adverse reaction resulting in discontinuation of study medication. The most common Grade 3 and 4 adverse reactions (NCI CTCAE v3.0) were diarrhea and palmar-plantar erythrodysesthesia.

Hormone receptor-positive, metastatic breast cancer

In a randomized, Phase 3 clinical trial of patients (N = 1,286) with hormone receptor-positive, metastatic breast cancer, who had not received chemotherapy for their metastatic disease, patients received letrozole with or without TYKERB. In this trial, the safety profile of TYKERB was consistent with previously reported results from trials of TYKERB in the advanced or metastatic breast cancer population.

Hormone receptor-positive, HER2+ metastatic breast cancer

In another randomized, Phase 3 clinical trial of postmenopausal patients (N = 355) with hormone receptor positive (HR+), HER2-positive metastatic breast cancer (MBC) which had progressed after prior trastuzumab-containing chemotherapy and endocrine therapies patients received TYKERB with trastuzumab and an aromatase inhibitor (AI) (letrozole, exemestane, or anastrozole), TYKERB with an AI, or trastuzumab with an AI. In this trial, the safety profile of the treatment groups was consistent with the known safety of these agents. The most frequent study treatment-related AEs (>10%) in each of the TYKERB-containing treatment arms were diarrhea, rash, paronychia, nausea, stomatitis, acneiform dermatitis, and decreased appetite, which were infrequent to absent in the trastuzumab treatment arm. The frequency of cardiac AEs (mostly decrease in ejection fraction) was 7% in the TYKERB+trastuzumab+AI group, 2% in the TYKERB+AI group and 3% in the trastuzumab+AI group.

Pediatric use

The safety and effectiveness of TYKERB in pediatric patients have not been established.

Geriatric use

Of the total number of metastatic breast cancer patients in clinical studies of TYKERB in combination with capecitabine (N = 198), 17% were 65 years of age and older, and 1% were 75 years of age and older. Of the total number of hormone receptor-positive, HER2-positive metastatic breast cancer patients in clinical studies of TYKERB in combination with letrozole (N = 642), 44% were 65 years of age and older, and 12% were 75 years of age and older. No overall differences in safety or effectiveness were observed between elderly subjects and younger subjects, and other reported clinical experience has not identified differences in responses between the elderly and younger patients, but greater sensitivity of some older individuals cannot be ruled out.

Renal impairment

Lapatinib pharmacokinetics have not been specifically studied in patients with renal impairment or in patients undergoing hemodialysis. There is no experience with TYKERB in patients with severe renal impairment. However, renal impairment is unlikely to affect the pharmacokinetics of lapatinib given that less than 2% (lapatinib and metabolites) of an administered dose is eliminated by the kidneys.

Hepatic impairment

The pharmacokinetics of lapatinib were examined in subjects with preexisting moderate (n = 8) or severe (n = 4) hepatic impairment (Child-Pugh Class B/C (Table 3), respectively) and in 8 healthy control subjects. Systemic exposure (AUC) to lapatinib after a single oral 100-mg dose increased approximately 14% and 63% in subjects with moderate and severe preexisting hepatic impairment, respectively.

Administration of TYKERB in patients with severe hepatic impairment should be undertaken with caution due to increased exposure to the drug. A dose reduction should be considered for patients with severe preexisting hepatic impairment. In patients who develop severe hepatotoxicity while on therapy, TYKERB should be discontinued, and patients should not be retreated with TYKERB.

OVERDOSAGE

There is no known antidote for overdoses of TYKERB. The maximum oral doses of lapatinib that have been administered in clinical trials are 1,800 mg once daily. More frequent ingestion of TYKERB could result in serum concentrations exceeding those observed in clinical trials and could result in increased toxicity. Therefore, missed doses should not be replaced and dosing should resume with the next scheduled daily dose. Asymptomatic and symptomatic cases of overdose have been reported. The doses ranged from 2,500 to 9,000 mg daily and where reported, the duration varied between 1 and 17 days. Symptoms observed include TYKERB-associated events and in some cases sore scalp, sinus tachycardia (with otherwise normal ECG), and/or mucosal inflammation. Because TYKERB is not significantly renally excreted and is highly bound to plasma proteins, hemodialysis would not be expected to be an effective method to enhance the elimination of lapatinib. Treatment of overdose with TYKERB should consist of general supportive measures

Pharmacodynamics

Cardiac electrophysiology

The effect of lapatinib on the QT-interval was evaluated in a single-blind, placebo-controlled, single sequence (placebo and active treatment) crossover study in patients with advanced solid tumors (N = 58). During the 4-day treatment period, three doses of matching placebo were administered 12 hours apart in the morning and evening on Day 1 and in the morning on Day 2. This was followed by three doses of lapatinib 2000 mg (1.3 – 1.6 times the recommended dosage) administered in the same way. Measurements, including ECGs and pharmacokinetic samples were done at baseline and at the same time points on Day 2 and Day 4. In the evaluable population of subjects who had complete dosing and ECG assessments (N = 37), the maximum mean ΔΔQTcF (90% CI) of 8.75 ms (4.08, 13.42) was observed 10 hours after ingestion of the third dose of lapatinib 2000 mg. The ΔΔQTcF exceeded the 5 ms threshold and the upper bound 90% CIs exceeded the 10 ms threshold at multiple time points. There was a concentration-dependent increase in QTcF effects.

Pharmacokinetics

Absorption

Absorption following oral administration of TYKERB is incomplete and variable. Serum concentrations appear after a median lag time of 0.25 hours (range 0 to 1.5 hours). Peak plasma concentrations (Cmax) of lapatinib are achieved approximately 4 hours after administration. Daily dosing of TYKERB results in achievement of steady state within 6 to 7 days, indicating an effective half-life of 24 hours. At the dose of 1,250 mg daily, steady-state geometric mean [95% confidence interval (CI)] values of Cmax were 2.43 mcg/mL (1.57 to 3.77 mcg/mL) and AUC were 36.2 mcg.h/mL (23.4 to 56 mcg.h/mL). Divided daily doses of TYKERB resulted in approximately 2-fold higher exposure at steady state (steady-state AUC) compared to the same total dose administered once daily. Systemic exposure to lapatinib is increased when administered with food. Lapatinib AUC values were approximately 3- and 4-fold higher (Cmax approximately 2.5- and 3-fold higher) when administered with a lowfat (5% fat-500 calories) or with a high-fat (50% fat-1,000 calories) meal, respectively.

Distribution

Lapatinib is highly bound (greater than 99%) to albumin and alpha-1 acid glycoprotein. In vitro studies indicate that lapatinib is a substrate for the transporters breast cancer-resistance protein (BCRP, ABCG2) and P-glycoprotein (P-gp, ABCB1). Lapatinib has also been shown to inhibit P-gp, BCRP, and the hepatic uptake transporter OATP 1B1, in vitro at clinically relevant concentrations.

Metabolism

Lapatinib undergoes extensive metabolism, primarily by CYP3A4 and CYP3A5, with minor contributions from CYP2C19 and CYP2C8 to a variety of oxidated metabolites, none of which accounts for more than 14% of the dose recovered in the feces or 10% of lapatinib concentration in plasma.

Elimination

At clinical doses, the terminal phase half-life following a single dose was 14.2 hours; accumulation with repeated dosing indicates an effective half-life of 24 hours.

Elimination of lapatinib is predominantly through metabolism by CYP3A4/5 with negligible (less than 2%) renal excretion. Recovery of parent lapatinib in feces accounts for a median of 27% (range 3% to 67%) of an oral dose.

Effects of age, gender, or race

Studies of the effects of age, gender, or race on the pharmacokinetics of lapatinib have not been performed.

Pharmacogenomics

The HLA alleles DQA1*02:01 and DRB1*07:01 were associated with hepatotoxicity reactions in a genetic substudy of a monotherapy trial with TYKERB (n = 1,194). Severe liver injury (ALT greater than 5 times the upper limit of normal, NCI CTCAE Grade 3) occurred in 2% of patients overall; the incidence of severe liver injury among DQA1*02:01 or DRBI*07:01 allele carriers was 8% versus 0.5% in non-carriers. These HLA alleles are present in approximately 15% to 25% of Caucasian, Asian, African, and Hispanic populations and 1% in Japanese populations. Liver function should be monitored in all patients receiving therapy with TYKERB regardless of genotype.

Therapeutic efficacy of lapatinib in the treatment of breast cancer

i). Within the past 2 years, four separate groups have reported marked improvement in relapse-free survival when trastuzumab was added to adjuvant chemotherapy in patients with HER2-overexpressing breast cancer. These results add further credence to the relevance of this receptor as a tumor target. Despite the significant benefits observed in early and advanced HER2-positive breast cancer, overexpression of the receptor is still associated with a poorer prognosis and an increased risk of disease relapse, even in patients with primary operable disease. Besides cytotoxic chemotherapy, and possibly hormonal therapy, patients whose tumors exhibit resistance to trastuzumab have few molecular-targeted options available. Recently, lapatinib, a small molecule dual inhibitor of both HER2 and EGF receptors, has been developed to expand the options for treating HER-positive breast cancer.

Higa, GM and Abraham J. (2007) Lapatinib in the treatment of breast cancer, Expert Review of Anticancer Therapy, 7:9, 1183-1192, DOI: 10.1586/14737140.7.9.1183.

ii). On the basis of the current evidence, our results reveal that the addition of lapatinib to trastuzumab can significantly improve pCR, EFS and OS with a tolerated toxicity in patients with HER2-positive breast cancer. Further well-conducted, large-scale trials are needed to validate these findings.

Xu Z, et al. Efficacy and safety of lapatinib and trastuzumab for HER2-positive breast cancer: a systematic review and meta-analysis of randomised controlled trials

BMJ Open 2017;7:e013053. doi: 10.1136/bmjopen-2016-013053.

9.13. OLAPARIB (LYNPARZA®)

LYNPARZA® (olaparib) tablets, for oral use. Initial U.S. Approval: 2014.

RECENT MAJOR CHANGES

Indications and Usage 5/2020; Dosage and Administration 5/2020; Warnings and Precautions, Venous Thromboembolic Events 5/2020.

Please note: Olaparib (Lynparza) is also FDA-approved for some types of ovarian cancer, prostate cancer and pancreatic cancer as well as breast cancer. Only its approval for breast cancer will be addressed in this book.

Breast cancer

- for the treatment of adult patients with deleterious or suspected deleterious germline BRCA mutated (gBRCAm), HER2-negative metastatic breast cancer who have been treated with chemotherapy in the neoadjuvant, adjuvant or metastatic setting. Patients with hormone receptor (HR)-positive breast cancer should have been treated with a prior endocrine therapy or be considered inappropriate for endocrine therapy.

MECHANISM OF ACTION

Olaparib is an inhibitor of poly (ADP-ribose) polymerase (PARP) enzymes, including PARP1, PARP2, and PARP3. PARP enzymes are involved in normal cellular functions, such as DNA transcription and DNA repair. Olaparib has been shown to inhibit growth of select tumor cell lines in vitro and decrease tumor growth in mouse xenograft models of human cancer, both as monotherapy or following platinum-based chemotherapy. Increased cytotoxicity and anti-tumor activity following treatment with olaparib were noted in cell lines and mouse tumor models with deficiencies in BRCA1/2, ATM, or other genes involved in the homologous recombination repair (HRR) of DNA damage and correlated with platinum response. In vitro studies have shown that olaparib-induced cytotoxicity may involve inhibition of PARP enzymatic activity and increased formation of PARP-DNA complexes, resulting in DNA damage and cancer cell death.

DESCRIPTION

Olaparib is a poly (ADP-ribose) polymerase (PARP) inhibitor. The chemical name is 4-[(3-{[4 (cyclopropylcarbonyl) piperazin-1-yl]carbonyl}-4-fluorophenyl)methyl]phthalazin-1(2H)-one. The empirical molecular formula for Lynparza is C24H23FN4O3 and the relative molecular mass is 434.46. It has the following chemical structure: olaparib is a crystalline solid, is non-chiral and shows pH-independent low solubility across the physiological pH range. Lynparza (olaparib) tablets for oral use contain 100 mg or 150 mg of olaparib.

DOSAGE AND ADMINISTRATION

- Recommended dosage is 300 mg taken orally twice daily with or without food
- For moderate renal impairment (CLcr 31-50 mL/min), reduce Lynparza dosage to 200 mg orally twice daily.

DOSAGE FORMS AND STRENGTHS

Tablets: 150 mg, 100 mg

CONTRAINDICATIONS: none.

WARNINGS AND PRECAUTIONS

- **Myelodysplastic Syndrome/Acute Myeloid Leukemia (MDS/AML):** occurred in <1.5% of patients exposed to Lynparza monotherapy and the majority of events had a fatal outcome. Monitor patients for hematological toxicity at baseline and monthly thereafter. Discontinue if MDS/AML is confirmed.

- Pneumonitis occurred in <1% of patients exposed to Lynparza, and some cases were fatal. Interrupt treatment if pneumonitis is suspected. Discontinue if pneumonitis is confirmed.

• Embryo-fetal toxicity

Can cause fetal harm. Advise of the potential risk to a fetus and to use effective contraception.

• Venous thromboembolic events including pulmonary embolism occurred in 7% of patients with metastatic castrate resistant prostate cancer (mCRPC). Monitor patients for signs and symptoms of venous thrombosis and pulmonary embolism and treat as medically appropriate.

Figure 106. Model of the inhibitor olaparib (dark gray) occupying the NAD+-binding site of PARP1.

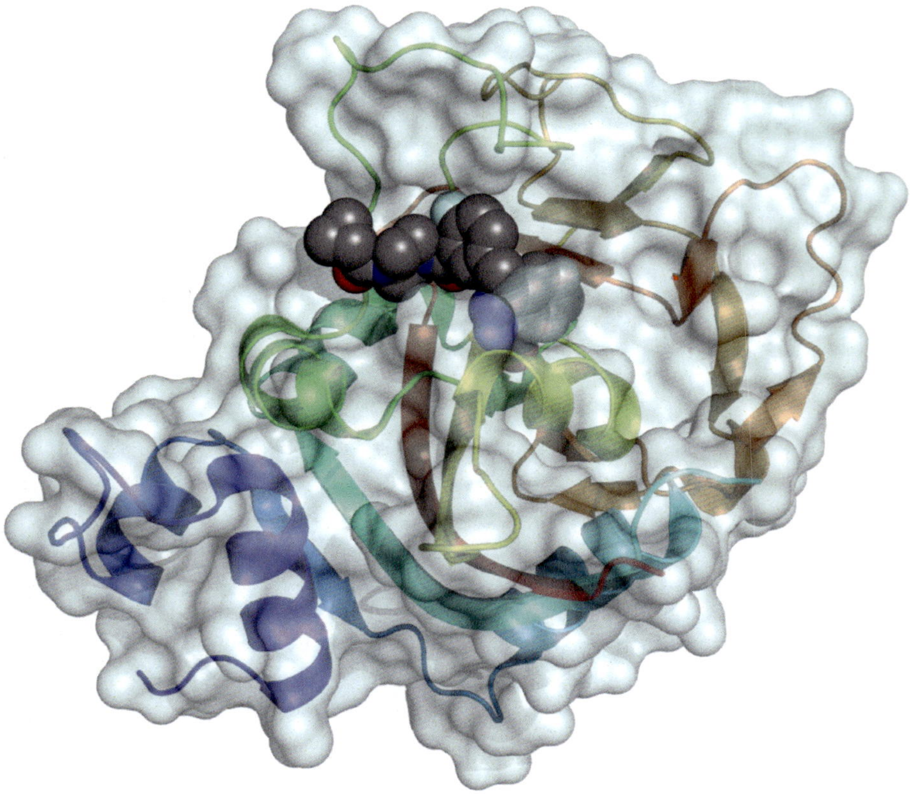

This image is by Fvasconcellos 10.013, Public Domain, https://commons.wikimedia.org/w/index.php?curid=61607160. https://en.wikipedia.org/wiki/PARP_inhibitor#/media/File:PARP1_binding_olaparib_5DS3.png. The copyrightholder of this image has released it intio the public domain. No changes were made to this image.

ADVERSE REACTIONS

The most common adverse reactions (≥10%) in clinical trials:

• as a single agent were nausea, fatigue (including asthenia), anemia, vomiting, diarrhea, decreased appetite, headache, neutropenia, dysgeusia, cough, dyspnea, dizziness, dyspepsia, leukopenia, thrombocytopenia, and abdominal pain upper.

• in combination with bevacizumab were nausea, fatigue (including asthenia), anemia, lymphopenia, vomiting, diarrhea, neutropenia, leukopenia, urinary tract infection, and headache. To report SUSPECTED ADVERSE REACTIONS, contact AstraZeneca at 1-800-236-9933 or FDA at 1-800-FDA-1088 or www.fda.gov/medwatch.

DRUG INTERACTIONS

• Strong or moderate CYP3A inhibitors

Avoid concomitant use. If concomitant use cannot be avoided, reduce Lynparza dosage.

• Strong or moderate CYP3A inducers

Avoid concomitant use

USE IN SPECIFIC POPULATIONS

Lactation

Advise women not to breastfeed.

FULL PRESCRIBING INFORMATION

INDICATIONS AND USAGE

Germline BRCA-mutated HER2-negative Metastatic Breast Cancer

Lynparza is indicated for the treatment of adult patients with deleterious or suspected deleterious gBRCAm, HER2-negative metastatic breast cancer, who have been treated with chemotherapy in the neoadjuvant, adjuvant, or metastatic setting. Patients with hormone receptor (HR)-positive breast cancer should have been treated with a prior endocrine therapy or be considered inappropriate for endocrine therapy. Select patients for therapy based on an FDA-approved companion diagnostic for Lynparza.

Continue treatment until disease progression or unacceptable toxicity for:

- Germline BRCA-mutated HER-2 negative metastatic breast cancer

Dosage modifications for adverse reactions

To manage adverse reactions, consider interruption of treatment or dose reduction. The recommended dose reduction is 250 mg taken twice daily. If a further dose reduction is required, then reduce to 200 mg taken twice daily.

Dosage modifications for concomitant use with strong or moderate cyp3a inhibitors

Avoid concomitant use of strong or moderate CYP3A inhibitors with Lynparza. If concomitant use cannot be avoided, reduce Lynparza dosage to:

• 100 mg twice daily when used concomitantly with a strong CYP3A inhibitor.

• 150 mg twice daily when used concomitantly with a moderate CYP3A inhibitor. After the inhibitor has been discontinued for 3 to 5 elimination half-lives, resume the Lynparza dose taken prior to initiating the CYP3A inhibitor.

Dosage modifications for renal impairment

Moderate renal impairment

In patients with moderate renal impairment (CLcr 31-50 mL/min), reduce the Lynparza dosage to 200 mg orally twice daily.

CONTRAINDICATIONS: none.

WARNINGS AND PRECAUTIONS

Myelodysplastic Syndrome/Acute Myeloid Leukemia

In clinical studies enrolling 2351 patients with various cancers who received Lynparza as a single agent, the incidence of Myelodysplastic Syndrome/Acute Myeloid Leukemia (MDS/AML was <1.5% (28/2351) and the majority of events had a fatal outcome.

A myelodysplastic syndrome (MDS) is one of a group of cancers in which immature blood cells in the bone marrow do not mature, so do not become healthy blood cells. Early on, no symptoms typically are seen. Later, symptoms may include feeling tired, shortness of breath, bleeding disorders, anemia, or frequent infections. Some types may develop into acute myeloid leukemia. (Figures 107 and 108).

Figure 107. *A blood smear from an adult female with a myelodysplastic syndrome related to radiotherapy and chemotherapy for Hodgkin disease. A hypogranular neutrophil with a pseudo-Pelger-Huet nucleus is shown. The red blood cells show marked poikilocytosis, in part related to post-splenectomy status. (Wright-Giemsa stain)*

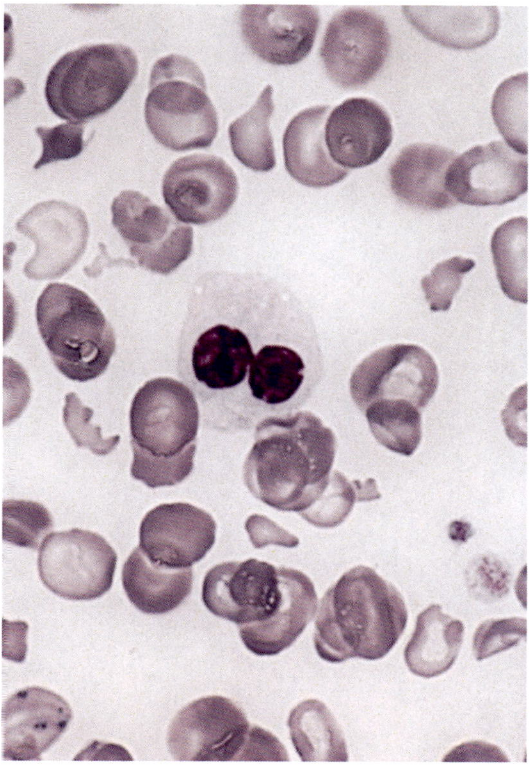

This image is byThe Armed Forces Institute of Pathology (AFIP) - PEIR Digital Library (Pathology image database). Image# 404814. Image and description are from the AFIP Atlas of Tumor Pathology.Declaration of PEIR: Public Domain, https://commons.wikimedia.org/w/index.php?curid=4345884. https://en.wikipedia.org/wiki/Myelodysplastic_syndrome#/media/File:Hypogranular_neutrophil_with_a_pseudo-Pelger-Huet_nucleus_in_MDS.jpg. This work is in the public domain in the United States because it is a work prepared by an officer or employee of the United States Government as part of that person's official duties under the terms of Title 17, Chapter 1, Section 105 of the US Code. No changes have been made to this image.

Figure 108. Enlarged spleen due to myelodysplastic syndrome; CT scan coronal section, spleen in red, left kidney in green.

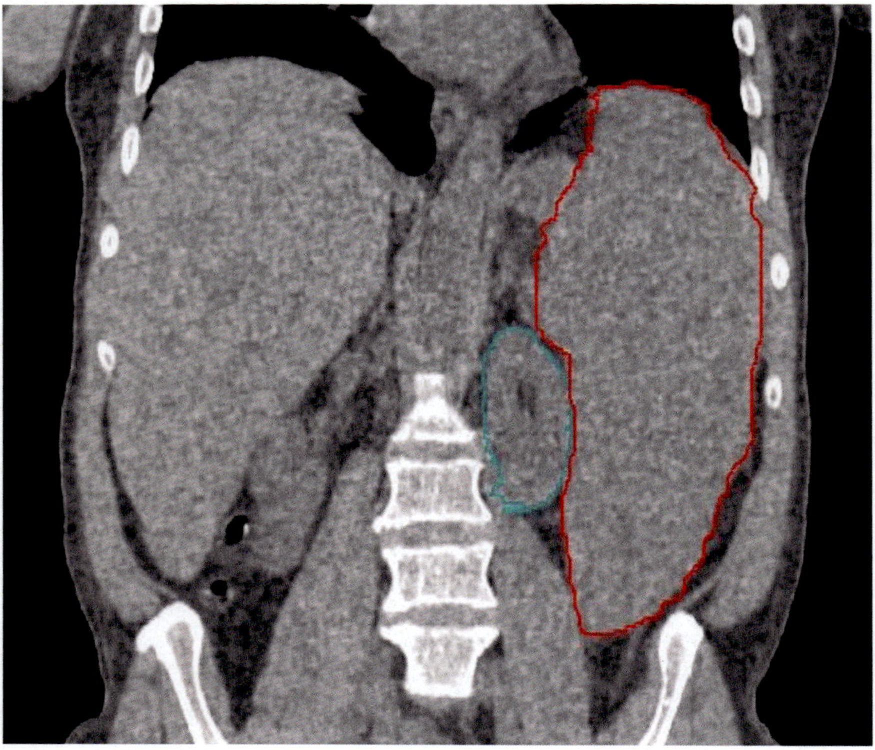

This image is by By Tdvorak - Own work, CC BY-SA 3.0, https://commons.wikimedia.org/w/index.php?curid=2819332. https://en.wikipedia.org/wiki/Myelodysplastic_syndrome#/media/File:Tumor_Myelodysplastic_Spleen.JPG. This file is licensed under the Creative Commons Attribution-

Acute myeloid leukemia (AML) is a cancer of the myeloid line of blood cells (Figure 109), characterized by the rapid growth of abnormal cells that build up in the bone marrow and blood and interfere with normal blood cell production. Symptoms may include feeling tired, shortness of breath, easy bruising and bleeding, and increased risk of infection. Occasionally, spread may occur to the brain, skin, or gums (Figure 110). As an acute leukemia, AML progresses rapidly and is typically fatal within weeks or months if left untreated.

Figure 109. Bone marrow aspirate showing acute myeloid leukemia. Several blast cells have Auer rods in the cytoplasm (red arrow).

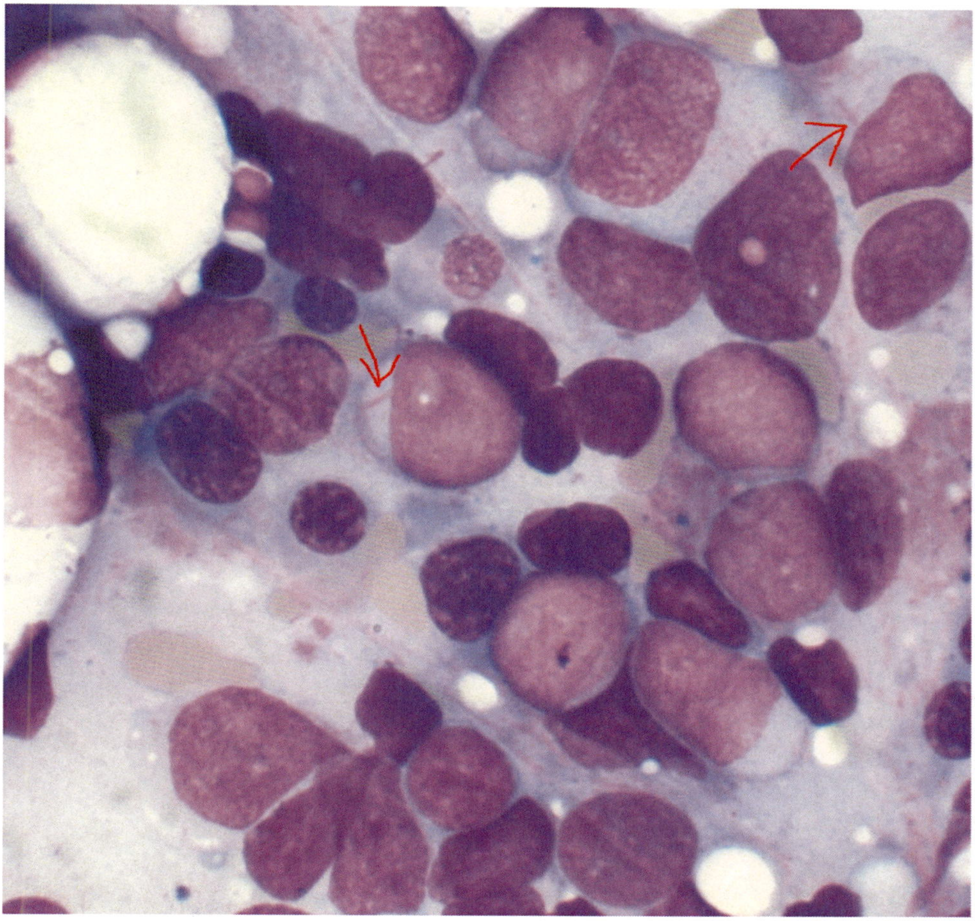

This image is by By VashiDonsk at the English-language Wikipedia, CC BY-SA 3.0, https://commons.wikimedia.org/w/index.php?curid=2571505. https://en.wikipedia.org/wiki/Acute_myeloid_leukemia#/media/File:Auer_rods.PNG. This file is licensed under the Creative Commons Attribution-Share Alike 3.0 Unported license. Attribution: VashiDonsk at the English-language Wikipedia. No changes have been made to this image.

Figure 110. Diffusely swollen gums due to infiltration by leukemic cells in a person with AML.

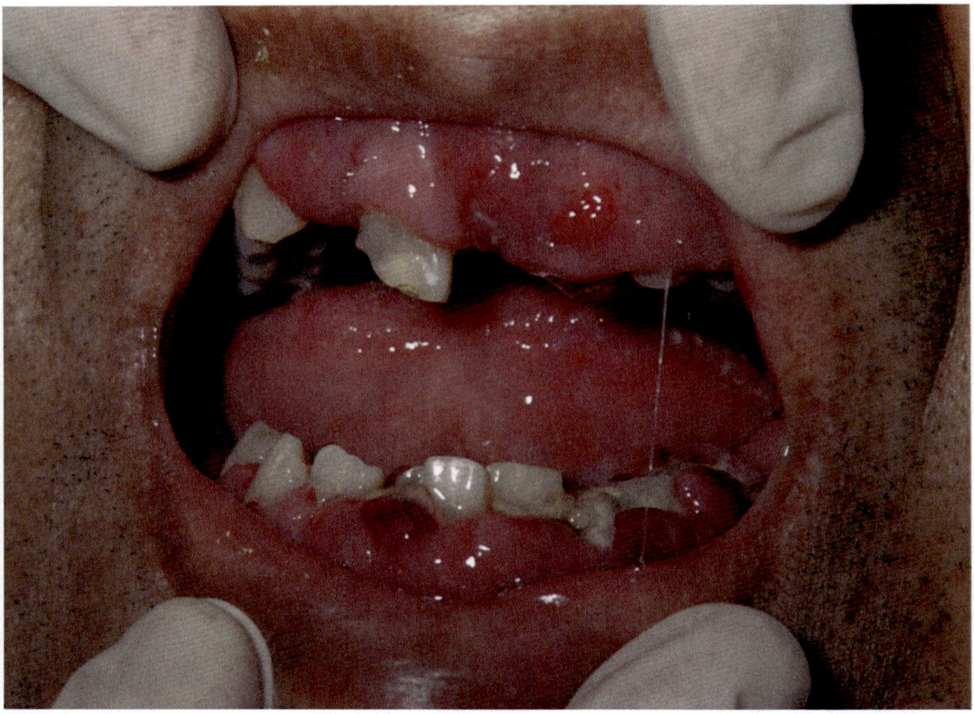

This image is by Herbert L. Fred, MD and Hendrik A. van Dijk - http://cnx.org/content/m14986/latest/, CC BY-SA 3.0, https://commons.wikimedia.org/w/index.php?curid=11893755. https://en.wikipedia.org/wiki/Acute_myeloid_leukemia#/media/File:AMLCase-66.jpg. This file is licensed under the Creative Commons Attribution-Share Alike 3.0 Unported license. No changes were made to this image.

Of these, 25/28 patients had a documented BRCA mutation, 2 patients had gBRCA wildtype and in 1 patient the BRCA mutation status was unknown. Additional cases of MDS/AML have been documented in patients treated with Lynparza in combination studies and in postmarketing reports. The duration of therapy with Lynparza in patients who developed secondary MDS/cancer-therapy related AML varied from 2 years. All of these patients had received previous chemotherapy with platinum agents and/or other DNA damaging agents including radiotherapy. Some of these patients also had a history of more than one primary malignancy or of bone marrow dysplasia. Do not start Lynparza until patients have recovered from hematological toxicity caused by previous chemotherapy (≤Grade 1). Monitor complete blood count for cytopenia at baseline and monthly thereafter for clinically significant changes during treatment. For prolonged hematological toxicities, interrupt Lynparza and monitor blood counts weekly until recovery. If the levels have not recovered to Grade 1 or less after 4 weeks, refer the patient to a hematologist for further investigations, including bone marrow analysis and blood sample for cytogenetics. If MDS/AML is confirmed, discontinue Lynparza.

Other adverse effects of Lynparza include pneumonitis which occurred in <1% of patients treated with Lynparza, including fatal cases, and Embryo-fetal toxicity.

Both of these complications are seen with many of the other targeted biologica agents for breast cancer and have previously been described in the sections of this book dealing with

- ado-trastuzumab emtansine (KADCYLA™)
- everolimus (AFINITOR)
- alpelisib (PIQRAY®)
- atezolizumab (TECENTRIQ®)
- fam-trastuzumab deruxtecan-nxki (ENHURTU)
- trastuzumab (Herceptin)
- pembrolizumab (Keytruda)
- palbociclib (IBRANCE)
- trastuzumab and hyaluronic acid (HERCEPTIN HYLECTA)
- lapatinib (TYKERB®)

Pharmacodynamics

Cardiac electrophysiology

The effect of olaparib on cardiac repolarization was assessed in 119 patients following a single dose of 300 mg and in 109 patients following multiple dosing of 300 mg twice daily. No clinically relevant effect of olaparib on QT interval was observed.

Pharmacokinetics

Lynparza is available as a tablet and capsule formulation. The oral bioavailability of the tablet formulation is higher than the capsule formulation. Population pharmacokinetic analyses have shown that the steady state exposure (AUC) following 300 mg tablet twice daily was 77% higher compared to that following 400 mg capsule twice daily. The olaparib geometric mean AUC and Cmax following a single 300 mg tablet dose were 42.0 µg*h/mL (n = 204) and 5.8 µg/mL (n = 204), respectively, and the steady state geometric mean AUC and Cmax following 300 mg tablet twice daily were 49.0 µg*h/mL (n = 227) and 7.7 µg/mL (n = 227), respectively. Olaparib showed time-dependent PK that the steady state clearance decreased by 15% after multiple dosing.

Absorption

Following oral administration of olaparib, absorption is rapid with median peak plasma concentrations typically achieved 1.5 hours after dosing. An AUC mean accumulation ratio of 1.8 is observed at steady state following multiple dosing of 300 mg tablets twice daily. Systemic exposure (single dose AUC) to olaparib increases approximately proportionally with doses over the dose range of 25 mg to 450 mg, Cmax increased slightly less than proportionally for the same dose range. Co-administration of a high fat meal with olaparib slowed the rate (tmax delayed by 2.5 hours) of absorption but did not significantly alter the extent of olaparib absorption (mean AUC increased by approximately 8%).

Distribution

Olaparib had a mean (± standard deviation) apparent volume of distribution of 158 ± 136 L after a single 300 mg dose of olaparib. The in vitro protein binding of olaparib is approximately 82%.

Metabolism

In vitro, CYP3A4/5 were shown to be the enzymes primarily responsible for the metabolism of olaparib. Following oral dosing of 14C-olaparib to female patients, unchanged olaparib accounted for the majority of the circulating radioactivity in plasma (70%). It was extensively metabolized with unchanged drug accounting for 15% and 6% of radioactivity in urine and feces, respectively. The majority of the metabolism is attributable to oxidation reactions with a number of the components produced undergoing subsequent glucuronide or sulfate conjugation.

Excretion

A mean (± standard deviation) terminal plasma half-life of 14.9 ± 8.2 hours and apparent plasma clearance of 7.4 ± 3.9 L/h were observed after a single 300 mg dose of olaparib. Following a single dose of 14C-olaparib, 86% of the dosed radioactivity was recovered within a 7-day collection period, 44% via the urine and 42% via the feces. The majority of the material was excreted as metabolites. Drug interactions

Based on the data from a drug-interaction trial (n=57), the AUC and Cmax of olaparib increased by 170% and 42%, respectively, when olaparib was administered in combination with itraconazole, a strong CYP3A inhibitor. Simulations suggested that a moderate CYP3A inhibitor (fluconazole) may increase the AUC and Cmax of olaparib by 121% and 14%, respectively. Based on the data from a drug-interaction trial (n=22), the AUC and Cmax of olaparib decreased by 87% and 71%, respectively, when olaparib was administered in combination with rifampicin, a strong CYP3A inducer. Simulations suggested that a moderate CYP3A inducer (efavirenz) may decrease the AUC and Cmax of olaparib by approximately 60% and 31%, respectively. In vitro studies have shown that olaparib is both an inhibitor and inducer of CYP3A and an inducer of CYP2B6. Olaparib is predicted to be a weak CYP3A inhibitor in humans. In vitro studies also indicated that olaparib is an inhibitor of UGT1A1, BCRP, OATP1B1, OCT1, OCT2, OAT3, MATE1 and MATE2K. The clinical relevance of these findings is unknown. In vitro, olaparib is a substrate of, and inhibits, the efflux transporter P-gp. The potential for olaparib to induce P-gp has not been evaluated.

Pharmacokinetics in specific populations

Hepatic impairment

In a hepatic impairment trial, the mean AUC increased by 15% and the mean Cmax by 13% when olaparib was dosed in patients with mild hepatic impairment (Child-Pugh classification A; n=9) compared with patients with normal hepatic function (n=13). Mild hepatic impairment had no effect on the protein binding of olaparib and therefore total plasma exposure was representative of free drug. There are no data in patients with moderate or severe hepatic impairment.

Renal impairment

In a renal impairment trial, the mean AUC increased by 24% and Cmax by 15%, when olaparib was dosed in patients with mild renal impairment (CLcr = 51-80 mL/min defined by the Cockcroft-Gault equation; n=13) and by 44% and 26%, respectively, when olaparib was dosed in patients with moderate renal impairment (CLcr = 31-50 mL/min; n=13), compared to those with normal renal function (CLcr ≥81 mL/min; n=12). There was no evidence of a relationship between the extent of plasma protein binding of olaparib and creatinine clearance. There are no data in patients with severe renal impairment or end-stage renal disease (CLcr ≤ 30 mL/min).

Clinical efficacy of olaparib in the treatment of breast cancer

i). Olaparib improves progression-free survival in germline BRCA mutated HER2 negative metastatic breast cancer patients as compared to standard chemotherapy, with a manageable toxicity profile. Efficacy is of clinical relevance especially in the context of triple negative breast cancer. However, several aspects, such as sequencing or combination of these agents with other anticancer agents and identification of appropriate biomarkers, still need to be clearly defined.

Griguolo G et al. Olaparib for the treatment of breast cancer. Expert Rev Anticancer Ther. 2018 Jun;18(6):519-530. doi: 10.1080/14737140.2018.1458613. Epub 2018 Mar 30. PMID: 29582690.

ii). This is a well-tolerated and effective treatment option for this patient population, particularly in patients with triple-negative breast cancer in which chemotherapy is the only alternative. More data are needed to understand the role of olaparib in combination with endocrine therapy, other targeted agents, and chemotherapy, as well as sequentially with platinum chemotherapy in the metastatic setting.

Le D, Gelmon KA. Olaparib tablets for the treatment of germ line BRCA-mutated metastatic breast cancer. Expert Rev Clin Pharmacol. 2018 Sep; 11(9):833-839. doi: 10.1080/17512433.2018.1513321. Epub 2018 Aug 30. PMID: 30118334.

9.14. MARGETUXIMAB-cmkb (MARGENZA)

MARGENZA™ (margetuximab-cmkb) injection, for intravenous use. Initial U.S. approval: 2020.

WARNING: LEFT VENTRICULAR DYSFUNCTION AND EMBRYO-FETAL TOXICITY

Left ventricular dysfunction

MARGENZA may lead to reductions in left ventricular ejection fraction (LVEF). Evaluate cardiac function prior to and during treatment. Discontinue MARGENZA treatment for a confirmed clinically significant decrease in left ventricular function.

Embryo-fetal toxicity

Exposure to MARGENZA during pregnancy can cause embryo-fetal harm. Advise patients of the risk and need for effective contraception.

MECHANISM OF ACTION

Margetuximab-cmkb binds to the extracellular domain of the human epidermal growth factor receptor 2 protein (HER2). Upon binding to HER2-expressing tumor cells, margetuximab-cmkb inhibits tumor cell proliferation, reduces shedding of the HER2 extracellular domain and mediates antibody-dependent cellular cytotoxicity (ADCC). In vitro, the modified Fc region of margetuximab-cmkb increases binding to activating Fc receptor FCGR3A (CD16A) and decreases binding to inhibitory Fc receptor FCGR2B (CD32B). These changes lead to greater in vitro ADCC and NK cell activation.

DESCRIPTION

Margetuximab-cmkb, a HER2/neu receptor antagonist, is a chimeric Fc-engineered IgG1 kappa monoclonal antibody. Margetuximab-cmkb is produced by recombinant DNA technology in a mammalian cell (Chinese Hamster Ovary) culture. Margetuximab-cmkb has an approximate molecular weight of 149 kDa. MARGENZA (margetuximab-cmkb) injection is a sterile, preservative-free, clear to slightly opalescent, colorless to pale yellow or pale brown solution that requires dilution for intravenous use. Some visible, translucent, inherent proteinaceous particles may be present. Each single-dose vial contains 250 mg of margetuximab-cmkb in 10 mL of solution. Each mL of solution contains 25 mg of margetuximab-cmkb, L-arginine hydrochloride (11 mg), polysorbate 80 (0.1 mg), sodium chloride (2.9 mg), sodium phosphate dibasic, heptahydrate (0.58 mg), sodium phosphate monobasic, monohydrate (1.1 mg), sucrose (30 mg), and Water for Injection, USP at a pH of approximately 6.1.

INDICATIONS AND USAGE

MARGENZA is a HER2/neu receptor antagonist indicated, in combination with chemotherapy, for the treatment of adult patients with metastatic HER2 positive breast cancer who have received two or more prior anti-HER2 regimens, at least one of which was for metastatic disease.

DOSAGE AND ADMINISTRATION

For intravenous infusion only. Administer MARGENZA as an intravenous infusion at 15 mg/kg over 120 minutes for the initial dose, then over a minimum of 30 minutes every 3 weeks for all subsequent doses. On days when both MARGENZA and chemotherapy are to be administered, MARGENZA may be administered immediately after chemotherapy completion.

DOSAGE FORMS AND STRENGTHS

Injection: 250 mg/10 mL (25 mg/mL) in a single-dose vial.

CONTRAINDICATIONS

• None.

WARNINGS AND PRECAUTIONS

• Infusion-Related Reactions (IRRs)

Monitor for signs and symptoms. If a significant infusion-associated reaction occurs, slow or interrupt the infusion and administer appropriate medical therapies.

ADVERSE REACTIONS

The most common adverse drug reactions (>10%) with MARGENZA in combination with chemotherapy are fatigue/asthenia, nausea, diarrhea, vomiting, constipation, headache, pyrexia, alopecia, abdominal pain, peripheral neuropathy, arthralgia/myalgia, cough, decreased appetite, dyspnea, infusion-related reactions, palmar-plantar erythrodysesthesia, and extremity pain.

To report SUSPECTED ADVERSE REACTIONS, contact MacroGenics at 1-844-633-6469 or FDA at 1-800-FDA-1088 or www.fda.gov/medwatch.

FULL PRESCRIBING INFORMATION

WARNING

LEFT VENTRICULAR DYSFUNCTION AND EMBRYO-FETAL TOXICITY

Left ventricular dysfunction

MARGENZA may lead to reductions in left ventricular ejection fraction (LVEF). Evaluate cardiac function prior to and during treatment. Discontinue MARGENZA treatment for a confirmed clinically significant decrease in left ventricular function.

Embryo-fetal toxicity

Exposure to MARGENZA during pregnancy can cause embryofetal harm. Advise patients of the risk and need for effective contraception.

INDICATIONS AND USAGE

MARGENZA is indicated, in combination with chemotherapy, for the treatment of adult patients with metastatic HER2-positive breast cancer who have received two or more prior anti-HER2 regimens, at least one of which was for metastatic diseas.

DOSAGE AND ADMINISTRATION

Recommended doses and schedules

The recommended dose of MARGENZA is 15 mg/kg, administered as an intravenous infusion every 3 weeks (21-day cycle) until disease progression or unacceptable toxicity. Administer MARGENZA as an intravenous infusion at 15 mg/kg over 120 minutes for the initial dose, then over a minimum of 30 minutes every 3 weeks for all subsequent doses. On days when both MARGENZA and chemotherapy are to be administered, MARGENZA may be administered immediately after chemotherapy completion

Dose modification or important dosing considerations

If a patient misses a dose of MARGENZA, administer the scheduled dose as soon as possible. Adjust the administration schedule to maintain a 3-week interval between doses.

Left ventricular dysfunction

Assess left ventricular ejection fraction (LVEF) before starting MARGENZA and regularly during treatment. Withhold MARGENZA dosing for at least 4 weeks for any of the following:

• ≥ 16% absolute decrease in LVEF from pre-treatment values

• LVEF below institutional limits of normal (or 50% if no limits are available) and ≥ 10% absolute decrease in LVEF from pretreatment values.

Left-sided heart failure

The left side of the heart receives oxygen-rich blood from the lungs and pumps it forward to the systemic circulation (the rest of the body except for the pulmonary circulation). Failure of the left side of the heart causes blood to back up (be congested) into the lungs, causing respiratory symptoms and fatigue due to insufficient supply of oxygenated blood. Common respiratory signs are increased rate of breathing and increased work of breathing (nonspecific signs of respiratory distress). Rales or crackles, heard initially in the lung bases, and when severe, throughout the lung fields suggest the development of pulmonary edema (fluid in the alveoli). Cyanosis, which suggests severe low blood oxygen, is a late sign of extremely severe pulmonary edema.

Left ventricular failure is described in more detail in the section of this book on ***ADO-TRASTUZUMAB EMTANSINE (KADCYLA™)***

Congestive cariac failure

Congestive heart failure (CHF) occurs when the heart (Figure 111) is unable to pump sufficiently to maintain blood flow to meet the body tissues' needs for metabolism. Signs and symptoms of heart failure commonly include shortness of breath, excessive tiredness, and leg swelling. The shortness of breath is usually worse with exercise or while lying down, and may wake the person at night. A limited ability to exercise is also a common feature.

Figure 111. The human heart: normal anterior exterior anatomy.

The heart is a muscular organ in most animals, which pumps blood through the blood vessels of the circulatory system. The pumped blood carries oxygen and nutrients to the body, while carrying metabolic waste such as carbon dioxide to the lungs. In humans, the heart is approximately the size of a closed fist and is located between the lungs, in the middle compartment of the chest.

This image is by Patrick J. Lynch, medical illustrator - Patrick J. Lynch, medical illustrator, CC BY 2.5, https://commons.wikimedia.org/w/index.php?curid=1492978. https://en.wikipedia.org/wiki/Heart#/media/File:Heart_anterior_exterior_view.jpg. This file is licensed under the Creative Commons Attribution 2.5 Generic license. No changes were made to this image.

Figure 111. The human heart: normal anterior exterior anatomy.

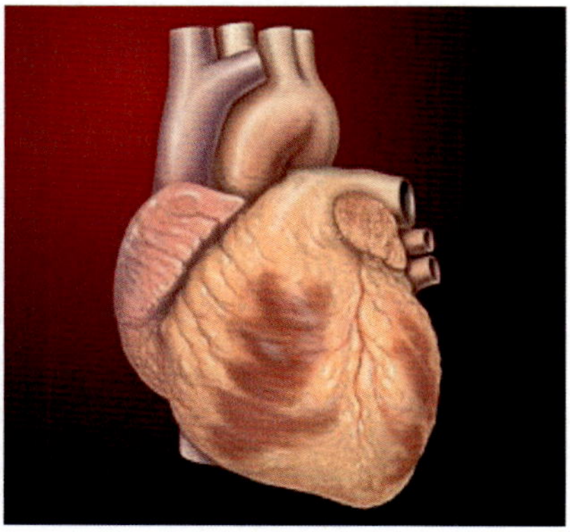

Figure 112. Signs and symptoms of severe heart failure

This image is by the National Heart, Lung, and Blood Institute, National Institutes of Health; originally uploaded by Wouterstomp at en.wikipedia. - http://www.nhlbi.nih.gov/health/dci/Diseases/Hf/HF_SignsAndSymptoms.html; transferred from en.wikipedia to Commons by Stevenfruitsmaak using CommonsHelper. Public Domain, https://commons.wikimedia.org/w/index.php?curid=4848343. https://en.wikipedia.org/wiki/Heart_failure#/media/File:Heartfailure.jpg. This image is a work of the National Institutes of Health, part of the United States Department of Health and Human Services. As a work of the U.S. federal government, the image is in the public domain. No changes were made to this image.

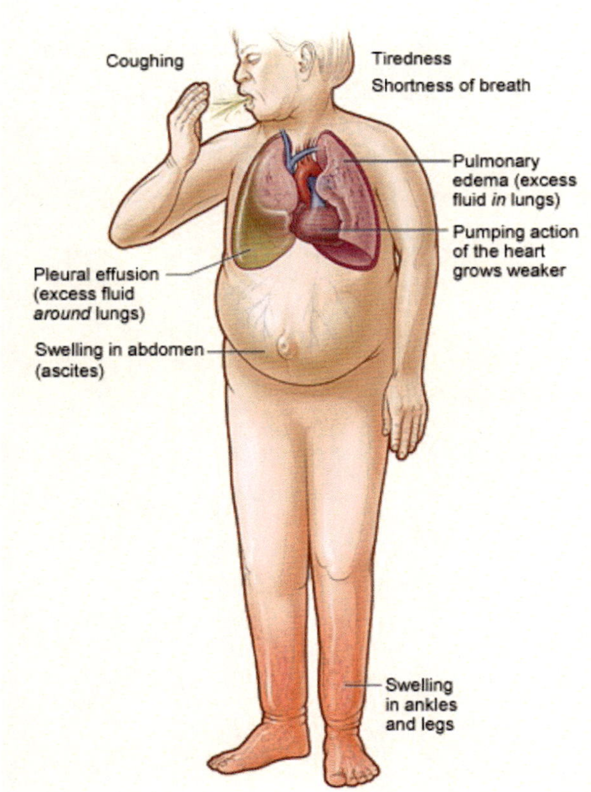

MARGENZA dosing may be resumed if, within 8 weeks, LVEF returns to normal limits and absolute decrease from baseline is ≤ 15%. Permanently discontinue MARGENZA if LVEF decline persists for greater than 8 weeks, or if dosing is interrupted on greater than 3 occasions for LVEF decline.

Infusion-related reactions

Decrease the rate of infusion for mild or moderate infusion-related reactions (IRRs). Interrupt the infusion for dyspnea or clinically significant hypotension. Permanently discontinue MARGENZA dosing in patients with severe or life-threatening IRRs.

DOSAGE FORMS AND STRENGTHS

Injection: 250 mg/10 mL (25 mg/mL) clear to slightly opalescent, colorless to pale yellow or pale brown solution in a single-dose vial.

CONTRAINDICATIONS: none.

WARNINGS AND PRECAUTIONS

Left ventricular dysfunction

Left ventricular cardiac dysfunction can occur with MARGENZA. *In the clinical trial* SOPHIA, left ventricular dysfunction occurred in 1.9% of patients treated with MARGENZA. MARGENZA has not been studied in patients with a pretreatment LVEF value of < 50%, a prior history of myocardial infarction or unstable angina within 6 months, or congestive heart failure NYHA class II-IV.

Withhold MARGENZA for ≥ 16% absolute decrease in LVEF from pre-treatment values or LVEF value below institutional limits of normal (or 50% if no limits are available) and ≥ 10% absolute decrease in LVEF from pretreatment values. Permanently discontinue MARGENZA if LVEF decline persists for greater than 8 weeks, or if dosing is interrupted on greater than 3 occasions due to LVEF decline).

Cardiac monitoring

Conduct thorough cardiac assessment, including history, physical examination, and determination of LVEF by echocardiogram or MUGA scan. The following schedule is recommended:

• Baseline LVEF measurement within 4 weeks prior to initiation of MARGENZA

• LVEF measurements (MUGA/echocardiogram) every 3 months during and upon completion of MARGENZA

• Repeat LVEF measurement at 4-week intervals if MARGENZA is withheld for significant left ventricular cardiac dysfunction.

Embryo-fetal toxicity

Based on findings in animals and mechanism of action, MARGENZA can cause fetal harm when administered to a pregnant woman. There are no available data on the use of MARGENZA in pregnant women to inform the drug-associated risk. In postmarketing reports, use of a HER2- directed antibody during pregnancy resulted in cases of oligohydramnios *(please see the section of this book on **ADO-TRASTUZUMAB EMTANSINE (KADCYLA™)** for further details on oligohydramnios)* and oligohydramnios sequence manifesting as pulmonary hypoplasia, skeletal abnormalities, and neonatal death. In an animal reproduction study, intravenous administration of margetuximab-cmkb to pregnant cynomolgus monkeys once every 3 weeks starting at gestational day (GD) 20 until delivery resulted in oligohydramnios and delayed infant kidney development. Animal exposures were ≥ 3 times the human exposures at the recommended dose, based on Cmax.

Verify pregnancy status of females of reproductive potential prior to initiation of MARGENZA. Advise pregnant women and females of reproductive potential that exposure to MARGENZA during pregnancy or within 4 months prior to conception can result in fetal harm. Advise females of reproductive potential to use effective contraception during treatment and for 4 months following the last dose of MARGENZA.

Infusion-related reactions

MARGENZA can cause infusion-related reactions (IRRs) Symptoms may include fever, chills, arthralgia, cough, dizziness, fatigue, nausea, vomiting, headache, diaphoresis, tachycardia, hypotension, pruritus, rash, urticaria, and dyspnea. In SOPHIA, IRRs were reported by 13% of patients on MARGENZA plus chemotherapy. Most of the IRRs occur during Cycle 1. Grade 3 IRRs were reported in 1.5% of MARGENZA-treated patients. All IRRs resolved within 24 hours, irrespective of severity. In SOPHIA, IRRs leading to interruption of treatment occurred in 9% in patients treated with MARGENZA and chemotherapy. One patient (0.4%) on MARGENZA discontinued treatment due to IRR. An infusion substudy in 88 patients in SOPHIA evaluated MARGENZA administered over 120 minutes for the initial dose, then 30 minutes from Cycle 2 forward. IRRs were ≤ Grade 2 and most occurred during the first (120 minutes) administration of MARGENZA. From Cycle 2 onward, one patient (1.1%) had an IRR (Grade 1). Monitor patients for IRRs during MARGENZA administration and as clinically indicated after completion of infusion.

Have medications and emergency equipment to treat IRRs available for immediate use. Monitor patients carefully until resolution of signs and symptoms. In patients who experience mild or moderate IRRs, consider premedications, including antihistamines, corticosteroids, and antipyretics. Decrease the rate of infusion for mild or moderate IRRs.

Interrupt MARGENZA infusion in patients experiencing dyspnea or clinically significant hypotension and intervene with medical therapy which may include epinephrine, corticosteroids, diphenhydramine, bronchodilators and oxygen. Patients should be evaluated and carefully monitored until complete resolution of signs and symptoms. Permanently discontinue MARGENZA in all patients with severe or life-threatening IRRs.

Immunogenicity

As with all therapeutic proteins, there is potential for immunogenicity with MARGENZA. The detection of antibody formation is highly dependent on assay sensitivity and specificity. Additionally, the observed incidence of antibody (including neutralizing antibody) positivity in an assay may be influenced by several factors including assay methodology, sample handling, timing of sample collection, concomitant medications, and underlying disease. For these reasons, comparison of the incidence of antibodies to MARGENZA in the studies described below with the incidence of antibodies in other studies or to other products may be misleading. In SOPHIA, samples were obtained from patients on MARGENZA for immunogenicity testing at baseline, every 2 cycles, and at end of study therapy. All patients enrolled in SOPHIA received trastuzumab previously, and treatment-emergent anti-margetuximab antibodies were observed in 4 patients (1.7%). Of these 4 patients, anti-margetuximab antibodies were detected prior to Cycle 7 of MARGENZA dosing in 1 patient, and more than 2 months after the last MARGENZA dose in 3 patients. In the infusion substudy, treatment-emergent anti-margetuximab antibodies were observed in 2 patients (3.8%). Of these 2 patients, anti-margetuximab antibodies were detected prior to Cycle 3 of MARGENZA dosing in 1 patient, and more than 6 months after the last MARGENZA dose in 1 patient. Due to the limited number of patients who developed antimargetuximab antibodies during treatment with MARGENZA, the impact of anti-margetuximab antibodies on the PK, safety and efficacy of MARGENZA is unknown.

DRUG INTERACTIONS

Anthracyclines

Patients who receive anthracyclines less than 4 months after stopping MARGENZA may be at increased risk of cardiac dysfunction. While this interaction has not been studied with MARGENZA, clinical data from other HER2-directed antibodies warrants consideration. Avoid anthracycline-based therapy for up to 4 months after stopping MARGENZA. If concomitant use is unavoidable, closely monitor patient's cardiac function.

USE IN SPECIFIC POPULATIONS

Pregnancy risk summary

Based on findings in animals and mechanism of action, MARGENZA can cause fetal harm when administered to a pregnant woman. There are no available data on use of MARGENZA in pregnant women to inform the drug-associated risk. In postmarketing reports, use of a HER2- directed antibody during pregnancy resulted in cases of oligohydramnios and oligohydramnios sequence manifesting as pulmonary hypoplasia, skeletal abnormalities, and neonatal death. In an animal reproduction study, intravenous administration of margetuximab-cmkb to pregnant cynomolgus monkeys once every 3 weeks, starting at gestational day (GD) 20 until delivery, resulted in oligohydramnios and delayed infant kidney development. Animal exposures were ≥ 3 times the human exposures at the recommended dose, based on Cmax (see Data). Advise patients of potential risks to a fetus. There are clinical considerations if MARGENZA is used during pregnancy or within 4 months prior to conception. Estimated background risk of major birth defects and miscarriage for the indicated population is unknown. In the U.S. general population, background risks of major birth defects and miscarriage in clinically recognized pregnancies are 2 - 4% and 15 - 20%, respectively.

Clinical considerations

Fetal/neonatal adverse reactions

Monitor women who received MARGENZA during pregnancy or within 4 months prior to conception for oligohydramnios. If oligohydramnios occurs, perform fetal testing that is appropriate for gestational age and consistent with community standards of care.

Data

Animal data

In an enhanced pre- and post-natal development study, pregnant cynomolgus monkeys received intravenous doses of 50 or 100 mg/kg margetuximab-cmkb once every 3 weeks starting on GD 20 and until delivery. Animal exposures at doses of 50 and 100 mg/kg were 3 and 6 times, respectively, the human exposures at the recommended dose, based on Cmax. Treatment with 50 and 100 mg/kg margetuximab-cmkb resulted in oligohydramnios beginning on GD 75. An infant mortality occurred on post-natal day 63 following maternal exposure to 100 mg/kg margetuximab-cmkb. Clinical findings included tubular degeneration/necrosis and tubular dilatation in the kidney. Maternal doses of 50 and 100 mg/kg resulted in decreased infant kidney weights and histologic immature nephrons. Measurable serum concentrations of margetuximabcmkb were observed in infant animals, which is consistent with margetuximab-cmkb crossing the placenta.

Lactation risk summary

There is no information regarding presence of MARGENZA in human milk, effects on the breastfed child, or effects on milk production. Published data suggest human IgG is present in human milk but does not enter neonatal or infant circulation in substantial amounts. Consider developmental and health benefits of breastfeeding along with the mother's clinical need for MARGENZA treatment and any potential adverse effects on the breastfed child from MARGENZA or from the underlying maternal condition. This consideration should also take into account the MARGENZA washout period of 4 months.

Females and males of reproductive potential

MARGENZA can cause fetal harm when administered to a pregnant woman.
Pregnancy testing

Verify pregnancy status of females of reproductive potential prior to initiation of MARGENZA.

Contraception

Females

Advise females of reproductive potential to use effective contraception during treatment and for 4 months following the last dose of MARGENZA

Pediatric use

Safety and effectiveness of MARGENZA have not been established in pediatric patients.

Geriatric use

Of the 266 patients treated with MARGENZA 20% were 65 years of age or older and 4% were 75 years or older. No overall differences in efficacy were observed between patients ≥65 years of age compared to younger patients. There was a higher incidence of Grade ≥ 3 adverse reactions observed in patients age 65 years or older (56%) compared to younger patients (47%), as well as adverse reactions associated with potential cardiotoxicity (35% vs 18%).

CLINICAL PHARMACOLOGY

Pharmacodynamics

The exposure-response relationship and time course of pharmacodynamic response for the safety and effectiveness of margetuximab-cmkb have not been fully characterized.

Pharmacokinetics

Following the approved recommended dosage, the steady-state geometric mean (% CV) Cmax of margetuximab-cmkb is 466 (20%) µg/mL and AUC0-21d is 4120 (21%) µg.day/mL in patients with HER2-positive relapsed or refractory advanced breast cancer. Margetuximab undergoes both linear and nonlinear elimination. After a single dose, margetuximab-cmkb Cmax and AUC0- 21d increase in an approximately dose proportional manner from 10 to 18 mg/kg (0.67 to 1.2 times the approved recommended dose). At the approved recommended dosage, time to steadystate was 2 months, and accumulation ratio was 1.65 based on AUC0-21d. No clinically significant differences in margetuximab-cmkb exposure were observed when infusion time was reduced from 120 minutes to 30 minutes.

Distribution

Margetuximab-cmkb geometric mean (%CV) steady-state volume of distribution is 5.47 L (22%).

Elimination

The geometric mean (%CV) terminal half-life of margetuximab-cmkb is 19.2 days (28%) and clearance is 0.22 L/day (24%). Four months after margetuximab-cmkb discontinuation, concentrations decrease to approximately 3% of the steady-state trough serum concentration.

Metabolism

Margetuximab-cmkb is expected to be metabolized into small peptides by catabolic pathways.

Specific populations

No clinically significant differences in margetuximab-cmkb PK were observed based on age (29 to 83 years), sex, race (Caucasian, Black, Asian), mild to moderate (CLcr 30 to 89 mL/min estimated using the Cockcroft-Gault equation) renal impairment, mild hepatic impairment bilirubin ≤ ULN and AST > ULN, or total bilirubin 1 to 1.5 ULN and any AST), HER2 expression level (0 to 3 by IHC), tumor burden (2 – 317 mm), ECOG score (0 to 2), albumin (24 to 50 g/L), FCGR3A (CD16A), FCGR2A (CD32A) and FCGR2B (CD32B) genotype, number of metastatic sites (≤ 2 or > 2), number of prior therapy lines (≤ 2 or > 2) or concurrent chemotherapies (capecitabine, gemcitabine, eribulin and vinorelbine).

The effect of severe renal impairment (CLcr 15 to 29 mL/min), end-stage renal disease with or without hemodialysis, and moderate (total bilirubin > 1.5 to ≤ 3 ULN and any AST) or severe hepatic impairment (total bilirubin >3 ULN and any AST) on margetuximab-cmkb PK is unknown.

Clinical efficacy of margetuximab-cmkb (MARGENZA) in the treatment of breast cancer

i).The investigators concluded: "In this phase III randomized clinical trial, margetuximab plus chemotherapy had acceptable safety and a statistically significant improvement in [progression-free survival] compared with trastuzumab plus chemotherapy in [HER2]-positive [advanced breast cancer] after progression on two or more prior anti-[HER2] therapies. Final [overall survival] analysis is expected in 2021.

Rugo HS et al: Efficacy of margetuximab vs trastuzumab in patients with pretreated ERBB2-positive advanced breast cancer: A phase 3 randomized clinical trial. JAMA Oncol 7:573-584, 2021.

9.15. NERATINIB (NERLYNX)

NERLYNX® (neratinib) tablets, for oral use. Initial U.S. Approval: 2017.

RECENT MAJOR CHANGES

Indications and usage

Advanced or metastatic breast cancer 2/2020

Dosage and administration,

Antidiarrheal prophylaxis 2/2020

Dosage and administration, recommended dose and schedule 2/2020

Dosage and administration, dose modifications 2/2020

Warnings and Precautions

Diarrhea 2/2020

Warnings and Precautions, Hepatotoxicity (5.2) 2/2020

MECHANISM OF ACTION

Neratinib is an intracellular kinase inhibitor that irreversibly binds to epidermal growth factor receptor (EGFR), HER2, and HER4. In vitro, neratinib reduces EGFR and HER2 autophosphorylation, downstream MAPK and AKT signaling pathways (Figure 113) and showed antitumor activity in EGFR and/or HER2 expressing carcinoma cell lines. Neratinib human metabolites M3, M6, M7 and M11 inhibited the activity of EGFR, HER2, and HER4 in vitro. In vivo, oral administration of neratinib inhibited tumor growth in mouse xenograft models with tumor cell lines expressing HER2 and EGFR.

Figure 113. Overview of signal transduction pathways involved in apoptosis, also known as "programmed cell death".

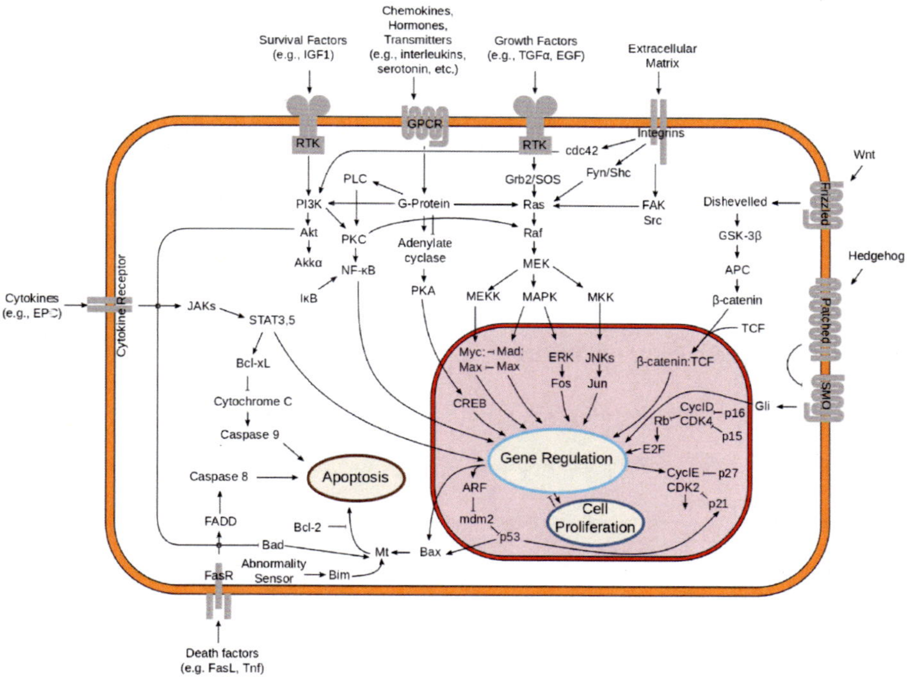

This image is by By cybertory - This file was derived from: Signal transduction v1.png, CC BY-SA 3.0, https://commons.wikimedia.org/w/index.php?curid=12081090. https://en.wikipedia.org/wiki/Cell_cycle#/media/File:Signal_transduction_pathways.svg. This file is licensed under the Creative Commons Attribution-Share Alike 3.0 Unported license. No changes were made to this image.

DESCRIPTION

NERLYNX (neratinib) immediate release, film-coated tablets for oral administration contain 40 mg of neratinib, equivalent to 48.31 mg neratinib maleate. Neratinib is a member of the 4-anilino quinolidine class of protein kinase inhibitors. The molecular formula for neratinib maleate is $C_{30}H_{29}ClN_6O_3 \cdot C_4H_4O_4$ and the molecular weight is 673.11 Daltons. The chemical name is (E)-N-{4-[3-chloro-4-(pyridin-2-yl methoxy)anilino]-3-cyano-7-ethoxyquinolin-6-yl}-4-(dimethylamino)but-2-enamide maleate. Neratinib maleate is an off-white to yellow powder with pKas of 7.65 and 4.66. The solubility of neratinib maleate increases dramatically as neratinib becomes protonated at acidic pH. Neratinib maleate is sparingly soluble at pH 1.2 (32.90 mg/mL) and insoluble at approximate pH 5.0 and above (0.08 mg/mL or less). Inactive ingredients: Tablet core: colloidal silicon dioxide, mannitol, microcrystalline cellulose, crospovidone, povidone, magnesium stearate, and purified water. Coating: red film coat: polyvinyl alcohol, titanium dioxide, polyethylene glycol, talc, and iron oxide red.

INDICATIONS AND USAGE

NERLYNX is a kinase inhibitor indicated:

- As a single agent, for the extended adjuvant treatment of adult patients with early stage HER2-positive breast cancer, to follow adjuvant trastuzumab-based therapy.

- In combination with capecitabine, for the treatment of adult patients with advanced or metastatic HER2-positive breast cancer who have received two or more prior anti-HER2 based regimens in the metastatic setting.

DOSAGE AND ADMINISTRATION

- Antidiarrheal prophylaxis

Initiate loperamide with the first dose of NERLYNX and continue during the first 56 days of treatment. After day 56, use loperamide to maintain 1-2 bowel movements per day.

• Extended adjuvant treatment of early-stage breast cancer

240 mg (6 tablets) given orally once daily, with food, continuously until disease recurrence for up to one year.

• Advanced or metastatic breast cancer

240 mg (6 tablets) given orally once daily with food on Days 1-21 of a 21-day cycle plus capecitabine (750 mg/m^2 given orally twice daily) on Days 1-14 of a 21-day cycle until disease progression or unacceptable toxicities.

• Dose interruptions and/or dose reductions are recommended based on individual safety and tolerability.

• Hepatic impairment

Reduce starting dose to 80 mg in patients with severe hepatic impairment.

DOSAGE FORMS AND STRENGTHS

Tablets: 40 mg.

CONTRAINDICATIONS

None.

Further information on **WARNINGS AND PRECAUTIONS**

• Diarrhea

Aggressively manage diarrhea. If diarrhea occurs despite recommended prophylaxis, treat with additional antidiarrheals, fluids, and electrolytes as clinically indicated. Withhold NERLYNX in patients experiencing severe and/or persistent diarrhea. Permanently discontinue NERLYNX in patients experiencing Grade 4 diarrhea or Grade ≥2 diarrhea that occurs after maximal dose reduction.

Electrolyte imbalance, or water-electrolyte imbalance, is an abnormality in the concentration of electrolytes in the body. Electrolytes play a vital role in maintaining homeostasis in the body. They help to regulate heart and neurological function, fluid balance, oxygen delivery, acid–base balance and much more. Electrolyte imbalances can develop by consuming too little or too much electrolyte as well as excreting too little or too much electrolyte (Figure 114).

Figure 114. Diagram of ion concentrations and charge across a semi-permeable cellular membrane.

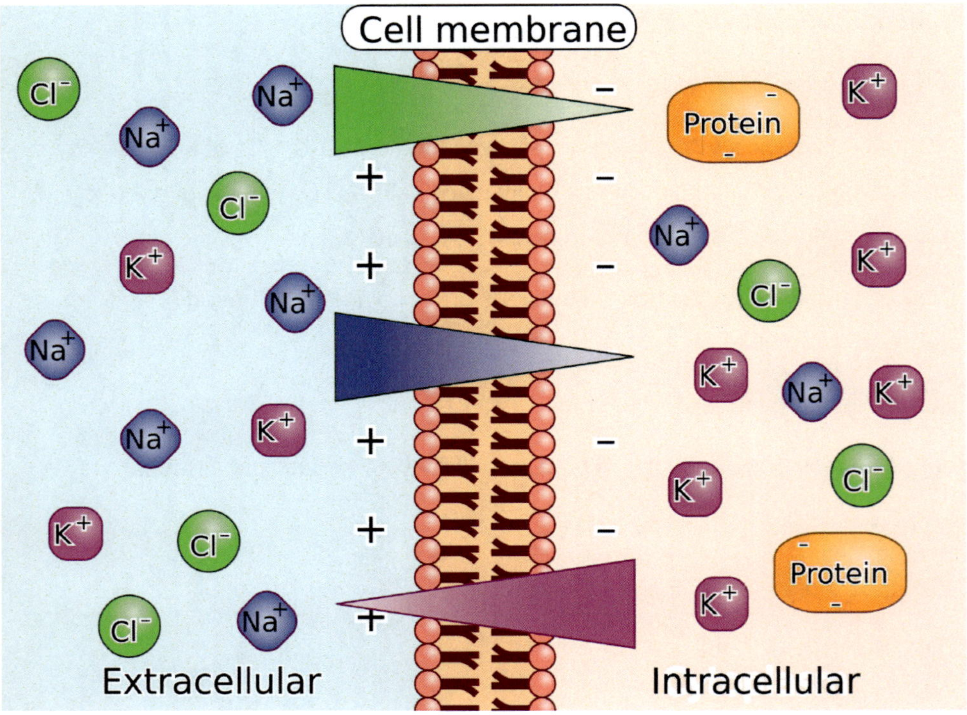

This image is by By Gibbs-donnan-en.svg: Biezlderivative work: Looie496 (talk) - Gibbs-donnan-en.svg, CC BY-SA 3.0, https://commons.wikimedia.org/w/index.php?curid=8969169. https://en.wikipedia.org/wiki/Electrolyte_imbalance#/media/File:Membrane_potential_ions_en.svg. This file is licensed under the Creative Commons Attribution-Share Alike 3.0 Unported license. No changes were made to this image.

- Hepatotoxicity

Monitor liver function tests monthly for the first 3 months of treatment, then every 3 months while on treatment and as clinically indicated. Withhold NERLYNX in patients experiencing Grade 3 liver abnormalities and permanently discontinue NERLYNX in patients experiencing Grade 4 liver abnormalities.

• Embryo-fetal toxicity

NERLYNX can cause fetal harm. Advise patients of potential risk to a fetus and to use effective contraception.

ADVERSE REACTIONS

The most common adverse reactions (reported in ≥5% of patients) were:

• NERLYNX as a single agent: diarrhea, nausea, abdominal pain, fatigue, vomiting, rash, stomatitis, decreased appetite, muscle spasms, dyspepsia, AST, or ALT increased, nail disorder, dry skin, abdominal distention, epistaxis, weight decreased, and urinary tract infection.

• NERLYNX in combination with capecitabine: diarrhea, nausea, vomiting, decreased appetite, constipation, fatigue/asthenia, weight decreased, dizziness, back pain, arthralgia, urinary tract infection, upper respiratory tract infection, abdominal distention, renal impairment, and muscle spasms.

To report SUSPECTED ADVERSE REACTIONS, contact Puma Biotechnology, Inc. at 1-844-NERLYNX (1-844-637-5969) or FDA at 1-800-FDA-1088 or www.fda.gov/medwatch.

DRUG INTERACTIONS

• Gastric acid reducing agents:

Avoid concomitant use with proton pump inhibitors.

Proton-pump inhibitors (PPIs) are a class of medications that cause a profound and prolonged reduction of stomach acid production. They do so by irreversibly inhibiting the stomach's H+/K+ ATPase proton pump. A proton pump is an integral membrane protein pump that builds up a proton gradient across a biological membrane.
A biological membrane, biomembrane or cell membrane is a selectively permeable membrane that separates cell from the external environment or creates intracellular compartments. Biological membranes, in the form of eukaryotic cell membranes, consist of a phospholipid bilayer with

embedded, integral and peripheral proteins used in communication and transportation of chemicals and ions. Examples are shown in Figure 115.

Figure 115. Cross-sectional view of the structures that can be formed by phospholipids in an aqueous solution.

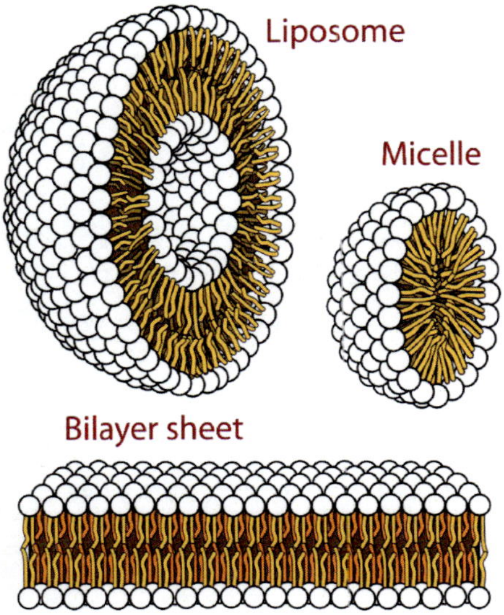

This image is by By Mariana Ruiz Villarreal ,LadyofHats - Own work, Public Domain, https://commons.wikimedia.org/w/index.php?curid=3032610. https://en.wikipedia.org/wiki/Biological_membrane#/media/File:Phospholipids_aqueous_solution_structures.svg. This work has been released into the public domain by its author, LadyofHats. This applies worldwide. No changes have been made to this image.

When patients require gastric acid reducing agents, use an H2 receptor antagonist or antacid. Separate NERLYNX by at least 3 hours with antacids. Separate NERLYNX by at least 2 hours before or 10 hours after H2-receptor antagonists.

• Strong CYP3A4 inhibitors

Avoid concomitant use.

Moderate CYP3A4 and P-gp dual inhibitors

Avoid concomitant use

Strong or moderate CYP3A4 inducers

Avoid concomitant use.

• P-glycoprotein (P-gp) substrates

Monitor for adverse reactions of narrow therapeutic agents that are P-gp substrates when used concomitantly with NERLYNX.

USE IN SPECIFIC POPULATIONS

Lactation

Advise women not to breastfeed.

FULL PRESCRIBING INFORMATION

INDICATIONS AND USAGE

Extended adjuvant treatment of early-stage breast cancer

NERLYNX as a single agent is indicated for the extended adjuvant treatment of adult patients with early-stage human epidermal growth factor receptor 2 (HER2)-positive breast cancer, to follow adjuvant trastuzumab based therapy.

Advanced or metastatic breast cancer

NERLYNX in combination with capecitabine is indicated for the treatment of adult patients with advanced or metastatic HER2-positive breast cancer who have received two or more prior anti-HER2 based regimens in the metastatic setting.

DOSAGE AND ADMINISTRATION

Antidiarrheal prophylaxis

Administer antidiarrheal prophylaxis during the first 2 cycles of treatment and initiate with the first dose of NERLYNX. Titrate loperamide to 1-2 bowel movements per day.

Recommended dose and schedule

Extended adjuvant treatment of early-stage breast cancer

The recommended dose of NERLYNX is 240 mg (six tablets) given orally once daily, with food, continuously until disease recurrence or for up to one year.

Advanced or metastatic breast cancer

The recommended dose of NERLYNX is 240 mg (six tablets) given orally once daily with food on Days 1-21 of a 21-day cycle plus capecitabine (750 mg/m^2 given orally twice daily) on Days 1-14 of a 21-day cycle until disease progression or unacceptable toxicities. Instruct patients to take NERLYNX at approximately the same time every day. NERLYNX tablets should be swallowed whole (tablets should not be chewed, crushed, or split prior to swallowing). If a patient misses a dose, do not replace missed dose, and instruct the patient to resume NERLYNX with the next scheduled daily dose.

Dose modifications

Dose modifications for adverse reactions

NERLYNX dose modification is recommended based on individual safety and tolerability. Management of some adverse reactions may require dose interruption and/or dose reduction as per the table below. Discontinue NERLYNX for patients with adverse reactions that fail to recover to Grade 0-1 or baseline, with toxicities that result in a treatment delay >3 weeks, or if unable to tolerate 120 mg daily. Additional clinical situations may result in dose adjustments as clinically indicated (e.g. intolerable toxicities, persistent Grade 2 adverse reactions, etc.).

Dose level	NERLYNX dose
Recommended starting dose	240 mg daily (six 40 mg tablets)
First dose reduction	200 mg daily (five 40 mg tablets)
Second dose reduction	160 mg daily (four 40 mg tablets)

Third dose reduction	120 mg daily (three 40 mg tablets)

When NERLYNX is used in combination with capecitabine, refer to the capecitabine prescribing information for dose modifications of capecitabine. *Please see the FDA approval label for further detailed recommendations for NERLYNX dose reduction when used with or withour capecitabine.*

Dose modifications for hepatic impairment

Reduce the NERLYNX starting dose to 80 mg in patients with severe hepatic impairment (Child Pugh C). No dose modifications are recommended for patients with mild to moderate hepatic impairment (Child Pugh A or B)

Dose modifications for hepatotoxicity

Patients who experience ≥Grade 3 diarrhea requiring IV fluid treatment or any signs or symptoms of hepatotoxicity, such as worsening of fatigue, nausea, vomiting, right upper quadrant pain or tenderness, fever, rash, or eosinophilia, should be evaluated for changes in liver function tests. Fractionated bilirubin and prothrombin time should also be collected during hepatotoxicity evaluation. *Again, please see the full FDA approval label for further information on dose reduction for hepatotoxicity.*

Concomitant use with gastric acid reducing agents

Proton pump inhibitors (PPI)

Avoid concomitant use with NERLYNX

H2-receptor antagonists

Take NERLYNX at least 2 hours before the next dose of the H2-receptor antagonist or 10 hours after the H2-receptor antagonist

Antacids

Separate dosing of NERLYNX by 3 hours after antacids

DOSAGE FORMS AND STRENGTHS

Tablets: 40 mg neratinib (equivalent to 48.31 mg of neratinib maleate). Film-coated, red, oval shaped and debossed with ‘W104’ on one side and plain on the other side.

CONTRAINDICATIONS: none.

Further information on **WARNINGS AND PRECAUTIONS**

Diarrhea

Severe diarrhea and sequelae, such as dehydration, hypotension, and renal failure occurred during treatment with NERLYNX. Diarrhea was reported in 95% of NERLYNX-treated patients in ExteNET, a randomized placebo-controlled trial in the extended adjuvant setting who were not required to receive antidiarrheal prophylaxis. In the NERLYNX arm, Grade 3 diarrhea occurred in 40% and Grade 4 diarrhea occurred in 0.1% of patients. The majority of patients (93%) had diarrhea in the first month of treatment, the median time to first onset of Grade ≥3 diarrhea was 8 days (range, 1-350), and the median cumulative duration of Grade ≥3 diarrhea was 5 days (range, 1-139).

Diarrhea was reported in 83% of NERLYNX plus capecitabine treated patients in NALA, a randomized placebo-controlled trial in the metastatic breast cancer setting who were required to receive anti-diarrheal prophylaxis in the first cycle. The majority of patients (70%) had diarrhea in the first cycle of treatment, the median time to first onset of Grade ≥3 diarrhea was 11 days (range, 2-728) and the median cumulative duration of Grade ≥3 diarrhea was 3 days (range, 1-21). In the NERLYNX plus capecitabine arm, Grade 3 diarrhea occurred in 24% of patients.

Antidiarrheal prophylaxis has been shown to lower the incidence and severity of diarrhea. Instruct patients to initiate antidiarrheal prophylaxis with loperamide along with the first dose of NERLYNX and continue during the first 56 days of treatment; after day 56 titrate dose to achieve 1-2 bowel movements per day and not to exceed 16 mg loperamide per day. Consider adding other agents to loperamide as clinically indicated. Monitor patients for diarrhea and treat with additional antidiarrheals as needed. When severe diarrhea with dehydration occurs, administer fluid and electrolytes as needed, interrupt NERLYNX, and reduce subsequent doses.

Perform stool cultures as clinically indicated to exclude infectious causes of Grade 3 or 4 diarrhea or diarrhea of any grade with complicating features (dehydration, fever, neutropenia).

Hepatotoxicity

NERLYNX has been associated with hepatotoxicity characterized by increased liver enzymes. In ExteNET, 10% of patients experienced an alanine aminotransferase (ALT) increase ≥2x ULN, 5% of patients experienced an aspartate aminotransferase (AST) increase ≥2x ULN, and 1.7% of patients experienced an AST or ALT elevation >5 x ULN (≥Grade 3). Hepatotoxicity or increases in liver transaminases led to drug discontinuation in 1.7% of NERLYNX-treated patients. In the NALA study, in NERLYNX and capecitabine-treated patients, 7% experienced an ALT or AST >3x ULN, 2% experienced ALT or AST >5x ULN, 7% experienced a bilirubin >1.5x ULN, and 1.3% experienced a bilirubin >3x ULN. Hepatotoxicity or increases in liver transaminases led to drug discontinuation in 0.3% of NERLYNX and capecitabine-treated patients. Total bilirubin, AST, ALT, and alkaline phosphatase should be measured prior to starting treatment with NERLYNX monthly for the first 3 months of treatment, then every 3 months while on treatment and as clinically indicated. These tests should also be performed in patients experiencing Grade 3 diarrhea or any signs or symptoms of hepatotoxicity, such as worsening of fatigue, nausea, vomiting, right upper quadrant tenderness, fever, rash, or eosinophilia *(Figure 116).*

Figure 116. Eosinophil under a microscope from a blood smear. (400x).

This image is by Bobjgalindo - Own work, CC BY-SA 4.0, https://commons.wikimedia.org/w/index.php?curid=7761793. https://en.wikipedia.org/wiki/Eosinophil#/media/File:Eosinophil_blood_smear.JPG. This file is licensed under the Creative Commons Attribution-Share Alike 4.0 International, 3.0 Unported, 2.5 Generic, 2.0 Generic and 1.0 Generic license. No changes were made to this image.

Figure 116. Eosinophil under a microscope from a blood smear. (400x).

Note the characteristic reddish granules in the cytoplasm when stained with eosin, a red dye, using the Romanowsky method.

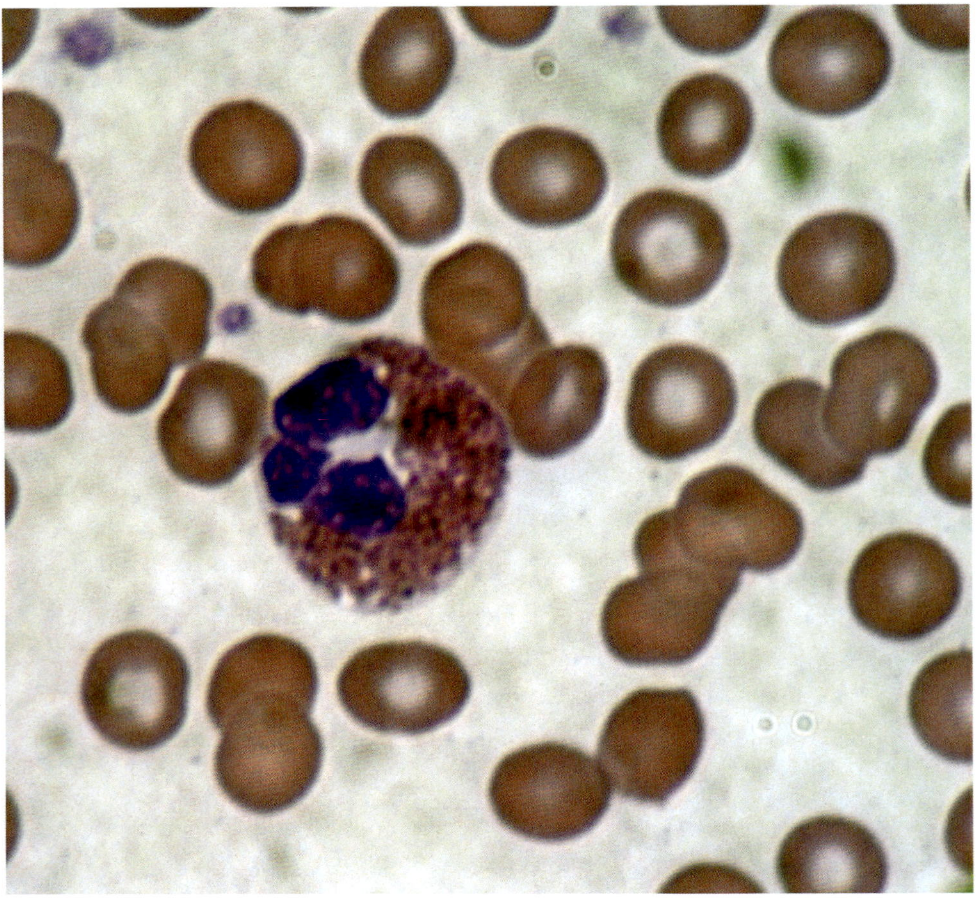

Embryo-fetal toxicity

Based on findings from animal studies and its mechanism of action, NERLYNX can cause fetal harm when administered to a pregnant woman. In animal reproduction studies, administration of neratinib to pregnant rabbits during organogenesis caused abortions, embryo-fetal death, and fetal abnormalities in rabbits at maternal AUCs approximately 0.2 times the AUC in patients receiving the recommended dose. Advise pregnant women of the potential risk to a fetus. Advise females of reproductive potential to use effective contraception during treatment and for at least 1 month after the last dose.

DRUG INTERACTIONS

Effect of Other Drugs on NERLYNX

Gastric acid reducing agents

Concomitant use of NERLYNX with a proton pump inhibitor, H2-receptor antagonist, or antacid may decrease neratinib plasma concentration. Decreased neratinib AUC may reduce NERLYNX activity. Lansoprazole (PPI) resulted in a decrease of neratinib Cmax by 71% and AUC by 65%.

Strong CYP3A4 Inhibitors

(Cytochrome P450 3A4 (abbreviated CYP3A4) (Figure 117) is an important enzyme in the body, mainly found in the liver and in the intestine. It oxidizes small foreign organic molecules (xenobiotics), such as toxins or drugs, so that they can be removed from the body.

While many drugs are deactivated by CYP3A4, there are also some drugs which are activated by the enzyme. Some substances, such as grapefruit juice and some drugs, interfere with the action of CYP3A4. These substances will therefore either amplify or weaken the action of those drugs that are modified by CYP3A4.

CYP3A4 is a member of the cytochrome P450 family of oxidizing enzymes. Several other members of this family are also involved in drug metabolism, but CYP3A4 is the most common and the most versatile one. Like all members of this family, it is a hemoprotein, i.e. a protein containing a heme group with an iron atom. In humans, the CYP3A4 protein is encoded by the CYP3A4 gene. This gene is part of a cluster of cytochrome P450 genes on chromosome 7q22.1

Figure 117. Cytochrome P450 3A4 homodimer + 2 HEM (green-red) + 2 D7J inhibitor (l.blue-red), Human. This image is by By Deposition authors: Sevrioukova, I.;visualization author: User:Astrojan - http://www.rcsb.org/pdb/explore/explore.do?structureId=6bd7, CC BY-SA 4.0, https://commons.wikimedia.org/w/index.php?curid=65226222. https://en.wikipedia.org/wiki/CYP3A4#/media/File:6bd7.jpg. This file is licensed

Figure 117. Cytochrome P450 3A4 homodimer + 2 HEM (green-red) + 2 D7J inhibitor (l.blue-red), Human.

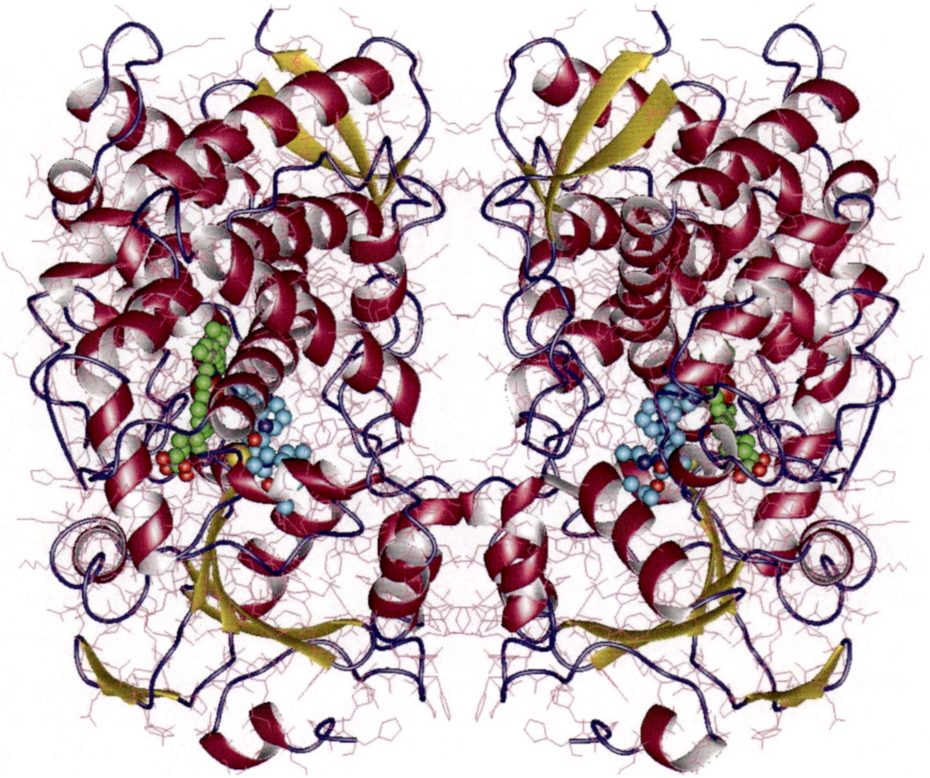

Concomitant use of NERLYNX with a strong CYP3A4 inhibitor (ketoconazole) increased neratinib Cmax by 221% and AUC by 381%

• Concomitant use of NERLYNX with other strong CYP3A4 inhibitors may increase neratinib concentrations.

• Increased neratinib concentrations may increase the risk of toxicity.

Strong or moderate CYP3A4 inducers

Concomitant use of NERLYNX with a strong CYP3A4 inducer (rifampin) reduced neratinib Cmax by 76% and AUC by 87%

• Concomitant use of NERLYNX with other strong or moderate CYP3A4 inducers may decrease NERLYNX concentrations.

• Decreased neratinib AUC may reduce NERLYNX activity.

P-glycoprotein (P-gp) substrates

Concomitant use of NERLYNX with digoxin, a P-gp substrate, increased digoxin concentrations. Increased concentrations of digoxin may lead to increased risk of adverse reactions including cardiac toxicity. Refer to the digoxin prescribing information for dosage adjustment recommendations due to drug interactions. NERLYNX may inhibit the transport of other P-gp substrates (e.g., dabigatran, fexofenadine)

P-glycoprotein 1 (permeability glycoprotein, abbreviated as P-gp or Pgp) also known as multidrug resistance protein 1 (MDR1) or ATP-binding cassette sub-family B member 1 (ABCB1) or cluster of differentiation 243 (CD243) (Figure 118) is an important protein of the cell membrane that pumps many foreign substances out of cells. More formally, it is an ATP-dependent efflux pump with broad substrate specificity. It exists in animals, fungi, and bacteria, and it likely evolved as a defense mechanism against harmful substances.

Figure 118. Structure of the mouse P-glycoprotein based on the 3g5u PDB coordinates. This image is by Boghog2 - Own work, Public Domain, https://commons.wikimedia.org/w/index.php?curid=8232615. https://en.wikipedia.org/wiki/P-glycoprotein#/media/File:MDR3_3g5u.png. The copyright holder of this work has released this work into the public domain. No changes have been made to this image.

Figure 118. Structure of the mouse P-glycoprotein based on the 3g5u PDB coordinates. Note that there is a significant overlap between mouse and human p-Gp.

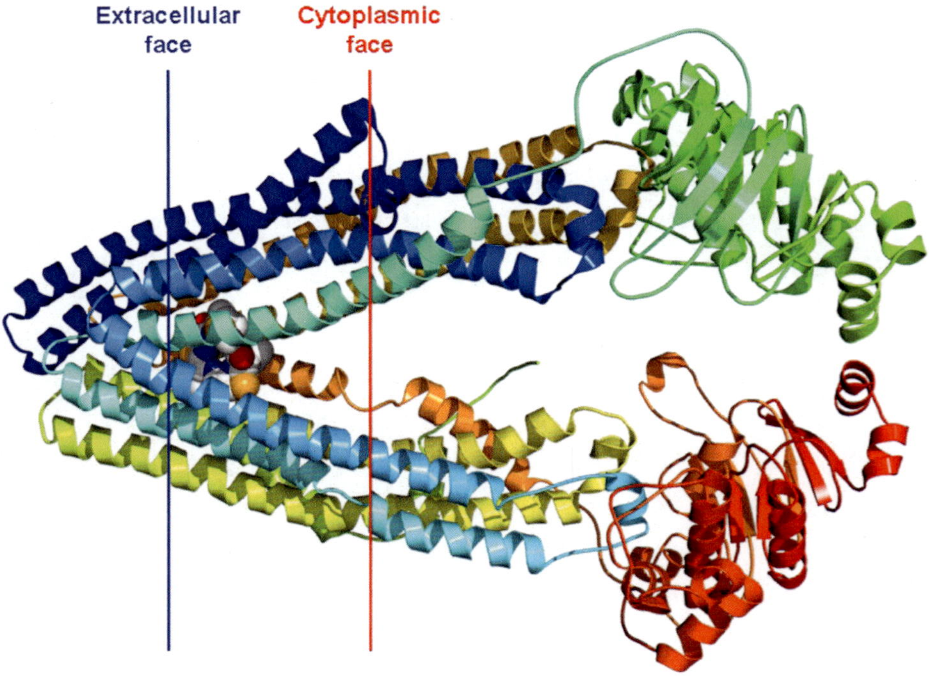

USE IN SPECIFIC POPULATIONS

Pregnancy risk summary

Based on findings from animal studies and the mechanism of action, NERLYNX can cause fetal harm when administered to a pregnant. There are no available data in pregnant women to inform the drug-associated risk. In animal reproduction studies, administration of neratinib to pregnant rabbits during organogenesis resulted in abortions, embryo-fetal death and fetal abnormalities in rabbits at maternal exposures (AUC) approximately 0.2 times exposures in patients at the recommended dose (see Data). Advise pregnant women of the potential risk to a fetus. The background risk of major birth defects and miscarriage for the indicated population is unknown. However, the background risk of major birth defects is 2%-

4% and of miscarriage is 15%-20% of clinically recognized pregnancies in the U.S. general population.

Data

Animal data

In a fertility and early embryonic development study in female rats, neratinib was administered orally for 15 days before mating to Day 7 of pregnancy, which did not cause embryonic toxicity at doses up to 12 mg/kg/day in the presence of maternal toxicity. A dose of 12 mg/kg/day in rats is approximately 0.5 times the maximum recommended dose of 240 mg/day in patients on a mg/m^2 basis. In an embryo-fetal development study in rats, pregnant animals received oral doses of neratinib up to 15 mg/kg/day during the period of organogenesis. No effects on embryo-fetal development or survival were observed. Maternal toxicity was evident at 15 mg/kg/day (approximately 0.6 times the AUC in patients receiving the maximum recommended dose of 240 mg/day). In an embryo-fetal development study in rabbits, pregnant animals received oral doses of neratinib up to 9 mg/kg/day during the period of organogenesis. Administration of neratinib at doses ≥6 mg/kg/day resulted in maternal toxicity, abortions, and embryo-fetal death (increased resorptions). Neratinib administration resulted in increased incidence of fetal gross external (domed head), soft tissue (dilation of the brain ventricles and ventricular septal defect), and skeletal (misshapen anterior fontanelles and enlarged anterior and/or posterior fontanelles) abnormalities at ≥3 mg/kg/day. The AUC (0-t) at 6 mg/kg/day and 9 mg/kg/day in rabbits were approximately 0.5 and 0.8 times, respectively, the AUCs in patients receiving the maximum recommended dose of 240 mg/day. In a peri- and postnatal development study in rats, oral administration of neratinib from gestation day 7 until lactation day 20 resulted in maternal toxicity at ≥10 mg/kg/day (approximately 0.4 times the maximum recommended dose of 240 mg/day in patients on a mg/m^2 basis) including decreased body weights, body weight gains, and food consumption. Effects on long-term memory were observed in male offspring at maternal doses ≥5 mg/kg/day (approximately 0.2 times the maximum recommended dose of 240 mg/day in patients on a mg/m^2 basis).

Lactation risk summary

No data are available regarding the presence of neratinib or its metabolites in human milk or its effects on the breastfed infant or on milk production. Because of the potential for serious adverse reactions in breastfed infants from NERLYNX, advise lactating women not to breastfeed while taking NERLYNX and for at least 1 month after the last dose.

Females and males of reproductive potential

Pregnancy

Based on animal studies, NERLYNX can cause fetal harm when administered to a pregnant woman. Females of reproductive potential should have a pregnancy test prior to starting treatment with NERLYNX.

Contraception

Females

Based on animal studies, NERLYNX can cause fetal harm when administered to a pregnant woman. Advise females of reproductive potential to use effective contraception during treatment with NERLYNX and for at least 1 month after the last dose.

Males

Based on findings in animal reproduction studies, advise male patients with female partners of reproductive potential to use effective contraception during treatment and for 3 months after the last dose of NERLYNX

Pediatric use

The safety and efficacy of NERLYNX in pediatric patients has not been established.

Geriatric use

In the ExteNET trial, in the NERLYNX arm; 1236 patients were <65 years, 172 patients were ≥65 years, of whom 25 patients were 75 years or older. There was a higher frequency of treatment discontinuations due to adverse reactions in the ≥65 years age group than in the <65 years age group; in the NERLYNX arm, the percentages were 45% compared with 25%, respectively, and in the placebo arm 6% and 5%, respectively. The incidence of serious adverse reactions in the NERLYNX arm vs. placebo arm was 7% vs. 6%. (<65 years old) and 10% vs. 8% (≥65 years old). The serious adverse reactions most frequently reported in the ≥65 years old group were vomiting (2.3%), diarrhea (1.7%), renal failure (1.7%), and dehydration (1.2%). In the NALA trial, in the NERLYNX plus capecitabine arm, 242 patients were <65 years, 61 patients were ≥65 years, of whom 12 patients were 75 years or older. The incidence of serious adverse reactions in the NERLYNX plus capecitabine arm in the ≥65 years age group was 36% and in the <65 years age group was 34%. The serious adverse reactions most frequently reported in the ≥65 years-old group were diarrhea (16%), acute kidney injury (8%), and dehydration (7%). No overall differences in effectiveness were observed between patients ≥65 years old and patients <65 years.

Pharmacodynamics

Cardiac electrophysiology

The effect of NERLYNX on the QTc interval was evaluated in a randomized, placebo, and positive-controlled, double-blind, single-dose, crossover study in 60 healthy subjects. At 140% the therapeutic exposures of NERLYNX, there was no clinically relevant effect on the QTc interval.

Pharmacokinetics

Neratinib exhibits a non-linear PK profile with less than dose proportional increase of AUC with the increasing daily dose over the range of 40 to 400 mg.

Absorption

The neratinib and major active metabolites M3, M6 and M7 peak concentrations are reached in the range of 2 to 8 hours after oral administration.

Effect of food

The food-effect assessment was conducted in healthy volunteers who received NERLYNX 240 mg under fasting conditions and with high-fat food (approximately 55% fat, 31% carbohydrate, and 14% protein) or standard breakfast (approximately 50% carbohydrate, 35% fat, and 15% protein). A high-fat meal increased neratinib Cmax and AUCinf by 70% (90% CI: 1.1–2.7) and 120% (90% CI: 1.4–3.5), respectively. A standard breakfast increased the Cmax and AUCinf by 20% (90% CI: 0.97–1.42) and 10% (90% CI: 1.02–1.24), respectively

Distribution

In patients, following multiple doses of NERLYNX, the mean (%CV) apparent volume of distribution at steady-state (Vss/F) was 6433 (19%) L. In vitro protein binding of neratinib in human plasma was greater than 99% and independent of concentration. Neratinib bound predominantly to human serum albumin and human alpha-1 acid glycoprotein.

Elimination

Following 7 days of daily 240 mg oral doses of NERLYNX in healthy subjects, the mean (%CV) plasma halflife of neratinib, M3, M6, and M7 was 14.6 (38%), 21.6 (77%), 13.8 (50%) and 10.4 (33%) hours, respectively. The mean elimination half-life of neratinib ranged from 7 to 17 hours following a single oral dose in patients. Following multiple doses of NERLYNX at once-daily 240 mg in cancer patients, the mean (%CV) CL/F after first dose and at steady state (day 21) were 216 (34%) and 281 (40%) L/hour, respectively.

Metabolism

Neratinib is metabolized primarily in the liver by CYP3A4 and to a lesser extent by flavin-containing monooxygenase (FMO). After oral administration of NERLYNX, neratinib represents the most prominent component in plasma. At steady state after 240 mg daily oral doses of NERLYNX in a healthy subject study (n=25), the systemic exposures (AUC) of the active metabolites M3, M6, M7 and M11were 15%, 33%, 22% and 4% of the systemic neratinib exposure (AUC) respectively.

Excretion

After oral administration of 200 mg (0.83 times of approved recommended dosage) radiolabeled neratinib oral formulation, fecal excretion accounted for approximately 97% and urinary excretion accounted for 1.1% of the total dose. Sixty-one percent of the excreted radioactivity was recovered within 96 hours and 98% was recovered after 10 days.

Specific populations

Age, gender, race, and renal function do not have a clinically significant effect on neratinib pharmacokinetics.

Patients with hepatic impairment

Neratinib is mainly metabolized in the liver. Single doses of 120 mg NERLYNX were evaluated in non-cancer patients with chronic hepatic impairment (n=6 each in Child Pugh Class A, B, and C) and in healthy subjects (n=9) with normal hepatic function. Neratinib exposures in the patients with Child Pugh Class A (mild impairment) and Child Pugh Class B (moderate impairment) were similar to that in normal healthy volunteers. Patients with severe hepatic impairment (Child Pugh Class C) had neratinib Cmax and AUC increased by 173% and 181%, respectively, as compared to the normal hepatic function controls.

Drug interaction studies

Gastric acid reducing agents

NERLYNX solubility decreases with increasing GI tract pH values. Drugs that alter the pH values of the GI tract may alter the solubility of neratinib and hence its absorption and systemic exposure. When multiple doses of lansoprazole (30 mg daily), a proton pump inhibitor, were co-administered with a single 240 mg oral dose of NERLYNX, the neratinib Cmax and AUC decreased by 71% and 65%, respectively. When a single oral dose of 240 mg NERLYNX was administered 2 hours following a daily dose of 300 mg ranitidine, an H2 receptor antagonist, the neratinib Cmax and AUC were reduced by 57% and 48%, respectively. When a single oral dose of 240 mg NERLYNX was administered 2 hours prior to 150 mg ranitidine twice daily (administered in the morning and evening, approximately 12 hours apart), the neratinib Cmax and AUC were reduced by 44% and 32%, respectively

Strong CYP3A4 inhibitors

Concomitant use of ketoconazole (400 mg once-daily for 5 days), a strong inhibitor of CYP3A4 and an inhibitor of P-gp, with a single oral 240 mg NERLYNX dose in healthy subjects (n=24) increased neratinib Cmax by 221% and AUC by 381%.

Moderate CYP3A4 and P-gp dual inhibitors

Simulations using physiologically based pharmacokinetic (PBPK) models suggested that a moderate CYP3A4 and P-gp dual inhibitor (verapamil) may increase the Cmax and AUC of neratinib by 203% and 299%, respectively.

Moderate CYP3A4 inhibitors

Simulations using PBPK models suggested that a moderate CYP3A4 inhibitor (fluconazole) may increase the Cmax and AUC of neratinib by 30% and 68%, respectively.

Strong and moderate CYP3A4 inducers

Concomitant use of rifampin, a strong inducer of CYP3A4, with a single oral 240 mg NERLYNX dose in healthy subjects (n=24) reduced neratinib Cmax by 76% and AUC by 87%. The AUC of active metabolites M6 and M7 were also reduced by 37-49% when compared to NERLYNX administered alone. Simulations using PBPK models suggested that a moderate CYP3A4 inducer (efavirenz) may decrease the Cmax and AUC of neratinib by 36% and 52%, respectively.

Effect of NERLYNX on P-gp transporters

Concomitant use of digoxin (a single 0.5 mg oral dose), a P-gp substrate, with multiple oral doses of NERLYNX 240 mg in healthy subjects (n=18) increased the mean digoxin Cmax by 54% and AUC by 32%.

Clinical efficacy of neratinib in the treatment of breast cancer

i). Neratinib is a potent, irreversible, pan-HER inhibitor that has shown promising activity in preclinical as well as clinical studies with an acceptable safety profile in humans. However, further elucidation is needed to determine when and in which combination this compound should be used. Although most studies showed that neratinib offers the greatest benefit to patients with HER2-positive breast cancer, some data indicate that some HER2-negative patients may also benefit. Moreover, neratinib is now being tested in many solid tumors carrying EGFR, HER2, or HER3 mutations, or EGFR amplification. It will be interesting to see where neratinib will be positioned in relation to other available HER-targeting antibodies as well as TKIs. Ongoing studies will help to better define patients likely to benefit most from neratinib-containing treatments and the associated predictive biomarkers.

Feldinger K, Kong A. Profile of neratinib and its potential in the treatment of breast cancer. Breast Cancer (Dove Med Press). 2015; 7:147-162. Published 2015 Jun 9. doi:10.2147/BCTT.S54414

ii). In this trial, neratinib yielded increased progression-free survival, response duration and a benefit in time to intervention for CNS progression. However, there was no overall survival benefit, no increase in overall response rate and no improvement in QoL. The most frequent adverse event in the neratinib arm was diarrhea, which was manageable with prophylactic treatment with loperamide. Conclusion: Neratinib is a valuable addition to the therapeutic armamentarium to treat metastatic, HER2-positive breast cancer. The current positioning of the combination of neratinib and capecitabine based on the results of the NALA trial needs to consider the rapidly evolving scenario due to the recent introduction of new drugs, like the pure-HER2 TKI tucatinib and the antibody drug-conjugate trastuzumab-deruxtecan.

Chilà G et al. The Clinical Efficacy and Safety of Neratinib in Combination with Capecitabine for the Treatment of Adult Patients with Advanced or Metastatic HER2-Positive Breast Cancer. Drug Des Devel Ther. 2021;15: 2711-2720 https://doi.org/10.2147/DDDT.S281599

9.16. PERTUZUMAB (PERJETA)

PERJETA® (pertuzumab) Injection, for intravenous use Initial U.S. Approval: 2012

WARNING: CARDIOMYOPATHY and EMBRYO-FETAL TOXICITY See full prescribing information for complete boxed warning.

Cardiomyopathy

PERJETA can result in subclinical and clinical **cardiac failure** manifesting as CHF, and decreased LVEF. Evaluate cardiac function prior to and during treatment. Discontinue PERJETA treatment for a confirmed clinically significant decrease in left ventricular function.

Embryo-fetal toxicity

Exposure to PERJETA can result in **embryo-fetal death and birth defects**. Studies in animals have resulted in oligohydramnios, delayed renal development, and death. Advise patients of these risks and the need for effective contraception.

RECENT MAJOR CHANGES

Indications and Usage 09/2013

Dosage and Administration 04/2013

Dosage and Administration 09/2013

Contraindications 09/2013

Warnings and Precautions 09/2013

INDICATIONS AND USAGE

PERJETA is a HER2/neu receptor antagonist indicated for:

- Use in combination with trastuzumab and docetaxel for treatment of patients with HER2-positive metastatic breast cancer (MBC) who have not received prior anti-HER2 therapy or chemotherapy for metastatic disease.

- Use in combination with trastuzumab and docetaxel as neoadjuvant treatment of patients with HER2-positive, locally advanced, inflammatory, or early stage breast cancer (either greater than 2 cm in diameter or node positive) as part of a complete treatment regimen for early breast cancer. This indication is based on demonstration of an improvement in pathological complete response rate. No data are available demonstrating improvement in event-free survival or overall survival.

Inflammatory breast cancer (IBC) is one of the most aggressive forms of breast cancer. It can occur at any age (and, extremely rarely, in men). It is referred to as "inflammatory" due to its frequent presentation with symptoms resembling a skin inflammation, such as erysipelas *(Figure 120).*

MECHANISM OF ACTION

Pertuzumab targets the extracellular dimerization domain (Subdomain II) of the human epidermal growth factor receptor 2 protein (HER2) and, thereby, blocks ligand-dependent heterodimerization of HER2 with other HER family members, including EGFR, HER3, and HER4. As a result, pertuzumab inhibits ligand-initiated intracellular signaling through two major signal pathways, mitogen-activated protein (MAP) kinase, and phosphoinositide 3-kinase (PI3K). Inhibition of these signaling pathways can result in cell growth arrest and apoptosis, respectively (Figure 119). In addition, pertuzumab mediates antibody-dependent cell-mediated cytotoxicity (ADCC).

Figure 119. A simplified representation of major signal transduction pathways in mammals.

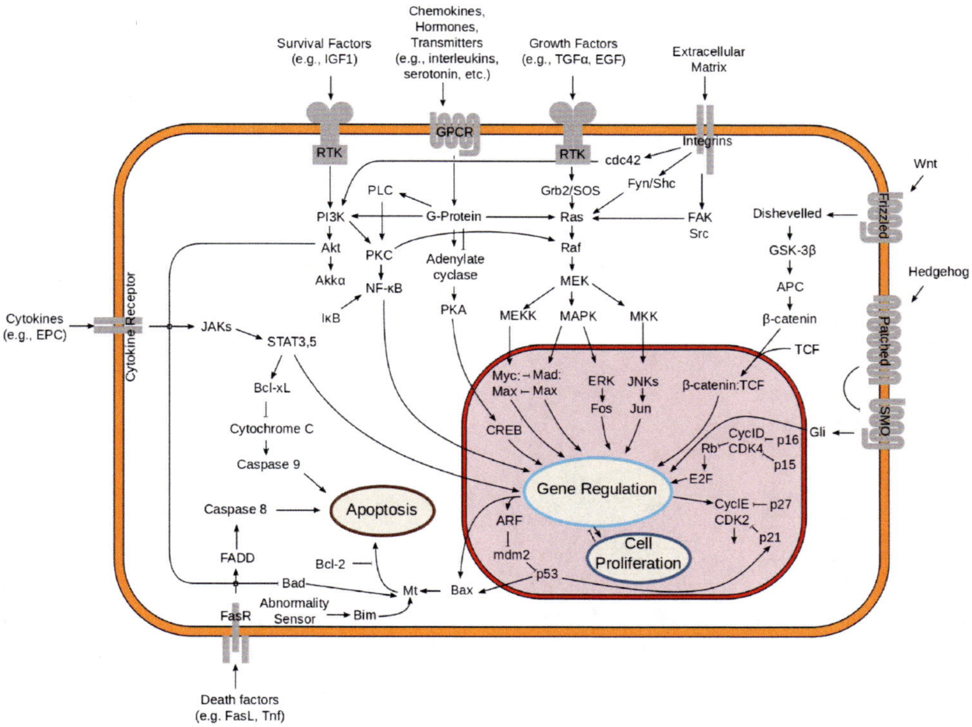

This image is reproduced here from Wikimedia Commons since permission has been granted by its creator, Cybertory, to copy, distribute and/or modify this document under the terms of the GNU Free Documentation License, Version 1.2 or any later version published by the Free Software Foundation; Author:

By Cybertory - This file was derived from: Signal transduction v1.png, CC BY-SA 3.0, https://commons.wikimedia.org/w/index.php?curid=12081090https://en.wikipedia.org/wiki/Creative_Commons_license. No change has been made to the image.

DESCRIPTION

Pertuzumab is a recombinant humanized monoclonal antibody that targets the extracellular dimerization domain (Subdomain II) of the human epidermal growth factor receptor 2 protein (HER2). Pertuzumab is produced by recombinant DNA technology in a mammalian cell (Chinese Hamster Ovary) culture containing the antibiotic, gentamicin. Gentamicin is not detectable in the final product. Pertuzumab has an approximate molecular weight of 148 kDa. PERJETA is a sterile, clear to slightly opalescent, colorless to pale brown liquid for intravenous infusion. Each single use vial contains 420 mg of pertuzumab at a concentration of 30 mg/mL in 20 mM L-histidine acetate (pH 6.0), 120 mM sucrose and 0.02% polysorbate 20.

Figure 120. Erysipas of the face due to invasive Streptococcus

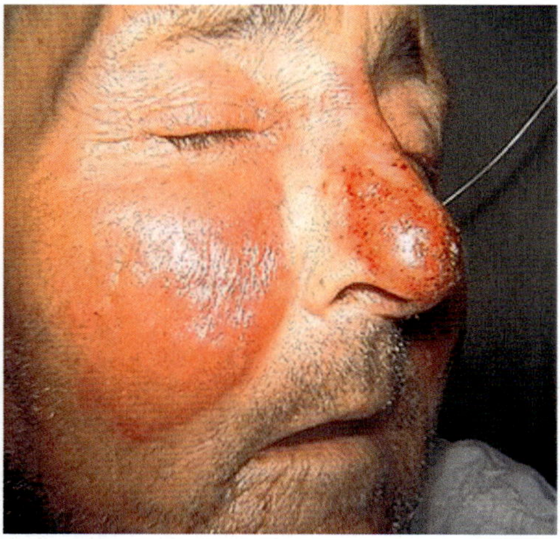

This image is by By CDC/Dr. Thomas F. Sellers/Emory University - This media comes from the Centers for Disease Control and Prevention's Public Health Image Library (PHIL), with identification number #2874.Note: Not all PHIL images are public domain; be sure to check copyright status and credit authors and content

providers. | Deutsch | English | македонски | slovenščina | +/−, Public Domain, https://commons.wikimedia.org/w/index.php?curid=6898976. https://en.wikipedia.org/wiki/Erysipelas#/media/File:Facial_erysipelas.jpg. This image is a work of the Centers for Disease Control and Prevention, part of the United States Department of Health and Human Services, taken or made as part of an employee's official duties. As a work of the U.S. federal government, the image is in the public domain. . No changes were made to this image.

Inflammatory breast cancer presents with variable signs and symptoms, frequently without detectable lumps or tumors; it therefore is often not detected by mammography or ultrasound. Typical presentation is rapid breast swelling, sometimes associated with skin changes (peau d'orange) *(Figure 121),* and nipple retraction. (*Peau d'orange (French for "orange peel skin" or, more literally, "skin of an orange") describes anatomy with the appearance and hair follicles get buried in the oedema and resemble an orange peel. Peau d'orange is caused by cutaneous lymphatic edema, which causes swelling. However, some parts of the edematous skin is tethered by the hair follicles and the sweat glands such that it cannot swell, leading to an appearance like orange skin).*

Figure 121. A facial eosinophilic granuloma demonstrating "peau d'orange". This image is by Sand, Michael, et al. - http://www.head-face-med.com/content/6/1/7, CC BY 2.0, https://commons.wikimedia.org/w/index.php?curid=19673622. https://en.wikipedia.org/wiki/Peau_d%27orange#/media/File:Facial_eosinophilic_granuloma.jpg. This file is licensed under the Creative Commons Attribution 2.0 Generic license. No changes were made to this image.

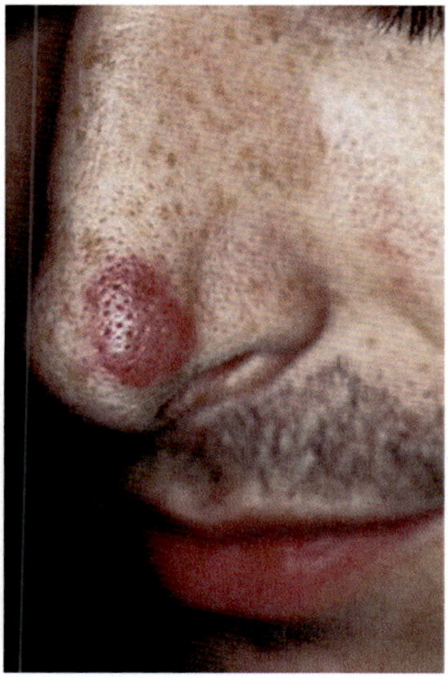

Other signs include redness, persistent itching, and unusually warm skin. IBC often initially resembles mastitis *(Figure 122).* Approximately 50% to 75% of cases have the typical presentation; an atypical presentation makes diagnosis more difficult. In some cases, a sign such as acute central venous thrombosis may be the sole presenting indication of the disease.

Figure 122. A drawing of mastitis invoving the left breast from the early 1900s.

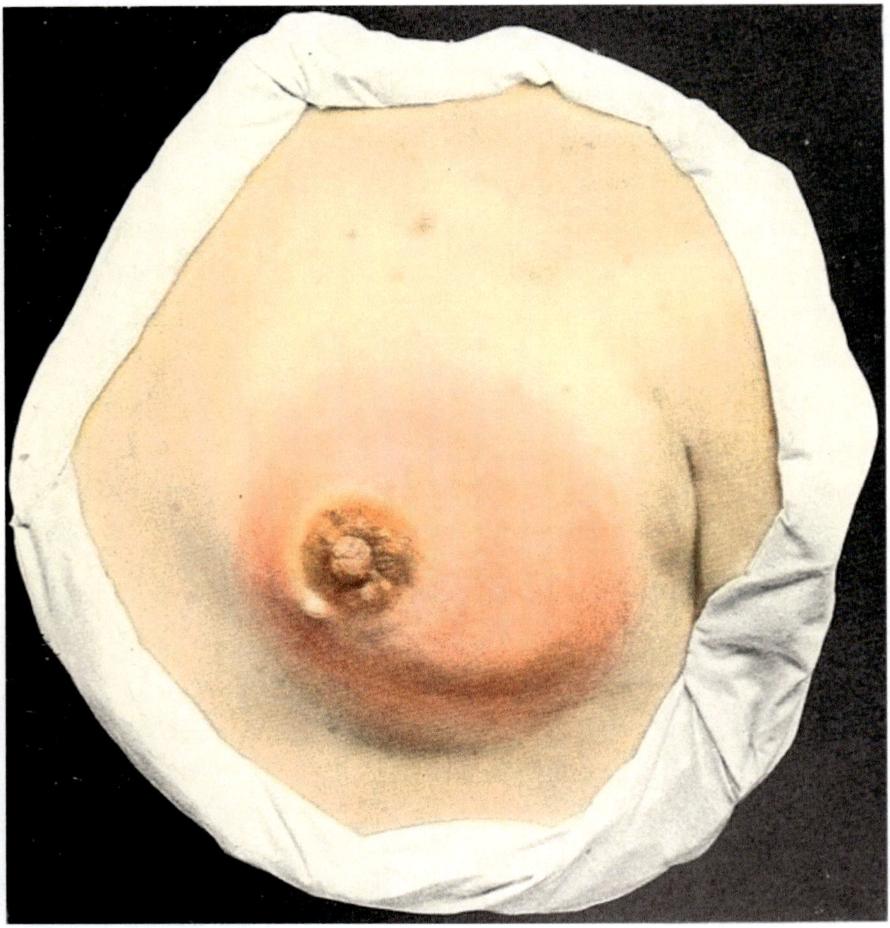

This image is by Internet Archive Book Images - https://www.flickr.com/photos/internetarchivebookimages/14768289625/Source book page: https://archive.org/stream/atlasofclinicals00bock/atlasofclinicals00bock#page/n342/mode/1up, No restrictions, https://commons.wikimedia.org/w/index.php?curid=43701179. https://en.wikipedia.org/wiki/Mastitis#/media/File:Atlas_of_clinical_surgery;_with_spe

cial_reference_to_diagnosis_and_treatment_for_practitioners_and_students_(1908)_(14768289625).jpg.

This image was originally posted to Flickr by Internet Archive Book Images at https://flickr.com/photos/126377022@N07/14768289625. It was reviewed on 27 September 2015 by FlickreviewR and was confirmed to be licensed under the terms of the No known copyright restrictions.

IBC comprises a small proportion of breast cancer cases (1% to 6% in the USA). African Americans are usually diagnosed with IBC at younger ages than are Caucasian women; they are also at higher risk for the disease. Recent advances in therapy have improved the prognosis considerably; at least one-third of women will survive with IBC for ten years or longer).

Limitations of use

• The safety of PERJETA as part of a doxorubicin-containing regimen has not been established.

• The safety of PERJETA administered for greater than 6 cycles for early breast cancer has not been established.

DOSAGE AND ADMINISTRATION

• For intravenous infusion only. Do not administer as an intravenous push or bolus.

• The initial PERJETA dose is 840 mg administered as a 60-minute intravenous infusion, followed every 3 weeks thereafter by 420 mg administered as a 30-to-60-minute intravenous infusion.

• MBC: administer PERJETA, trastuzumab, and docetaxel by intravenous infusion every 3 weeks.

• Neoadjuvant: administer PERJETA, trastuzumab, and docetaxel by intravenous infusion preoperatively every 3 weeks for 3 to 6 cycles.

DOSAGE FORMS AND STRENGTHS

• 420 mg/14 mL single-use vial.

CONTRAINDICATIONS

PERJETA is contraindicated in patients with known hypersensitivity to pertuzumab or to any of its excipients.

WARNINGS AND PRECAUTIONS

• Embryo-fetal toxicity

Fetal harm can occur when administered to a pregnant woman.

• Left ventricular dysfunction

Monitor LVEF and withhold dosing as appropriate.

• Infusion-related reactions

Monitor for signs and symptoms. If a significant infusion-associated reaction occurs, slow or interrupt the infusion and administer appropriate medical therapies.

• Hypersensitivity reactions/anaphylaxis

Monitor for signs and symptoms. If a severe hypersensitivity reaction/anaphylaxis *(Figures 123 and 124)* occurs, discontinue the infusion immediately and administer appropriate medical therapies.

Figure 123. Urticaria and flushing on the back of a person with anaphylaxis.

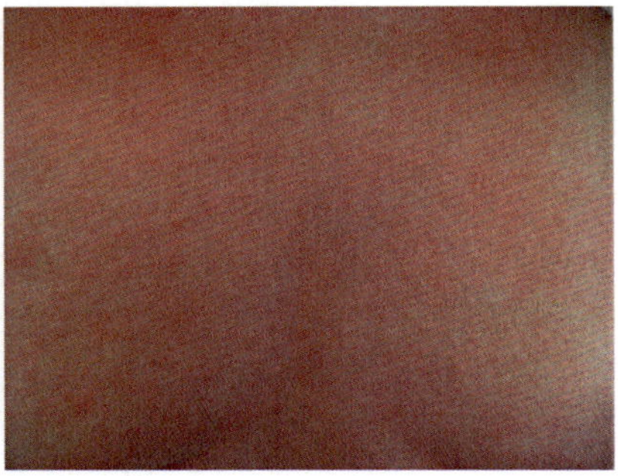

This image is by James Heilman, MD - Own work, CC BY-SA 3.0, https://commons.wikimedia.org/w/index.php?curid=8756708. https://en.wikipedia.org/wiki/Anaphylaxis#/media/File:Rash_on_the_chest_of_a_person_with_anaphylaxis.jpg. This file is licensed under the Creative

Figure 124. Signs and symptoms of anaphylaxis.

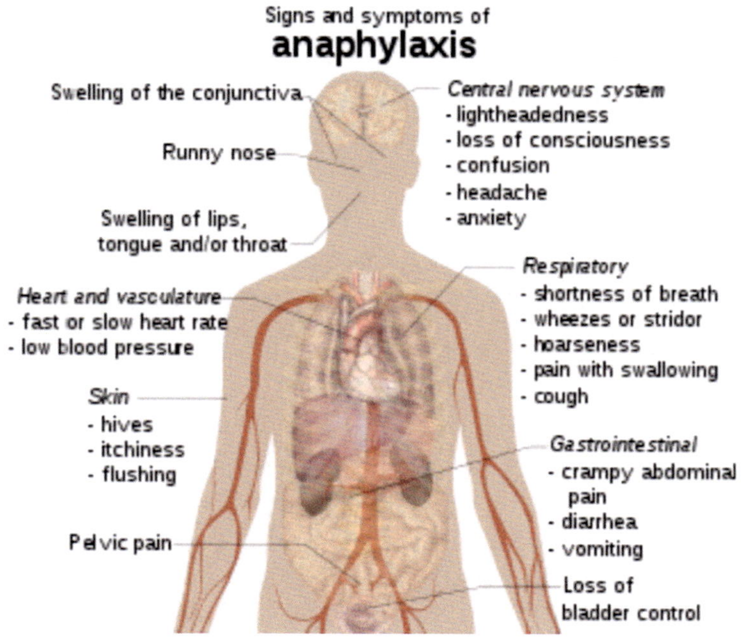

• HER2 testing: perform using FDA-approved tests by laboratories with demonstrated proficiency.

ADVERSE REACTIONS

Metastatic breast cancer

• The most common adverse reactions (> 30%) with PERJETA in combination with trastuzumab and docetaxel were diarrhea, alopecia, neutropenia, nausea, fatigue, rash, and peripheral neuropathy

Neoadjuvant treatment of breast cancer

- The most common adverse reactions (> 30%) with PERJETA in combination with trastuzumab and docetaxel were alopecia, diarrhea, nausea, and neutropenia.

- The most common adverse reactions (>30%) with PERJETA in combination with trastuzumab and docetaxel when given for 3 cycles following 3 cycles of FEC were fatigue, alopecia, diarrhea, nausea, vomiting, and neutropenia.

- The most common adverse reactions (>30%) with PERJETA in combination with docetaxel, carboplatin, and trastuzumab (TCH) were fatigue, alopecia, diarrhea, nausea, vomiting, neutropenia, thrombocytopenia, and anemia. To report SUSPECTED ADVERSE REACTIONS, contact Genentech at 1-888-835-2555 or FDA at 1-800-FDA-1088 or www.fda.gov/medwatch.

FULL PRESCRIBING INFORMATION

WARNING: CARDIOMYOPATHY AND EMBRYO-FETAL TOXICITY

Cardiomyopathy

PERJETA administration can result in subclinical and clinical cardiac failure. Evaluate left ventricular function in all patients prior to and during treatment with PERJETA. Discontinue PERJETA treatment for a confirmed clinically significant decrease in left ventricular function. *Please see the section on ado-trastuzumab emtansine for more information on cardiac failure.*

Embryo-fetal toxicity

Exposure to PERJETA can result in embryo-fetal death and birth defects. Studies in animals have resulted in oligohydramnios, delayed renal development, and death. Advise patients of these risks and the need for effective contraception.

INDICATIONS AND USAGE

Metastatic breast cancer (MBC)

PERJETA is indicated for use in combination with trastuzumab and docetaxel for the treatment of patients with HER2-positive metastatic breast cancer who have not received prior anti-HER2 therapy or chemotherapy for metastatic disease.

Neoadjuvant treatment of breast cancer

PERJETA is indicated for use in combination with trastuzumab and docetaxel for the neoadjuvant treatment of patients with HER2-positive, locally advanced, inflammatory, or early stage breast cancer (either greater than 2 cm in diameter or node positive) as part of a complete treatment regimen for early breast cancer. This indication is based on demonstration of an improvement in pathological complete response rate. No data are available demonstrating improvement in event-free survival or overall survival

Limitations of use

- The safety of PERJETA as part of a doxorubicin-containing regimen has not been established.

- The safety of PERJETA administered for greater than 6 cycles for early breast cancer has not been established.

DOSAGE AND ADMINISTRATION

Recommended doses and schedules

The initial dose of PERJETA is 840 mg administered as a 60-minute intravenous infusion, followed every 3 weeks by a dose of 420 mg administered as an intravenous infusion over 30 to 60 minutes. When administered with PERJETA, the recommended initial dose of trastuzumab is 8 mg/kg administered as a 90-minute intravenous infusion, followed every 3 weeks by a dose of 6 mg/kg administered as an intravenous infusion over 30 to 90 minutes. PERJETA, trastuzumab, and docetaxel should be administered sequentially. PERJETA and trastuzumab can be given in any order. Docetaxel should be administered after PERJETA and trastuzumab. An observation period of 30 to 60 minutes is recommended after each PERJETA infusion and before commencement of any subsequent infusion of trastuzumab or docetaxel

Metastatic breast cancer (MBC)

When administered with PERJETA, the recommended initial dose of docetaxel is 75 mg/m^2 administered as an intravenous infusion. The dose may be escalated to 100 mg/m^2 administered every 3 weeks if the initial dose is well tolerated.

Neoadjuvant treatment of breast cancer

PERJETA should be administered every 3 weeks for 3 to 6 cycles as part of one of the following treatment regimens for early breast cancer

- Four preoperative cycles of PERJETA in combination with trastuzumab and docetaxel followed by 3 postoperative cycles of fluorouracil, epirubicin, and cyclophosphamide (FEC) as given in Study 2
- Three preoperative cycles of FEC alone followed by 3 preoperative cycles of PERJETA in combination with docetaxel and trastuzumab as given in Study 3
- Six preoperative cycles of PERJETA in combination with docetaxel, carboplatin, and trastuzumab (TCH) (escalation of docetaxel above 75 mg/m^2 is not recommended) as given in Study 3.

Following surgery, patients should continue to receive trastuzumab to complete 1 year of treatment. There is insufficient evidence to recommend continued use of PERJETA for greater than 6 cycles for early breast cancer. There is insufficient evidence to recommend concomitant administration of an anthracycline with PERJETA, and there are no safety data to support sequential use of doxorubicin with PERJETA.

Dose modification

For delayed or missed doses, if the time between two sequential infusions is less than 6 weeks, the 420 mg dose of PERJETA should be administered. Do not wait until the next planned dose. If the time between two sequential infusions is 6 weeks or more, the initial dose of 840 mg PERJETA should be re-administered as a 60-minute intravenous infusion followed every 3 weeks thereafter by a dose of 420 mg administered as an intravenous infusion over 30 to 60 minutes. PERJETA should be discontinued if trastuzumab treatment is discontinued. Dose reductions are not recommended for PERJETA. For docetaxel dose modifications, see relevant prescribing information.

Left ventricular ejection fraction (LVEF)

Withhold PERJETA and trastuzumab dosing for at least 3 weeks for either:

- a drop in LVEF to less than 45%

or

- LVEF of 45% to 49% with a 10% or greater absolute decrease below pretreatment values. PERJETA may be resumed if the LVEF has recovered to greater than 49% or to 45% to 49% associated with less than a 10% absolute decrease below pretreatment values. If after a repeat assessment within approximately 3 weeks, the LVEF has not improved, or has declined further, PERJETA and trastuzumab should be discontinued, unless the benefits for the individual patient are deemed to outweigh the risks

Infusion-related reactions

The infusion rate of PERJETA may be slowed or interrupted if the patient develops an infusion-related reaction.

Hypersensitivity reactions/anaphylaxis

The infusion should be discontinued immediately if the patient experiences a serious hypersensitivity reaction.

DOSAGE FORMS AND STRENGTHS

PERJETA (pertuzumab) 420 mg/14 mL (30 mg/mL) in a single-use vial.

CONTRAINDICATIONS

PERJETA is contraindicated in patients with known hypersensitivity to pertuzumab or to any of its excipients.

WARNINGS AND PRECAUTIONS

Embryo-fetal toxicity PERJETA can cause fetal harm when administered to a pregnant woman. Treatment of pregnant cynomolgus monkeys with pertuzumab resulted in oligohydramnios, delayed fetal kidney development, and embryo-fetal death. If PERJETA is administered during pregnancy, or if the patient becomes pregnant while receiving this drug, the patient should be apprised of the potential hazard to a fetus

Verify pregnancy status prior to the initiation of PERJETA. Advise patients of the risks of embryo-fetal death and birth defects and the need for contraception during and after treatment. Advise patients to contact their healthcare provider immediately if they suspect they may be pregnant. If PERJETA is administered during pregnancy or if a patient becomes pregnant while receiving PERJETA, immediately report exposure to the Genentech Adverse Event Line at 1-888-835-2555. Encourage women who may be exposed during pregnancy to enroll in the U.S. BLA: Perjeta® (pertuzumab) – Genentech, Inc. by contacting 1-800-690-6720.

Monitor patients who become pregnant during PERJETA therapy for oligohydramnios. If oligohydramnios occurs, perform fetal testing that is appropriate for gestational age and consistent with community standards of care. The efficacy of intravenous hydration in the management of oligohydramnios due to PERJETA exposure is not known.

Left ventricular dysfunction

Decreases in LVEF have been reported with drugs that block HER2 activity, including PERJETA. In Study 1, for patients with MBC, PERJETA in combination with trastuzumab and docetaxel was not associated with increases in the incidence of symptomatic left ventricular systolic dysfunction (LVSD) or decreases in LVEF compared with placebo in combination with trastuzumab and docetaxel *(Significant left ventricular systolic dysfunction is defined as an LVEF less than 40%.)*

Left ventricular dysfunction occurred in 4.4% of patients in the PERJETA-treated group and 8.3% of patients in the placebo-treated group. Symptomatic left ventricular systolic dysfunction (congestive heart failure) occurred in 1.0% of patients in the PERJETA-treated group and 1.8% of patients in the placebo-treated group. Patients who have received prior anthracyclines or prior radiotherapy to the chest area may be at higher risk of decreased LVEF. In patients receiving neoadjuvant treatment in Study 2, the incidence of LVSD was higher in the PERJETA-treated groups compared to the trastuzumab- and docetaxel-treated group. An increased incidence of LVEF declines was observed in patients treated with PERJETA in combination with trastuzumab and docetaxel. In the overall treatment period, LVEF decline $>$ 10% and a drop to less than 50% occurred in 1.9% of patients treated with neoadjuvant trastuzumab and docetaxel as compared to 8.4% of patients treated with neoadjuvant PERJETA in combination with trastuzumab and docetaxel. Symptomatic LVSD occurred in 0.9% of patients treated with neoadjuvant PERJETA in combination with trastuzumab and no patients in the other 3 arms. LVEF recovered to ≥ 50% in all patients. In patients receiving neoadjuvant PERJETA in Study 3, in the overall treatment period, LVEF decline > 10% and a drop to less than 50% occurred in 6.9% of patients treated with PERJETA plus trastuzumab and FEC followed by PERJETA plus trastuzumab and docetaxel, 16.0% of patients treated with PERJETA plus trastuzumab and docetaxel following FEC, and 10.5% of patients treated with PERJETA in combination with TCH. Symptomatic LVSD occurred in 4.0% of patients treated with PERJETA plus trastuzumab and docetaxel following FEC, 1.3% of patients treated with PERJETA in combination with TCH, and none of the patients treated with PERJETA plus trastuzumab and FEC followed by PERJETA plus trastuzumab and docetaxel. LVEF recovered to ≥ 50% in all but one patient. PERJETA has not been studied in patients with a pretreatment LVEF value of ≤ 50%, a prior history of CHF, decreases in LVEF to < 50% during prior trastuzumab therapy, or conditions that could impair left ventricular function such as uncontrolled hypertension, recent myocardial infarction, serious cardiac arrhythmia requiring treatment or a cumulative prior anthracycline exposure to > 360 mg/m^2 of doxorubicin or its equivalent. Assess LVEF prior to initiation of PERJETA and at regular intervals (e.g., every three months in the metastatic setting and every six weeks in the neoadjuvant setting) during treatment to ensure that LVEF is within the institution's normal limits. If LVEF is < 45% or is 45% to 49% with a 10% or greater absolute decrease below the pretreatment value, withhold PERJETA and trastuzumab and repeat LVEF assessment within approximately 3 weeks. Discontinue PERJETA and trastuzumab if the LVEF has not improved or has declined further unless the benefits for the individual patient outweigh the risks.

Infusion-related reactions

PERJETA has been associated with infusion

An infusion reaction was defined in Study 1 as any event described as hypersensitivity, anaphylactic reaction, acute infusion reaction, or cytokine release syndrome *(see Section 11)* occurring during an infusion or on the same day as the infusion. The initial dose of PERJETA was given the day before trastuzumab and docetaxel to allow for the examination of PERJETA-associated reactions. On the first day, when only PERJETA was administered, the overall frequency of infusion reactions was 13.0% in the PERJETA-treated group and 9.8% in the placebo-treated group. Less than 1% were Grade 3 or 4. The most common infusion reactions (≥ 1.0%) were pyrexia, chills, fatigue, headache, asthenia, hypersensitivity, and vomiting. During the second cycle when all drugs were administered on the same day, the most common infusion reactions in the PERJETA-treated group (≥ 1.0%) were fatigue, dysgeusia, hypersensitivity, myalgia, and vomiting. In Study 2 and Study 3, PERJETA was administered on the same day as the other study treatment drugs. Infusion reactions were consistent with those observed in Study 1, with a majority of reactions being National Cancer Institute - Common Terminology Criteria for Adverse Events (NCI - CTCAE v3.0) Grade 1 – 2. Observe patients closely for 60 minutes after the first infusion and for 30 minutes after subsequent infusions of PERJETA. If a significant infusion-related reaction occurs, slow or interrupt the infusion, and administer appropriate medical therapies. Monitor patients carefully until complete resolution of signs and symptoms. Consider permanent discontinuation in patients with severe infusion reactions.

Cytokine release syndrome *(CRS) is a form of systemic inflammatory response syndrome (SIRS) that can be triggered by a variety of factors such as infections and certain drugs (and see Section 11). It refers to cytokine storm syndromes (CSS) and occurs when large numbers of white blood cells are activated and release inflammatory cytokines, which in turn activate yet more white blood cells. CRS is also an adverse effect of some monoclonal antibody medications, as well as adoptive T-cell therapies.*

The term ***cytokine storm*** *is often used interchangeably with CRS but, despite the fact that they have similar clinical phenotype, their characteristics are different. When occurring as a result of a therapy, CRS symptoms may be delayed until days or weeks after treatment. Immediate-onset CRS is a cytokine storm, although severe cases of CRS have also been called cytokine storms.*

Treatment for less severe CRS is supportive, addressing the symptoms like fever, muscle pain, or fatigue. Moderate CRS requires oxygen therapy and giving fluids and antihypotensive agents to raise blood pressure.

For moderate to severe CRS, the use of immunosuppressive agents like ***corticosteroids*** *may be necessary, but judgment must be used to avoid negating the effect of drugs intended to activate the immune system.*

Tocilizumab, an anti-IL-6 monoclonal antibody, was FDA-approved for steroid-refractory CRS based on retrospective case study data.

Lenzilumab, an anti-GM-CSF monoclonal antibody, may also be effective at managing cytokine release by reducing activation of myeloid cells and decreasing the production of IL-1, IL-6, MCP-1, MIP-1, and IP-10. Additionally, as a soluble cytokine blockade, it will not increase serum levels of GM-CSF (a phenomenon seen with tocilizumab and IL-6).

Hypersensitivity reactions/anaphylaxis

In Study 1, the overall frequency of hypersensitivity/anaphylaxis reactions was 10.8% in the PERJETA-treated group and 9.1% in the placebo-treated group. The incidence of Grade 3 – 4 hypersensitivity/anaphylaxis reactions was 2.0% in the PERJETA-treated group and 2.5% in the placebo-treated group according to NCI - CTCAE v3.0. Overall, 4 patients in PERJETA-treated group and 2 patients in the placebo-treated group experienced anaphylaxis. In Study 2 and Study 3, hypersensitivity/anaphylaxis events were consistent with those observed in Study 1. In Study 2, two patients in the PERJETA- and docetaxel-treated group experienced anaphylaxis. In Study 3, the overall frequency of hypersensitivity/anaphylaxis was highest in the PERJETA plus TCH treated group (13.2%), of which 2.6% were NCI-CTCAE (version 3) Grade 3 – 4. Patients should be observed closely for hypersensitivity reactions. Severe hypersensitivity, including anaphylaxis, has been observed in clinical trials with treatment of PERJETA. Medications to treat such reactions, as well as emergency equipment, should be available for immediate use. PERJETA is contraindicated in patients with known hypersensitivity to pertuzumab or to any of its excipients.

HER2 testing

Detection of HER2 protein overexpression is necessary for selection of patients appropriate for PERJETA therapy because these are the only patients studied and for whom benefit has been shown.

Assessment of HER2 status should be performed by laboratories using FDA-approved tests with demonstrated proficiency in the specific technology being utilized. Improper assay performance, including use of sub-optimally fixed tissue, failure to utilize specified reagents, deviation from specific assay instructions, and failure to include appropriate controls for assay validation, can lead to unreliable results.

ADVERSE REACTIONS

These are discussed in detail in other sections of the label.

Immunogenicity

As with all therapeutic proteins, there is the potential for an immune response to PERJETA. Patients in Study 1 were tested at multiple time-points for antibodies to PERJETA. Approximately 2.8% (11/386) of patients in the PERJETA-treated group and 6.2% (23/372) of patients in the placebo-treated group tested positive for anti-PERJETA antibodies. Of these 34 patients, none experienced anaphylactic/hypersensitivity reactions that were clearly related to the anti-therapeutic antibodies (ATA). The presence of pertuzumab in patient serum at the levels expected at the time of ATA sampling can interfere with the ability of this assay to detect anti-pertuzumab antibodies. In addition, the assay may be detecting antibodies to trastuzumab. As a result, data may not accurately reflect the true incidence of anti-pertuzumab antibody development. Immunogenicity data are highly dependent on the sensitivity and specificity of the test methods used. Additionally, the observed incidence of a positive result in a test method may be influenced by several factors, including sample handling, timing of sample collection, drug interference, concomitant medication, and the underlying disease. For these reasons, comparison of the incidence of antibodies to PERJETA with the incidence of antibodies to other products may be misleading.

DRUG INTERACTIONS

No drug-drug interactions were observed between pertuzumab and trastuzumab, or between pertuzumab and docetaxel.

USE IN SPECIFIC POPULATIONS

Pregnancy

Pregnancy Category D risk summary

There are no adequate and well-controlled studies of PERJETA in pregnant women. Based on findings in animal studies, PERJETA can cause fetal harm when administered to a pregnant woman. The effects of PERJETA are likely to be present during all trimesters of pregnancy. Pertuzumab administered to pregnant cynomolgus monkeys resulted in oligohydramnios, delayed fetal kidney development, and embryo-fetal deaths at clinically relevant exposures of 2.5 to 20-fold greater than the recommended human dose, based on Cmax. If PERJETA is administered during pregnancy, or if a patient becomes pregnant while receiving PERJETA, the patient should be apprised of the potential hazard to the fetus.

If PERJETA is administered during pregnancy or if a patient becomes pregnant while receiving PERJETA, immediately report exposure to the Genentech Adverse Event Line at 371 1-888-835-2555. Encourage women who may be exposed during pregnancy to enroll in the 372 MotHER Pregnancy Registry by contacting 1-800-690-6720.

Animal data

Reproductive toxicology studies have been conducted in cynomolgus monkeys. Pregnant monkeys were treated on Gestational Day (GD) 19 with loading doses of 30 to 150 mg/kg 377 pertuzumab, followed by bi-weekly doses of 10 to 100 mg/kg. These dose levels resulted in 378 clinically relevant exposures of 2.5 to 20-fold greater than the recommended human dose, based 379 on Cmax. Intravenous administration of pertuzumab from GD19 through GD50 (period of 380 organogenesis) was embryotoxic, with dose-dependent increases in embryo-fetal death between GD25 to GD70. The incidences of embryo-fetal loss were 33, 50, and 85% for dams treated with bi-weekly pertuzumab doses of 10, 30, and 100 mg/kg, respectively (2.5 to 20-fold greater than the recommended human dose, based on Cmax). At Caesarean section on GD100, oligohydramnios, decreased relative lung and kidney weights, and microscopic evidence of renal hypoplasia consistent with delayed renal development were identified in all pertuzumab dose 386 groups. Pertuzumab exposure was reported in offspring from all treated groups, at levels of 29% to 40% of maternal serum levels at GD100.

Renal hypoplasia is a congenital abnormality in which one or both of the kidneys are smaller than normal (hypoplastic) but with normal structure. It is defined as abnormally small kidneys, where the size is less than two standard deviations below the expected mean for the corresponding demographics, and the morphology is normal. Disease severity depends on whether hypoplasia is unilateral of bilateral, and the degree of reduction in the number of nephrons. Hypoplastic kidneys are prone to infection and kidney stone formation (Figure 125) have a reduced nephron number (Figure 126) but normal corticomedullary differentiation.

Figure 125. A kidney stone, 8 millimeters (0.3 in) in diameter.

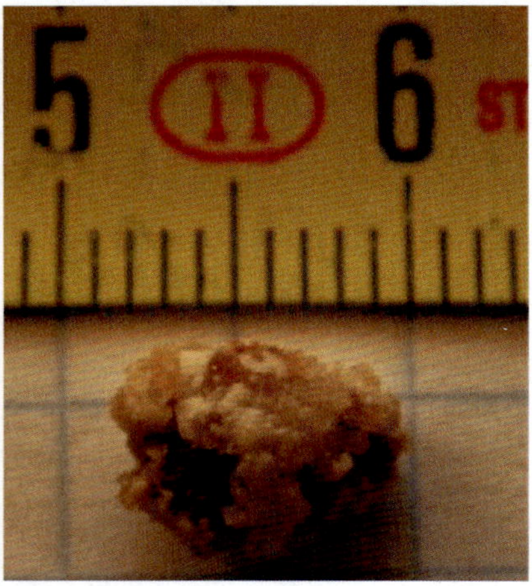

This image is by Robert R. Wal - http://en.wikipedia.org/wiki/Kidney_stone, Public Domain, https://commons.wikimedia.org/w/index.php?curid=3101185. https://en.wikipedia.org/wiki/Kidney_stone_disease#/media/File:Nefrolit.jpg. This work has been released into the public domain by its author, Robert R. Wal. This applies worldwide. No changes have been made to this image.

Figure 126. Diagram (left) of a long juxtamedullary nephron and (right) of a short cortical nephron. The left nephron is labelled with six named nephron segments. Also labelled is the collecting duct, mislabelled the "collection duct"; it is the last part of the nephron.

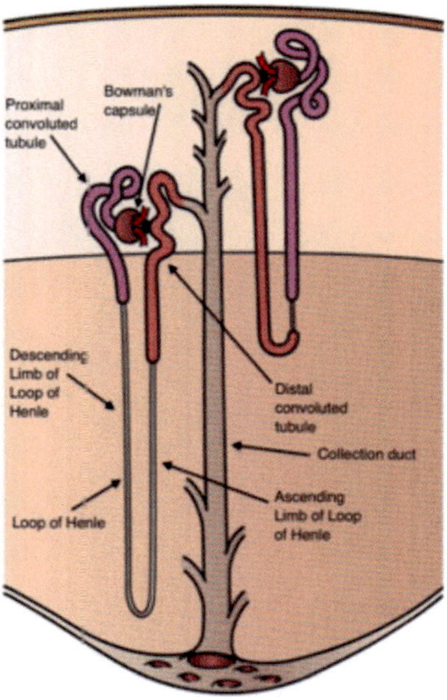

This image is by Artwork by Holly Fischer - http://open.umich.edu/education/med/resources/second-look-series/materials - Urinary Tract Slide 20, 26, CC BY 3.0, https://commons.wikimedia.org/w/index.php?curid=24367127. https://en.wikipedia.org/wiki/Nephron#/media/File:Kidney_Nephron.png. This file is licensed under the Creative Commons Attribution 3.0 Unported license. No changes have been made to this image.

Nursing mothers

It is not known whether PERJETA is excreted in human milk, but human IgG is excreted in human milk. Because many drugs are secreted in human milk and because of the potential for serious adverse reactions in nursing infants from PERJETA, a decision should be made whether to discontinue nursing, or discontinue drug, taking into account the elimination half-life of PERJETA and the importance of the drug to the mother

Pediatric use

The safety and effectiveness of PERJETA have not been established in pediatric patients.

Geriatric use

Of 402 patients who received PERJETA in Study 1, 60 patients (15%) were ≥ 65 years of age 399 and 5 patients (1%) were ≥ 75 years of age. No overall differences in efficacy and safety of PERJETA were observed between these patients and younger patients. Based on a population pharmacokinetic analysis, no significant difference was observed in the 402 pharmacokinetics of pertuzumab between patients < 65 years (n=306) and patients ≥ 65 years 403 (n=175).

Females of reproductive potential

PERJETA can cause embryo-fetal harm when administered during pregnancy. Counsel patients regarding pregnancy prevention and planning. Advise females of reproductive potential to use effective contraception while receiving PERJETA and for 6 months following the last dose of PERJETA. If PERJETA is administered during pregnancy or if a patient becomes pregnant while receiving PERJETA, immediately report exposure to the Genentech Adverse Event Line at 1-888-835-2555. Encourage women who may be exposed during pregnancy to enroll in the MotHER Pregnancy Registry by contacting1-800-690-6720.

Renal impairment

Dose adjustments of PERJETA are not needed in patients with mild (creatinine clearance [CLcr] 60 to 90 mL/min) or moderate (CLcr 30 to 60 mL/min) renal impairment. No dose adjustment can be recommended for patients with severe renal impairment (CLcr less than 30 mL/min) because of the limited pharmacokinetic data available.

Hepatic impairment

No clinical studies have been conducted to evaluate the effect of hepatic impairment on the pharmacokinetics of pertuzumab.

OVERDOSAGE

No drug overdoses have been reported with PERJETA to date.

Pharmacokinetics

Pertuzumab demonstrated linear pharmacokinetics at a dose range of 2 – 25 mg/kg. Based on a population PK analysis that included 481 patients, the median clearance (CL) of pertuzumab was 0.24 L/day and the median half-life was 18 days. With an initial dose of 840 mg followed by a maintenance dose of 420 mg every three weeks thereafter, the steady-state concentration of pertuzumab was reached after the first maintenance dose. The population PK analysis suggested no PK differences based on age, gender, and ethnicity (Japanese vs. non-Japanese). Baseline serum albumin level and lean body weight as covariates only exerted a minor influence on PK parameters. Therefore, no dose adjustments based on body weight or baseline albumin level are needed. No drug-drug interactions were observed between pertuzumab and trastuzumab, or between pertuzumab and docetaxel in a sub-study of 37 patients in the randomized trial. No dedicated renal impairment trial for PERJETA has been conducted. Based on the results of the population pharmacokinetic analysis, pertuzumab exposure in patients with mild (CLcr 60 to 90 mL/min, n=200) and moderate renal impairment (CLcr 30 to 60 mL/min, n=71) were similar to those in patients with normal renal function (CLcr greater than 90 mL/min, n=200). No relationship between CLcr and pertuzumab exposure was observed over the range of observed CLcr (27 to 244 mL/min).

Cardiac electrophysiology

The effect of pertuzumab with an initial dose of 840 mg followed by a maintenance dose of 420 mg every three weeks on QTc interval was evaluated in a subgroup of 20 patients with HER2-positive breast cancer in the randomized trial. No large changes in the mean QT interval (i.e., greater than 20 ms) from placebo based on Fridericia correction method were detected in the trial. A small increase in the mean QTc interval (i.e., less than 10 ms) cannot be excluded because of the limitations of the trial design.

Clinical efficacy of pertuzumab in the treatment of breast cancer

i). Patients given pertuzumab and trastuzumab plus docetaxel (group B) had a significantly improved pathological complete response rate compared with those given trastuzumab plus docetaxel, without substantial differences in tolerability. Pertuzumab and trastuzumab without chemotherapy eradicated tumours in a proportion of women and showed a favourable safety profile. These findings justify further exploration in adjuvant trials and support the neoadjuvant approach for accelerating drug assessment in early breast cancer.

Gianni, MD et al. The Lancet Oncology: 1470-2045, Vol: 13, 25-32, 2012. Efficacy and safety of neoadjuvant pertuzumab and trastuzumab in women with locally advanced, inflammatory, or early HER2-positive breast cancer (NeoSphere): a randomised multicentre, open-label, phase 2 trial.

9.17. PERTUZUMAB, TRASTUZUMAB, AND HYALURONIDASE-ZZXF (PHESGO)

PHESGO (pertuzumab, trastuzumab, and hyaluronidase-zzxf) injection, for subcutaneous use

Initial U.S. Approval: 2020

WARNING: CARDIOMYOPATHY, EMBRYO-FETAL TOXICITY, and PULMONARY TOXICITY See full prescribing information for complete boxed warning.

Cardiomyopathy

PHESGO administration can result in subclinical and clinical cardiac failure manifesting as CHF, and decreased LVEF, with greatest risk when administered concurrently with anthracyclines. Evaluate cardiac function prior to and during treatment. Discontinue PHESGO for cardiomyopathy.

Embryo-fetal toxicity

Exposure to PHESGO can result in embryo-fetal death and birth defects. Advise patients of these risks and the need for effective contraception.

Pulmonary toxicity

Discontinue PHESGO for anaphylaxis, angioedema, interstitial pneumonitis, or acute respiratory distress syndrome.

INDICATIONS AND USAGE

PHESGO is a combination of pertuzumab and trastuzumab, HER2/neu receptor antagonists, and hyaluronidase, an endoglycosidase, indicated for:

• Use in combination with chemotherapy as:

o neoadjuvant treatment of patients with HER2-positive, locally advanced, inflammatory, or early stage breast cancer (either greater than 2 cm in diameter or node positive) as part of a complete treatment regimen for early breast cancer.

o adjuvant treatment of patients with HER2-positive early breast cancer at high risk of recurrence

• Use in combination with docetaxel for treatment of patients with HER2 positive metastatic breast cancer (MBC) who have not received prior anti-HER2 therapy or chemotherapy for metastatic disease.

MECHANISM OF ACTION

Pertuzumab targets the extracellular dimerization domain (subdomain II) of HER2 and, thereby, blocks ligand-dependent heterodimerization of HER2 with other HER family members, including EGFR, HER3 and HER4. As a result, pertuzumab inhibits ligand-initiated intracellular signaling through two major signaling pathways, mitogen-activated protein (MAP) kinase and phosphoinositide 3-kinase (PI3K) (Figure 119). Inhibition of these signaling pathways can result in cell growth arrest and apoptosis, respectively. Trastuzumab binds to subdomain IV of the extracellular domain of the HER2 protein to inhibit the ligand-independent, HER2 mediated cell proliferation and PI3K signaling pathway in human tumor cells that overexpress HER2. Both pertuzumab and trastuzumab-mediated antibody-dependent cell-mediated cytotoxicity (ADCC) have been shown to be preferentially exerted on HER2-overexpressing cancer cells compared with cancer cells that do not overexpress HER2. While pertuzumab alone inhibited the proliferation of human tumor cells, the combination of pertuzumab and trastuzumab augmented anti-tumor activity in HER2-overexpressing xenograft models. Hyaluronan is a polysaccharide found in the extracellular matrix of the subcutaneous tissue. It is depolymerized by the naturally occurring enzyme hyaluronidase. Unlike the stable structural components of the interstitial matrix, hyaluronan has a half-life of approximately 0.5 days. Hyaluronidase increases permeability of the subcutaneous tissue by depolymerizing hyaluronan. In the doses administered, hyaluronidase in PHESGO acts transiently and locally. The effects of hyaluronidase are reversible and permeability of the subcutaneous tissue is restored within 24 to 48 hours. Hyaluronidase has been shown to increase the absorption rate of a trastuzumab product into the systemic circulation when given in the subcutis of Göttingen Minipigs (*Figure 127).*

Figure 127. A young Göttingen minipig.

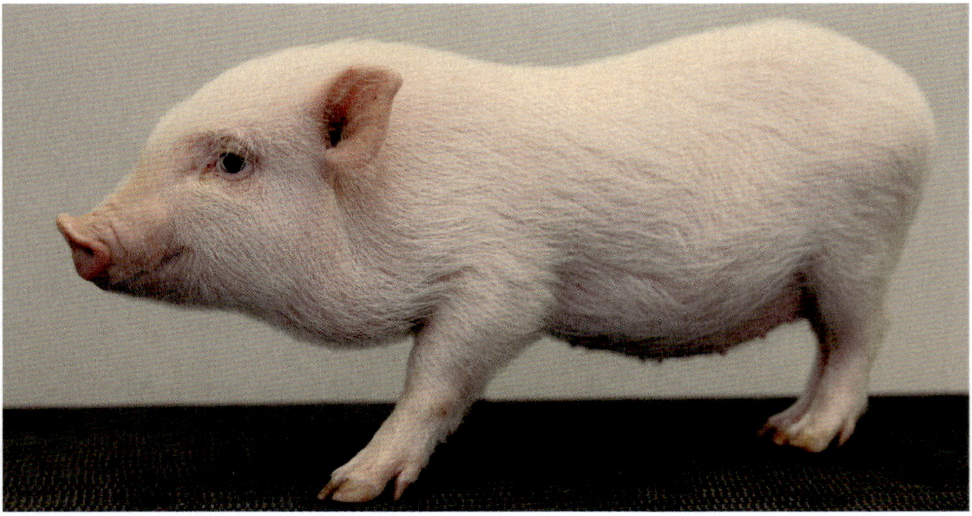

The Göttingen minipig (also known as the Göttinger or Goettingen minipig) is a breed of small swine. The Göttingen minipig is the smallest domestic pig breed known in the world; as an adult, they weigh around 35 kg (77 lb). Besides being known for their exceptionally small size, the Göttingen minipigs are known for their docile nature and very clean and well-characterized health status. Raising of this breed began in the late 1960s at the Institute of Animal Breeding and Genetics (Institut für Tierzucht und Haustiergenetik) at the University of Göttingen, Germany, by crossbreeding the Minnesota mini-pig, the Vietnamese pot-bellied pig, and the German Landrace pig. Göttingen minipigs are highly favored as pets; however, the breed was specifically developed for biomedical research.

DESCRIPTION

PHESGO is a combination of pertuzumab, trastuzumab, and hyaluronidase. Pertuzumab is a recombinant humanized monoclonal antibody that targets the extracellular dimerization domain (Subdomain II) of the human epidermal growth factor receptor 2 protein (HER2). Pertuzumab is produced by recombinant DNA technology in a mammalian cell (Chinese Hamster Ovary) culture. Pertuzumab has an approximate molecular weight of 148 kDa. Trastuzumab is a humanized IgG1 kappa monoclonal antibody that selectively binds with high affinity to the extracellular domain of the human epidermal growth factor receptor 2 protein, HER2. Trastuzumab is produced by recombinant DNA technology in a mammalian cell (Chinese Hamster Ovary) culture. Trastuzumab has a molecular weight of approximately 148 kDa. Hyaluronidase (recombinant human) is an endoglycosidase used to increase the dispersion and absorption of co-administered drugs when administered subcutaneously. It is a glycosylated single-chain protein produced by mammalian (Chinese Hamster Ovary) cells containing a DNA plasmid encoding for a soluble fragment of human hyaluronidase (PH20). Hyaluronidase (recombinant human) has a molecular weight of approximately 61 kDa. PHESGO (pertuzumab, trastuzumab, and hyaluronidase-zzxf) injection is a sterile, preservative-free, clear to opalescent, and colorless to slightly brownish solution supplied in single-dose vials for subcutaneous administration. PHESGO injection is supplied as two different configurations:

• PHESGO is supplied in a 15 mL single-dose vial containing 1,200 mg of pertuzumab, 600 mg of trastuzumab, and 30,000 units of hyaluronidase, and α,α-trehalose (397 mg), L-histidine (6.75 mg), L-histidine hydrochloric monohydrate (53.7 mg), L-methionine (22.4 mg), polysorbate 20 (6 mg), and sucrose (685 mg) with a pH of 5.5.

• PHESGO is supplied in a 10 mL single-dose vial containing 600 mg of pertuzumab, 600 mg of trastuzumab, and 20,000 units of hyaluronidase, and α, α-trehalose (397 mg), Lhistidine (4.4 mg), L-histidine hydrochloric monohydrate (36.1 mg), L-methionine (14.9 mg), polysorbate 20 (4 mg), and sucrose (342 mg) with a pH of 5.5.

DOSAGE AND ADMINISTRATION

• For subcutaneous use in the thigh only.

• PHESGO has different dosage and administration instructions than intravenous pertuzumab and trastuzumab products.

• Do not administer intravenously.

• Perform HER2 testing using FDA-approved tests by laboratories with demonstrated proficiency.

• The initial dose of PHESGO is 1,200 mg pertuzumab, 600 mg trastuzumab, and 30,000 units hyaluronidase administered subcutaneously over approximately 8 minutes, followed every 3 weeks by a dose of 600 mg pertuzumab, 600 mg trastuzumab, and 20,000 units hyaluronidase administered subcutaneously over approximately 5 minutes.

• Neoadjuvant: administer PHESGO by subcutaneous injection every 3 weeks and chemotherapy by intravenous infusion preoperatively for 3 to 6 cycles.

• Adjuvant: administer PHESGO by subcutaneous injection every 3 weeks and chemotherapy by intravenous infusion postoperatively for a total of 1 year (up to 18 cycles).

• MBC: administer PHESGO by subcutaneous injection and docetaxel by intravenous infusion every 3 weeks.

DOSAGE FORMS AND STRENGTHS

Injection

• 1,200 mg pertuzumab, 600 mg trastuzumab, and 30,000 units hyaluronidase/15 mL (80 mg, 40 mg, and 2,000 units/mL) of solution in a single-dose vial.

• 600 mg pertuzumab, 600 mg trastuzumab, and 20,000 units hyaluronidase/10 mL (60 mg, 60 mg, and 2,000 units/mL) of solution in a single-dose vial.

CONTRAINDICATIONS

PHESGO is contraindicated in patients with known hypersensitivity to pertuzumab, or trastuzumab, or hyaluronidase, or to any of its excipients.

WARNINGS AND PRECAUTIONS

• Exacerbation of chemotherapy-induced neutropenia.

• Hypersensitivity and administration-related reactions (ARRs)

Monitor patients for systemic hypersensitivity reactions. Permanently discontinue PHESGO in patients who experience anaphylaxis or severe hypersensitivity reactions.

ADVERSE REACTIONS

Neoadjuvant and adjuvant treatment of breast cancer

• The most common adverse reactions (>30%) with PHESGO were alopecia, nausea, diarrhea, anemia, and asthenia.

Metastatic breast cancer (based on intravenous pertuzumab)

• The most common adverse reactions (> 30%) with pertuzumab in combination with trastuzumab and docetaxel were diarrhea, alopecia, neutropenia, nausea, fatigue, rash, and peripheral neuropathy.

To report SUSPECTED ADVERSE REACTIONS, contact Genentech at 1-888-835-2555 or FDA at 1-800-FDA-1088 or www.fda.gov/medwatch.

USE IN SPECIFIC POPULATIONS

Females and males of reproductive potential

Verify the pregnancy status of females prior to initiation of PHESGO.

FULL PRESCRIBING INFORMATION WARNING: CARDIOMYOPATHY, EMBRYO-FETAL TOXICITY, and PULMONARY TOXICITY

Cardiomyopathy

PHESGO administration can result in subclinical and clinical cardiac failure. The incidence and severity was highest in patients receiving PHESGO with anthracycline-containing chemotherapy regimens *(Figure 128).*

Figure 128. Cartoon diagram of two doxorubicin molecules (shown as space-filling models) intercalating a strand of DNA.

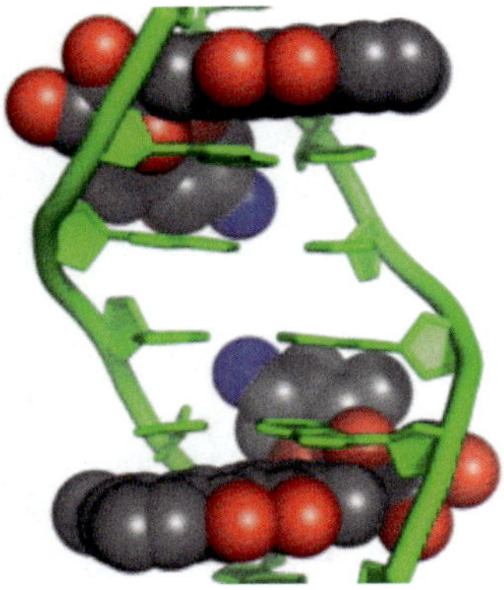

This image is by By Fvasconcellos 19:11, 28 November 2007 (UTC) - From PDB entry 1D12.More information:Frederick CA, Williams LD, Ughetto G, et al. (1990). "Structural comparison of anticancer drug-DNA complexes: adriamycin and daunomycin". Biochemistry 29 (10): 2538–49. PMID 2334681., Public Domain, https://commons.wikimedia.org/w/index.php?curid=3158967. https://en.wikipedia.org/wiki/Anthracycline#/media/File:Doxorubicin%E2%80%93DNA_complex_1D12.png. The copyright holder of this work, release this work into the public domain. No changes were made to this image

Anthracyclines are a class of drugs used in cancer chemotherapy that are extracted from Streptomyces bacterium. These compounds are used to treat many cancers, including leukemias, lymphomas, breast, stomach, uterine, ovarian, bladder cancer, and lung cancers. The first anthracycline discovered was daunorubicin (trade name Daunomycin), which is produced naturally by Streptomyces peucetius, a species of actinobacteria. Clinically the most important anthracyclines are doxorubicin, daunorubicin, epirubicin and idarubicin.

Evaluate cardiac function prior to and during treatment with PHESGO. Discontinue PHESGO treatment in patients receiving adjuvant therapy and withhold PHESGO in patients with metastatic disease for clinically significant decrease in left ventricular function. *Please see the section on* ***ADO-TRASTUZUMAB EMTANSINE*** *for further information on drug-induced cardiac failure.*

Embryo-fetal toxicity

Exposure to PHESGO can result in embryo-fetal death and birth defects, including oligohydramnios and oligohydramnios sequence manifesting as pulmonary hypoplasia, skeletal abnormalities, and neonatal death. Advise patients of these risks and the need for effective contraception

Pulmonary toxicity

PHESGO administration can result in serious and fatal pulmonary toxicity. Discontinue PHESGO for anaphylaxis, angioedema, interstitial pneumonitis, or acute respiratory distress syndrome *(Figure 129).* Monitor patients until symptoms completely resolve

Figure 129. Two chest x-rays; the left shows ARDS, the right shows the same patient's chest after recovery

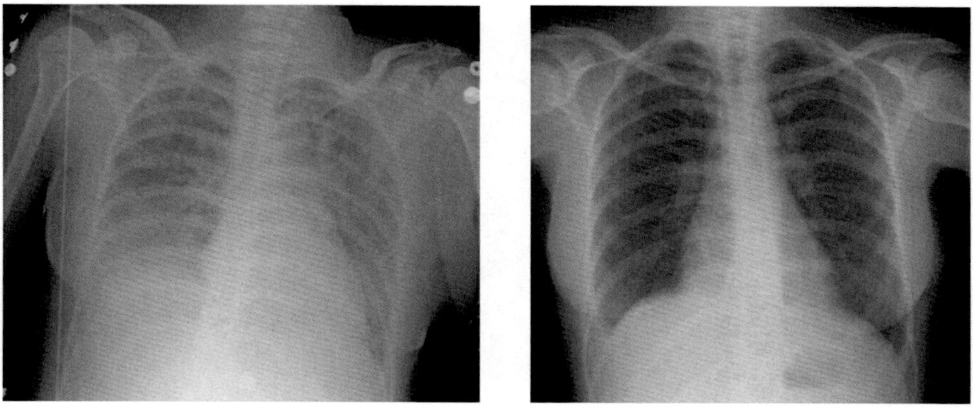

This image is by By Altaf Gauhar Haji, Shekhar Sharma, DK Vijaykumar and Jerry Paul. - Transfusion related acute lung injury presenting with acute dyspnoea: a case report. Journal of Medical Case Reports 2008, 2:336. doi:10.1186/1752-1947-2-336, CC BY 2.0, https://commons.wikimedia.org/w/index.php?curid=5898904. https://en.wikipedia.org/wiki/Acute_respiratory_distress_syndrome#/media/File:Transfusion-related_acute_lung_injury_chest_X-ray.gif. This file is licensed under the Creative Commons Attribution 2.0 Generic license. No changes were made to this image.

Figure 130. *Micrograph of hyaline membranes, as seen in diffuse alveolar damage (DAD), the histologic correlate of adult respiratory distress syndrome (ARDS), transfusion related acute lung injury (TRALI), acute interstitial pneumonia (AIP).*

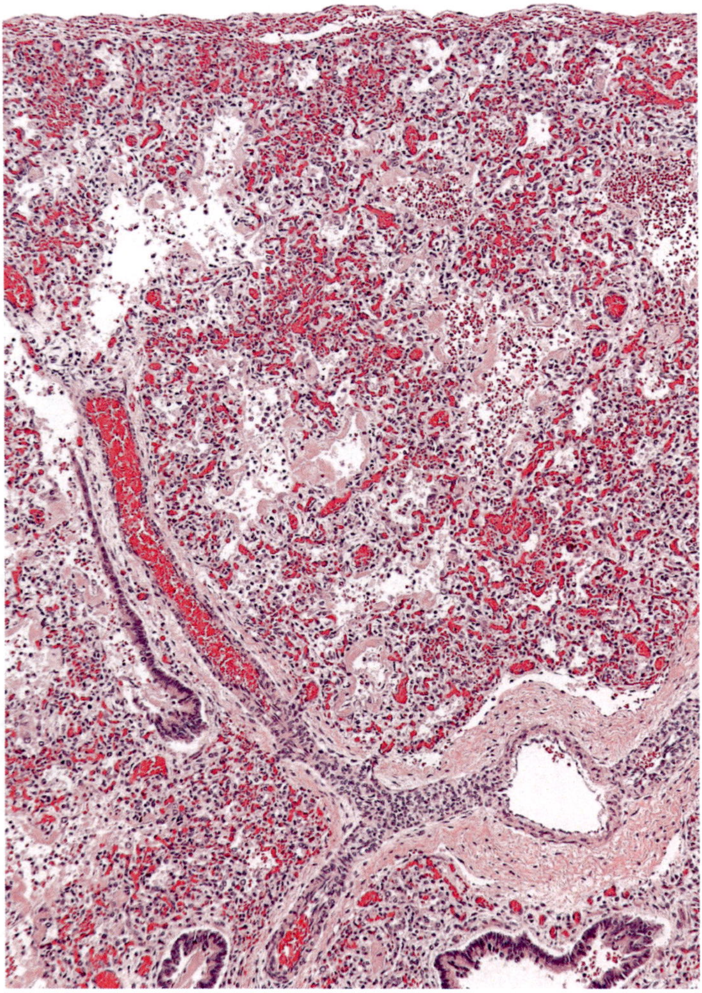

This image is by By Nephron - Own work, CC BY-SA 3.0, https://commons.wikimedia.org/w/index.php?curid=14967283. n.wikipedia.org/wiki/Acute_respiratory_distress_syndrome#/media/File:Hyaline_membranes_-_intermed_mag.jpg. This file is licensed under the Creative Commons Attribution-Share Alike 3.0 Unported license. No changes have been made to this image.

INDICATIONS AND USAGE

Early breast cancer (EBC)

PHESGO is indicated for use in combination with chemotherapy for

• the neoadjuvant treatment of adult patients with HER2-positive, locally advanced, inflammatory, or early stage breast cancer (either greater than 2 cm in diameter or node positive) as part of a complete treatment regimen for early breast cancer

• the adjuvant treatment of adult patients with HER2-positive early breast cancer at high risk of recurrence. Select patients for therapy based on an FDA-approved companion diagnostic test

Metastatic breast cancer (MBC)

PHESGO is indicated for use in combination with docetaxel for the treatment of adult patients with HER2-positive metastatic breast cancer who have not received prior anti-HER2 therapy or chemotherapy for metastatic disease Select patients for therapy based on an FDA-approved companion diagnostic test.

DOSAGE AND ADMINISTRATION

Patient Selection

Select patients based on HER2 protein overexpression or HER2 gene amplification in tumor specimens. Assessment of HER2 protein overexpression and HER2 gene amplification should be performed using FDA-approved tests specific for breast cancer by laboratories with demonstrated proficiency. Information on the FDA-approved tests for the detection of HER2 protein overexpression and HER2 gene amplification is available at: http://www.fda.gov/CompanionDiagnostics. Improper assay performance, including use of suboptimally fixed tissue, failure to utilize specified reagents, deviation from specific assay instructions, and failure to include appropriate controls for assay validation, can lead to unreliable results.

Important dosage and administration information

PHESGO is for subcutaneous use only in the thigh. Do not administer intravenously. PHESGO has different dosage and administration instructions than intravenous pertuzumab, intravenous trastuzumab, and subcutaneous trastuzumab when administered alone. Do not substitute PHESGO for or with pertuzumab, trastuzumab, ado-trastuzumab emtansine, or fam-trastuzumab deruxtecan. PHESGO must always be administered by a healthcare professional. In patients receiving an anthracycline-based regimen for early breast cancer, administer PHESGO following completion of the anthracycline. In patients receiving PHESGO for early breast cancer with docetaxel or paclitaxel, administer docetaxel or paclitaxel after PHESGO. In patients receiving PHESGO for metastatic breast cancer with docetaxel, administer docetaxel after PHESGO. Observe patients for a minimum of 30 minutes after initial dose of PHESGO and 15 minutes after each maintenance dose of PHESGO for signs or hypersensitivity symptoms or administration-related reactions. Medications to treat such reactions, as well as emergency equipment, should be available for immediate use.

Recommended doses and schedules

The recommended dosage and administration schedule for PHESGO are shown here.

Dose	Strength	Administration instructions
Initial dose	1,200 mg pertuzumab, 600 mg trastuzumab, and 30,000 units hyaluronidase in 15 mL (1,200 mg, 600 mg, and 30,000 units/15 mL)	Administer subcutaneously over approximately 8 minutes
Maintenance dose	600 mg pertuzumab, 600 mg trastuzumab, and 20,000 units hyaluronidase in 10 mL (600 mg, 600 mg, and 20,000 units/10 mL)	Administer subcutaneously over approximately 5 minutes every 3 weeks

No dose adjustments for PHESGO are required for patient body weight or for concomitant chemotherapy regimen. Patients currently receiving intravenous pertuzumab and trastuzumab can transition to PHESGO. In patients receiving intravenous pertuzumab and trastuzumab with < 6 weeks since their last dose, administer PHESGO as a maintenance dose of 600 mg pertuzumab/600 mg trastuzumab and every 3 weeks for subsequent administrations. In patients receiving intravenous pertuzumab and trastuzumab with ≥ 6 weeks since their last dose, administer PHESGO as an initial dose of 1,200 mg pertuzumab/600 mg trastuzumab, followed by a maintenance dose of 600 mg pertuzumab/600 mg trastuzumab every 3 weeks for subsequent administrations.

Neoadjuvant treatment of breast cancer

Administer PHESGO every 3 weeks for 3 to 6 cycles as part of a treatment regimen for early breast cancer. Refer to the prescribing information for pertuzumab, administered in combination with trastuzumab and chemotherapy, for recommended dose and dosage modifications. Following surgery, patients should continue to receive PHESGO to complete 1 year of treatment (up to 18 cycles) or until disease recurrence or unmanageable toxicity, whichever occurs first, as a part of a complete regimen for early breast cancer.

Adjuvant treatment of breast cancer

Administer PHESGO every 3 weeks for a total of 1 year (up to 18 cycles) or until disease recurrence or unmanageable toxicity, whichever occurs first, as part of a complete regimen for early breast cancer, including standard anthracycline- and/or **taxane**-based chemotherapy *(Figure 131)*. Start PHESGO on Day 1 of the first taxane-containing cycle.

Figure 131. Taxane structure with numbering.

This image is by By Mykhal - Own work, Public Domain, https://commons.wikimedia.org/w/index.php?curid=92454092. https://en.wikipedia.org/wiki/Taxane#/media/File:Taxane_numbering.svg. This image of a simple structural formula is ineligible for copyright and therefore in the public domain, because it consists entirely of information that is common property and contains no original authorship. No changes have been made to this image.

Figure 131. Taxane structure with numbering.

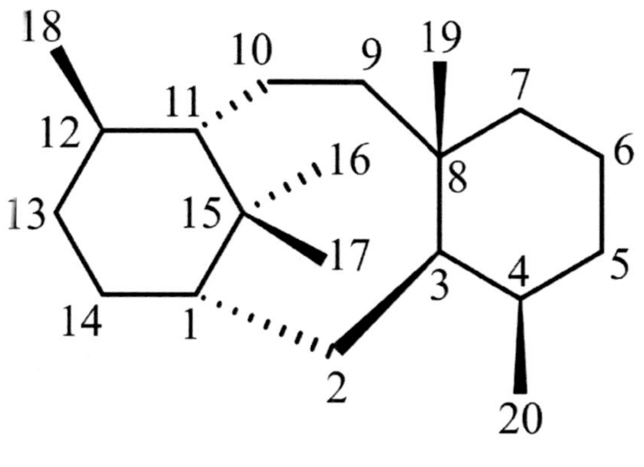

Taxanes were originally identified from plants of the genus Taxus (yew trees), and feature a taxadiene core. Paclitaxel (Taxol) and docetaxel (Taxotere) are widely used as chemotherapy agents. The principal mechanism of action of the taxane class of drugs is the disruption of microtubule function. Microtubules are essential to cell division, and taxanes stabilize GDP-bound tubulin in the microtubule, thereby inhibiting the process of cell division as depolymerization is prevented. Thus, in essence, taxanes are mitotic inhibitors.

Metastatic breast cancer (MBC)

When administered with PHESGO, the recommended initial dose of docetaxel is 75 mg/m^2 administered as an intravenous infusion. The dose may be escalated to 100 mg/m^2 administered every 3 weeks if the initial dose is well tolerated. Administer PHESGO until disease progression or unmanageable toxicity, whichever occurs first.
Dose modification for delayed or missed doses

For delayed or missed doses of PHESGO, if the time between two sequential injections is less than 6 weeks, administer the maintenance dose of 600 mg, 600 mg, and 20,000 units/10 mL. Do not wait until the next planned dose. If the time between two sequential injections is 6 weeks or more, re-administer the initial dose of 1,200 mg, 600 mg, and 30,000 units/15 mL, followed every 3 weeks thereafter by a maintenance dose of 600 mg, 600 mg, and 20,000 units/10 mL. For chemotherapy dose modifications, see relevant prescribing information.

Dose modifications for left ventricular dysfunction.

	Pretreatment LVEF:	Monitor LVEF every:	Withhold PHESGO for at least 3 weeks for an LVEF decrease to:	Resume PHESGO after 3 weeks if LVEF has recovered to:
Early	Equal to, or greater than, 55%*	~12 weeks (once during neo-adjuvant therapy)	<50% with a fall of ≥10%-points below pretreatment value	Either >50% or with a fall of ≥10%-points below pretreatment value
Metastatic	Equal to, or	~12 weeks	Either <40%	Either >45%

	greater than, 50%		or 40%-45% with a fall of ≥10% points below pre-treatment value	or 40%-45% with a fall of <10% points below pretreatment value

* For patients receiving anthracycline-based chemotherapy, a LVEF of ≥ 50% is required after completion of anthracyclines, before starting PHESGO. If after a repeat assessment within approximately 3 weeks, the LVEF has not improved, has declined further, and/or the patient is symptomatic, permanently discontinue PHESGO.

Hypersensitivity and administration-related reactions

Discontinue the injection immediately if the patient experiences a serious hypersensitivity reaction (e.g. anaphylaxis).

CONTRAINDICATIONS

PHESGO is contraindicated in patients with known hypersensitivity to pertuzumab, or trastuzumab, or hyaluronidase, or to any of its excipients.

Further information on **WARNINGS AND PRECAUTIONS**

Cardiomyopathy

PHESGO can cause hypertension, arrhythmias, left ventricular cardiac dysfunction, disabling cardiac failure, cardiomyopathy, and cardiac death [see Boxed Warning: Cardiomyopathy].

PHESGO can cause asymptomatic decline in LVEF. An increased incidence of LVEF decline has been observed in patients treated with intravenous pertuzumab, intravenous trastuzumab, and docetaxel.

A 4-6-fold increase in the incidence of symptomatic myocardial dysfunction has been reported among patients receiving trastuzumab, with the highest absolute incidence occurring when trastuzumab was administered with an anthracycline. Patients who receive anthracycline after stopping PHESGO may also be at increased risk of cardiac dysfunction.

Cardiac monitoring

Prior to initiation of PHESGO, conduct a thorough cardiac assessment, including history, physical examination, and determination of LVEF by echocardiogram or MUGA scan. During treatment with PHESGO, assess LVEF at regular intervals. If after a repeat assessment within approximately 3 weeks, the LVEF has not improved, has declined further, and/or the patient is symptomatic, permanently discontinue PHESGO. Following completion of PHESGO, continue to monitor for cardiomyopathy and assess LVEF measurements every 6 months for at least 2 years as a component of adjuvant therapy.

In the FeDeriCa study, the percentage of patients with at least one cardiac disorder was 22% in the PHESGO arm. The most frequent cardiac adverse reaction in the PHESGO arm was ejection fraction decreased. The incidence of cardiac failure (NYHA Class III/IV) with a LVEF decline ≥ 10% and a drop to less than 50% was 0.8% in the PHESGO arm. Confirmed asymptomatic or mildly symptomatic (NYHA Class II) declines in LVEF ≥ 10% and a drop to less than 50% was 1.2% in the PHESGO arm.

PHESGO and/or intravenous pertuzumab and trastuzumab have not been studied in patients with a pretreatment LVEF value of < 55% (EBC) or 360 mg/m^2 of doxorubicin or its equivalent.

Embryo-fetal toxicity

PHESGO can cause fetal harm when administered to a pregnant woman. In post-marketing reports, use of intravenous trastuzumab during pregnancy resulted in cases of oligohydramnios and oligohydramnios sequence manifesting as pulmonary hypoplasia, skeletal abnormalities, and neonatal death. In an animal reproduction study, administration of intravenous pertuzumab to pregnant cynomolgus monkeys during the period of organogenesis resulted in oligohydramnios, delayed fetal kidney development, and embryo-fetal death at exposures 2.5 to 20 times the exposure in humans at the recommended dose, based on Cmax.

Verify the pregnancy status of females of reproductive potential prior to the initiation of PHESGO. Advise pregnant women and females of reproductive potential that exposure to PHESGO during pregnancy or within 7 months prior to conception can result in fetal harm. Advise females of reproductive potential to use effective contraception during treatment and for 7 months following the last dose of PHESGO

Pulmonary toxicity

PHESGO can cause serious and fatal pulmonary toxicity. These adverse reactions have been reported with intravenous trastuzumab. Pulmonary toxicity includes dyspnea, interstitial pneumonitis, pulmonary infiltrates, pleural effusions *(Figure 132)*, non-cardiogenic pulmonary edema, pulmonary insufficiency and hypoxia, acute respiratory distress syndrome, and pulmonary fibrosis *(Figure 133)*. Patients with symptomatic intrinsic lung disease or with extensive tumor involvement of the lungs, resulting in dyspnea at rest, appear to have more severe toxicity.

Figure 132. A large left sided pleural effusion as seen on an upright chest X-ray This image is by James Heilman, MD - Own work, CC BY-SA 3.0, https://commons.wikimedia.org/w/index.php?curid=14634441. https://en.wikipedia.org/wiki/Pleural_effusion#/media/File:Effusionhalf.PNG.

Figure 132. A large left sided pleural effusion as seen on an upright chest X-ray.

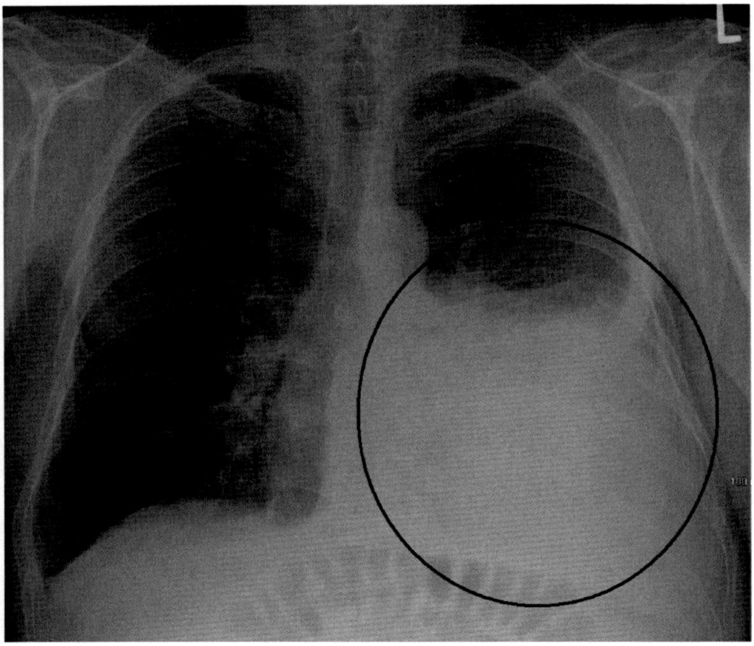

Figure 133. High resolution CT of lung showing extensive fibrosis possibly from usual interstitial pneumonitis. There is also a large emphysematous bulla.

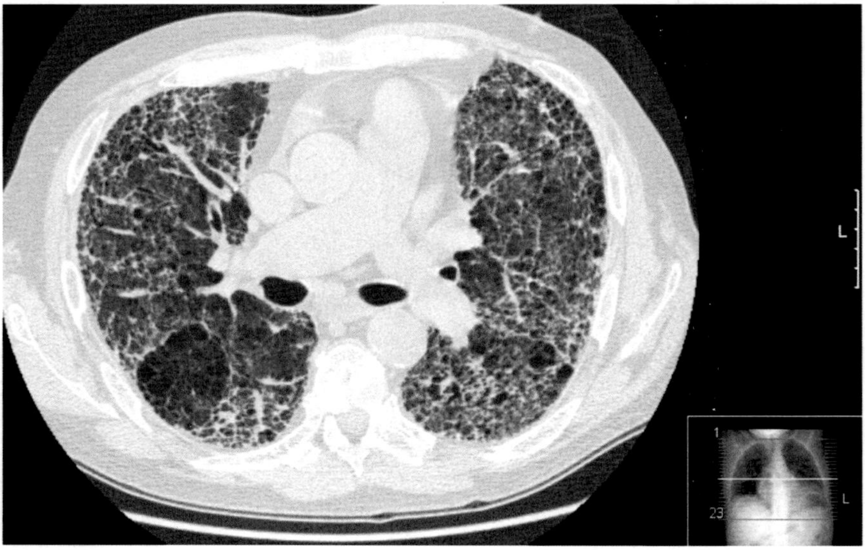

This image is by By Drriad - Own work, CC BY-SA 3.0, https://commons.wikimedia.org/w/index.php?curid=2868154. HRCT of lung showing extensive fibrosis possibly from usual interstitial pneumonitis. There is also a

large emphysematous bulla. This file is licensed under the Creative Commons Attribution-Share Alike 3.0 Unported, 2.5 Generic, 2.0 Generic and 1.0 Generic license. No changes have been made to this image.

Exacerbation of chemotherapy-induced neutropenia

PHESGO may exacerbate chemotherapy-induced neutropenia. In randomized controlled clinical trials with intravenous trastuzumab, Grade 3-4 neutropenia and febrile neutropenia were higher in patients receiving trastuzumab in combination with myelosuppressive chemotherapy as compared to those who received chemotherapy alone. The incidence of septic death was similar among patients who received trastuzumab and those who did not.

Hypersensitivity and administration-related reactions

Severe administration-related reactions (ARRs), including hypersensitivity, anaphylaxis, and events with fatal outcomes, have been associated with intravenous pertuzumab and trastuzumab. Patients experiencing dyspnea at rest due to complications of advanced malignancy and comorbidities may be at increased risk of a severe or of a fatal ARR.

In the FeDeriCa study, the incidence of hypersensitivity was 1.2% in the PHESGO arm. Administration-related reactions occurred in 21% of patients who received PHESGO. In the PHESGO arm, the most common administration-related reactions were injection site reaction (15%) and injection site pain (2%). Closely monitor patients during and for 30 minutes after the injection of initial dose and during and for 15 minutes following subsequent injections of maintenance dose of PHESGO. If a significant injection-related reaction occurs, slow down or pause the injection and administer appropriate medical therapies. Evaluate and carefully monitor patients until complete resolution of signs and symptoms.

Permanently discontinue with PHESGO in patients who experience anaphylaxis or severe injection-related reactions. Medications to treat such reactions, as well as emergency equipment, should be available for immediate use. For patients experiencing reversible Grade 1 or 2 hypersensitivity reactions, consider pre-medication with an analgesic, antipyretic, or an antihistamine prior to readministration of PHESGO. PHESGO is contraindicated in patients with known hypersensitivity to pertuzumab, trastuzumab, hyaluronidase or to any of its excipients.

Immunogenicity

As with all therapeutic proteins, there is potential for immunogenicity with PHESGO. The detection of antibody formation is highly dependent on the sensitivity and specificity of the assay. Additionally, the observed incidence of antibody (including neutralizing antibody) positivity in an assay may be influenced by several factors including assay methodology, sample handling, timing of sample collection, concomitant medications, and underlying disease. For these reasons, comparison of the incidence of antibodies to PHESGO and intravenous pertuzumab and trastuzumab in the FeDeriCa study with the incidence of antibodies in other studies or to other products may be misleading. In the FeDeriCa study, the incidence of treatment-emergent anti-pertuzumab and antitrastuzumab antibodies in most patients completing 1-4 cycles of therapy was 3% (7/237) and 0.4% (1/237), respectively, in patients treated with intravenous pertuzumab and trastuzumab. The incidence of treatment-emergent anti-pertuzumab, anti-trastuzumab, and anti-recombinant human hyaluronidase PH20 antibodies in most patients completing 1-4 cycles of therapy was 4.8% (11/231), 0.9% (2/232), and 0.9% (2/225), respectively, in patients treated with PHESGO. Among patients who tested positive to anti-pertuzumab antibodies, neutralizing anti-pertuzumab antibodies□□□ were detected in one patient treated with intravenous pertuzumab and trastuzumab and in one patient treated with PHESGO. Among patients who tested positive to anti-trastuzumab antibodies, neutralizing anti-trastuzumab antibodies were detected in one patient treated with PHESGO. The clinical relevance of the development of anti-pertuzumab, anti-trastuzumab or antirecombinant human hyaluronidase PH20 antibodies after treatment with PHESGO is unknown.

□*A neutralizing antibody is an antibody that defends a cell from a pathogen or infectious particle by neutralizing any effect it has biologically. Neutralization renders the particle no longer infectious or pathogenic. Neutralizing antibodies are part of the humoral response of the adaptive immune system against viruses, intracellular bacteria and microbial toxin. By binding specifically to surface structures (antigen) on an infectious particle, neutralizing antibodies prevent the particle from interacting with its host cells it might infect and destroy. Immunity due to neutralizing antibodies is also known as sterilizing immunity, as the immune system eliminates the infectious particle before any infection takes place. (Figure 134).*

Figure 134. Covering an antigen in antibodies make it less infectious and less pathogenic. In the image on the right, virus entry to the cell is prevented by neutralizing antibodies binding to the virus.

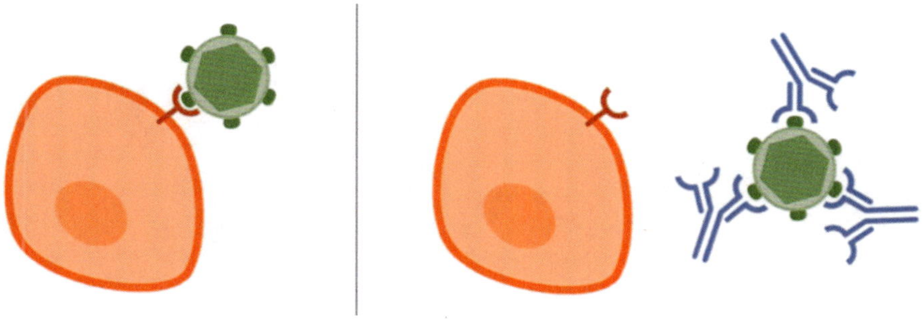

This image is by xspareta - Producció pròpia, CC BY-SA 4.0, https://commons.wikimedia.org/w/index.php?curid=37832961. https://en.wikipedia.org/wiki/Neutralizing_antibody#/media/File:NAb_esquema.jpg. This file is licensed under the Creative Commons Attribution-Share Alike 4.0 International, 3.0 Unported, 2.5 Generic, 2.0 Generic and 1.0 Generic license. No changes were made to the image.

Postmarketing experience

The following adverse reactions have been identified with the use of intravenous pertuzumab and trastuzumab. Because these reactions are reported voluntarily from a population of uncertain size, it is not always possible to reliably estimate their frequency or establish a causal relationship to drug exposure.

• Glomerulopathy

Glomerulopathy is a set of diseases affecting the glomeruli of the nephron. Such diseases can include processes that are inflammatory or noninflammatory. Because the term glomerulitis exists for inflammatory conditions, glomerulopathy sometimes carries a noninflammatory implication.

• Immune thrombocytopenia

Immune thrombocytopenia, is a type of thrombocytopenic purpura defined as an isolated low platelet count with a normal bone marrow in the absence of other causes of low platelets. It causes a characteristic red or purple bruise-like rash, petechiae/purpura (Figure 135) and an increased tendency to bleed.

Figure 135. Oral petechiae/purpura – lower lip.

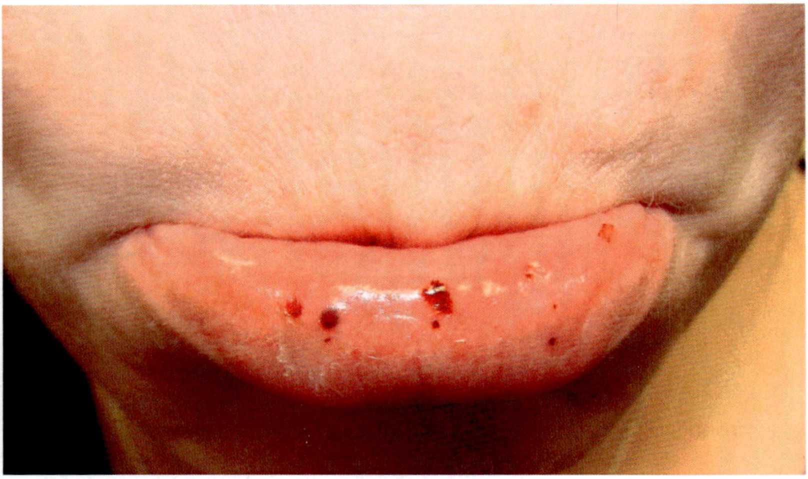

• Tumor lysis syndrome (TLS)

Patients with significant tumor burden (e.g. bulky metastases) may be at a higher risk. Patients could present with hyperuricemia, hyperphosphatemia, and acute renal failure which may represent possible TLS. Providers should consider additional monitoring and/or treatment as clinically indicated.

Tumor lysis syndrome is a group of metabolic abnormalities that can occur as a complication during the treatment of cancer, where large amounts of tumor cells are killed off (lysed) at the same time by the treatment, releasing their contents into the bloodstream. Tumor lysis syndrome is characterized by high blood potassium (hyperkalemia), high blood phosphate (hyperphosphatemia), low blood calcium (hypocalcemia), high blood uric acid (hyperuricemia), and higher than normal levels of blood urea nitrogen (BUN) and other nitrogen-containing compounds (azotemia). These changes in blood electrolytes and metabolites are a result of the release of cellular contents of dying cells into the bloodstream from breakdown of cells. The metabolic abnormalities seen in tumor lysis syndrome can result in nausea and vomiting, but more seriously acute uric acid nephropathy, acute kidney failure, seizures, cardiac arrhythmias, and death.

DRUG INTERACTIONS

Patients who receive anthracycline after stopping PHESGO may be at increased risk of cardiac dysfunction because of PHESGO's long washout period. If possible, avoid anthracycline-based therapy for up to 7 months after stopping PHESGO. If anthracyclines are used, carefully monitor the patient's cardiac function.

USE IN SPECIFIC POPULATIONS

Pregnancy pregnancy pharmacovigilance program

There is a pregnancy pharmacovigilance program for PHESGO. If PHESGO is administered during pregnancy, or if a patient becomes pregnant while receiving PHESGO or within 7 months following the last dose of PHESGO, health care providers and patients should immediately report PHESGO exposure to Genentech at 1-888-835-2555.

Risk summary

PHESGO can cause fetal harm when administered to a pregnant woman. In post-marketing reports, use of intravenous trastuzumab during pregnancy resulted in cases of oligohydramnios and oligohydramnios sequence manifesting as pulmonary hypoplasia, skeletal abnormalities, and neonatal death (see Data). In an animal reproduction study, administration of pertuzumab to pregnant cynomolgus monkeys during the period of organogenesis resulted in oligohydramnios, delayed fetal kidney development, and embryo-fetal deaths at clinically relevant exposures that were 2.5 to 20-fold greater than exposures in humans receiving the recommended dose, based on Cmax (see Data). Apprise the patient of the potential risks to a fetus. There are clinical considerations if PHESGO is used during pregnancy or within 7 months prior to conception. The estimated background risk of major birth defects and miscarriage for the indicated population is unknown. In the U.S. general population, the estimated background risk of major birth defects and miscarriage in clinically recognized pregnancies is 2-4% and 15-20%, respectively.

Clinical Considerations

Fetal/neonatal adverse reactions

Monitor women who received PHESGO during pregnancy or within 7 months prior to conception for oligohydramnios. If oligohydramnios occurs, perform fetal testing that is appropriate for gestational age and consistent with community standards of care.

Data

Human data

In post-marketing reports, use of trastuzumab during pregnancy resulted in cases of oligohydramnios and of oligohydramnios sequence, manifesting in the fetus as pulmonary hypoplasia, skeletal abnormalities, and neonatal death. These case reports described oligohydramnios in pregnant women who received trastuzumab either alone or in combination with chemotherapy. In some case reports, amniotic fluid index increased after trastuzumab was stopped. In one case, trastuzumab therapy resumed after amniotic index improved and oligohydramnios recurred.

Animal data

PHESGO for subcutaneous injection contains pertuzumab, trastuzumab, and hyaluronidase.

Pertuzumab

Pregnant cynomolgus monkeys were treated on Gestational Day (GD) 19 with loading doses of 30 to 150 mg/kg pertuzumab, followed by bi-weekly doses of 10 to 100 mg/kg. These dose levels resulted in clinically relevant exposures of 2.5 to 20-fold greater than exposures in humans receiving the recommended dose, based on Cmax. Intravenous administration of pertuzumab from GD19 through GD50 (period of organogenesis) was embryotoxic, with dose-dependent increases in embryo-fetal death between GD25 to GD70. The incidences of embryo-fetal loss were 33, 50, and 85%. At Caesarean section on GD100, oligohydramnios, decreased relative lung and kidney weights, and microscopic evidence of renal hypoplasia consistent with delayed renal development were identified in all pertuzumab dose groups. Pertuzumab exposure was reported in offspring from all treated groups, at levels of 29% to 40% of maternal serum levels at GD100.

Trastuzumab

In studies where intravenous trastuzumab was administered to pregnant cynomolgus monkeys during the period of organogenesis at doses up to 25 mg/kg given twice weekly (up to 25 times the recommended weekly human dose of 2 mg/kg), trastuzumab crossed the placental barrier during the early (Gestation Days 20 to 50) and late (Gestation Days 120 to 150) phases of gestation. The resulting concentrations of trastuzumab in fetal serum and amniotic fluid were approximately 33% and 25%, respectively, of those present in the maternal serum but were not associated with adverse developmental effects.

Hyaluronidase

In an embryo-fetal study, mice have been dosed daily by subcutaneous injection during the period of organogenesis with hyaluronidase (recombinant human) at dose levels up to 2,200,000 U/kg, which is >2,400 and 3,600, based on loading and maintenance doses, respectively, times higher than the human dose. The study found no evidence of teratogenicity. Reduced fetal weight and increased numbers of fetal resorptions were observed, with no effects found at a daily dose of 360,000 U/kg, which is >400 and 600, based on loading and maintenance doses, respectively, times higher than the human dose. In a peri-and post-natal reproduction study, mice have been dosed daily by subcutaneous injection, with hyaluronidase (recombinant human) from implantation through lactation and weaning at dose levels up to 1,100,000 U/kg, which is >1,200 and 1,800, based on loading and maintenance doses, respectively, times higher than the human dose. The study found no adverse effects on sexual maturation, learning and memory or fertility of the offspring.

Lactation risk summary

There is no information regarding the presence of pertuzumab, trastuzumab or hyaluronidase in human milk, the effects on the breastfed infant, or the effects on milk production. Published data suggest that human IgG is present in human milk but does not enter the neonatal and infant circulation in substantial amounts. Trastuzumab was present in the milk of lactating cynomolgus monkeys but not associated with neonatal toxicity (see Data). Consider the developmental and health benefits of breast feeding along with the mother's clinical need for PHESGO treatment and any potential adverse effects on the breastfed child from PHESGO or from the underlying maternal condition. This consideration should also take into account the elimination half-life of pertuzumab and the trastuzumab wash out period of 7 months. Data In lactating cynomolgus monkeys, trastuzumab was present in breast milk at about 0.3% of maternal serum concentrations after pre- (beginning Gestation Day 120) and post-partum (through post-partum Day 28) doses of 25 mg/kg administered twice weekly (25 times the recommended weekly human dose of 2 mg/kg of intravenous trastuzumab). Infant monkeys with detectable serum levels of trastuzumab did not exhibit any adverse effects on growth or development from birth to 1 month of age.

Females and males of reproductive potential

PHESGO can cause embryo-fetal harm when administered during pregnancy. Pregnancy Testing

Verify the pregnancy status of females of reproductive potential prior to the initiation of PHESGO.

Contraception

Females

Advise females of reproductive potential to use effective contraception during treatment and for 7 months following the last dose of PHESGO.

Pediatric use

The safety and effectiveness of PHESGO in pediatric patients have not been established.

Geriatric use

Of the total number of patients in the FeDeriCa study (n=500) treated with PHESGO, 11% were 65 and over, while 1.6% were 75 and over. Clinical studies of PHESGO did not include sufficient numbers of patients age 65 years and older to determine whether they respond differently from younger patients. In the intravenous trastuzumab trials, the risk of cardiac dysfunction was increased in geriatric patients as compared to younger patients, in both those receiving treatment for adjuvant therapy or metastatic disease. Other differences in safety or effectiveness were not observed between elderly patients and younger patients. In the intravenous pertuzumab in combination with trastuzumab trials, the risk of decreased appetite, anemia, weight decreased, asthenia, dysgeusia, peripheral neuropathy and hypomagnesemia was increased in patients 65 years of age and older compared to patients less than 65 years of age. (*Dysgeusia, also known as parageusia, is a distortion of the sense of taste. Dysgeusia is also often associated with ageusia, which is the complete lack of taste, and hypogeusia, which is a decrease in taste sensitivity).*

Pharmacodynamics

Cardiac electrophysiology

The effect of intravenous pertuzumab with an initial dose of 840 mg followed by a maintenance dose of 420 mg every three weeks on QTc interval was evaluated in a subgroup of 20 patients with HER2-positive breast cancer (NCT00567190). No large changes in the mean QT interval (i.e., greater than 20 ms) from placebo based on Fridericia correction method were detected in the trial. A small increase in the mean QTc interval (i.e., less than 10 ms) cannot be excluded because of the limitations of the trial design. The effects of trastuzumab on electrocardiographic (ECG) endpoints, including QTc interval duration, were evaluated in patients with HER2 positive solid tumors. Trastuzumab had no clinically relevant effect on the QTc interval duration and there was no apparent relationship between serum trastuzumab concentrations and change in QTcF interval duration in patients with HER2 positive solid tumors.

Pharmacokinetics

The pharmacokinetics (PK) of pertuzumab and trastuzumab was characterized in the FeDeriCa study following subcutaneous administration of PHESGO (1200 mg pertuzumab/600 mg trastuzumab initial dose followed by 600 mg pertuzumab/600 mg trastuzumab every 3 weeks) and intravenous administration of pertuzumab and trastuzumab (840 mg pertuzumab/8 mg/kg trastuzumab initial dose followed by 420 mg pertuzumab/6 mg/kg trastuzumab every 3 weeks). Trastuzumab is estimated to reach concentrations that are < 1 mcg/mL by 7 months in at least 95% patients. Pertuzumab Cycle 7 Ctrough (i.e., pre-dose cycle 8) showed non-inferiority of pertuzumab within PHESGO (88.7 mcg/mL) to intravenous pertuzumab (72.4 mcg/mL), with a geometric mean ratio of 1.22 (90% CI: 1.14–1.31). Trastuzumab Cycle 7 Ctrough showed non-inferiority of trastuzumab within PHESGO (58.7 mcg/mL) to intravenous trastuzumab (44.1 mcg/mL), with a geometric mean ratio of 1.33 (90% CI: 1.24–1.43).

A population PK analysis reported that, following subcutaneous administration of PHESGO, the mean Cycle 7 Cmax and AUC0-21 days of pertuzumab were 34% lower and 5% higher, respectively, than that following intravenous administration of pertuzumab. The mean Cycle 7 Cmax and AUC0-21 days of trastuzumab were 31% lower and 9% higher, respectively, than that following intravenous administration of trastuzumab.

Specific populations

Lean body weight and baseline serum albumin level were included as significant covariates in the pertuzumab population PK model. However, no dose adjustments based on body weight or baseline albumin level are needed, as the exposure changes are not considered clinically relevant. Body weight showed a statistically significant influence on trastuzumab PK. In patients with a body weight < 58 kg, mean Cycle 7 AUC0-21 days of trastuzumab was about 34% higher after PHESGO than after intravenous trastuzumab treatment, whereas in the highest BW group (> 77 kg) Cycle 7 AUC0-21 days was 24% lower after PHESGO than after intravenous trastuzumab treatment. However, no body weight-based dose adjustments are needed, as the exposure changes are not considered clinically relevant. No clinically significant differences in the pharmacokinetics of pertuzumab and trastuzumab were observed based on age (25 to 80 years), race (Asian and non-Asian) and renal impairment (creatinine clearance determined by Cockcroft-Gault 30 mL/min or greater).

The effects of hepatic impairment on the pharmacokinetics of pertuzumab and trastuzumab are unknown.

Drug interaction studies

There have been no formal drug interaction studies performed with PHESGO in humans. Clinically significant interactions among pertuzumab, trastuzumab, and concomitant medications used in clinical trials have not been observed.

Clinical efficacy of PHESGO in the treatment of breast cancer

FDA NEWS RELEASE

FDA Approves Breast Cancer Treatment That Can Be Administered At Home By Health Care Professional

"Currently, most patients with HER2-positive breast cancer receive trastuzumab and pertuzumab at infusion centers. With a new administration route, Phesgo offers an out-patient option for patients to receive trastuzumab and pertuzumab," said Richard Pazdur, M.D., director of the FDA's Oncology Center of Excellence and acting director of the Office of Oncologic Diseases in the FDA's Center for Drug Evaluation and Research. "As part of the FDA's ongoing commitment to address the novel coronavirus pandemic, we continue to keep a strong focus on patients with cancer who constitute a vulnerable population at risk of contracting the disease. At this critical time, we continue to expedite oncology product development. This application was approved about four months ahead of the FDA goal date."

9.18. SACITUZUMAB GOVITECAN-hziy (TRODELVY™)

TRODELVY™ (sacituzumab govitecan-hziy) for injection, for intravenous use. Initial U.S. Approval: 2020.

WARNING: NEUTROPENIA AND DIARRHEA

• Severe neutropenia may occur. Withhold TRODELVY for absolute neutrophil count below 1500/mm^3 or neutropenic fever. Monitor blood cell counts periodically during treatment. Consider G-CSF for secondary prophylaxis. Initiate anti-infective treatment in patients with febrile neutropenia without delay.

• Severe diarrhea may occur. Monitor patients with diarrhea and give fluid and electrolytes as needed. Administer atropine, if not contraindicated, for early diarrhea of any severity. At the onset of late diarrhea, evaluate for infectious causes and, if negative, promptly initiate loperamide. If severe diarrhea occurs, withhold TRODELVY until resolved to < Grade 1 and reduce subsequent doses.

MECHANISM OF ACTION

Sacituzumab govitecan-hziy is a Trop-2-directed antibody-drug conjugate. Sacituzumab is a humanized antibody that recognizes Trop-2□. The small molecule, SN-38, is a topoisomerase I inhibitor, which is covalently attached to the antibody by a linker. Pharmacology data suggest that sacituzumab govitecan-hziy binds to Trop-2-expressing cancer cells and is internalized with the subsequent release of SN-38 via hydrolysis of the linker. SN-38 interacts with topoisomerase I and prevents re-ligation of topoisomerase I-induced single strand breaks. The resulting DNA damage leads to apoptosis and cell death. Sacituzumab govitecan-hziy decreased tumor growth in mouse xenograft models of triple-negative breast cancer.

□*Tumor-associated calcium signal transducer 2, also known as Trop-2 and as epithelial glycoprotein-1 antigen (EGP-1), is a protein that in humans is encoded by the TACSTD2 gene. This intronless gene encodes a carcinoma-associated antigen. This antigen is a member of a family including at least two type I membrane proteins. It transduces an intracellular calcium signal and acts as a cell surface receptor.This antigen is the target of sacituzumab govitecan, an antibody-drug conjugate.*

DESCRIPTION

Sacituzumab govitecan-hziy is a Trop-2 directed antibody and topoisomerase inhibitor conjugate, composed of the following three components

• the humanized monoclonal antibody, hRS7 IgG1κ (also called sacituzumab), which binds to Trop-2 (the trophoblast cell-surface antigen-2).

• the drug SN-38, a topoisomerase inhibitor.

• a hydrolysable linker (called CL2A), which links the humanized monoclonal antibody to SN-38. The recombinant monoclonal antibody is produced by mammalian (murine myeloma) cells, while the small molecule components SN-38 and CL2A are produced by chemical synthesis. Sacituzumab govitecan-hziy contains on average 7 to 8 molecules of SN-38 per antibody molecule. Sacituzumab govitecan-hziy has a molecular weight of approximately 160 kilodaltons.

INDICATIONS AND USAGE

TRODELVY is a Trop-2-directed antibody and topoisomerase inhibitor conjugate indicated for the treatment of adult patients with metastatic triple-negative breast cancer (mTNBC) who have received at least two prior therapies for metastatic disease.

This indication is approved under accelerated approval based on tumor response rate and duration of response. Continued approval for this indication may be contingent upon verification and description of clinical benefit in confirmatory trials.

DOSAGE AND ADMINISTRATION

• Do NOT substitute TRODELVY for or use with other drugs containing irinotecan or its active metabolite SN-38.

• For intravenous infusion only. Do not administer as an intravenous push or bolus.

• The recommended dose is 10 mg/kg once weekly on Days 1 and 8 of continuous 21-day treatment cycles until disease progression or unacceptable toxicity.

•Premedication for prevention of infusion reactions and prevention of chemotherapy-induced nausea and vomiting is recommended.

• Monitor patients during the infusion and for at least 30 minutes after completion of infusion. Treatment interruption and/or dose reduction may be needed to manage adverse reactions.

• See Full Prescribing Information for preparation and administration instructions.

DOSAGE FORMS AND STRENGTHS

For injection: 180 mg lyophilized powder in single-dose vials for reconstitution.

CONTRAINDICATIONS

Severe hypersensitivity reaction to TRODELVY.

WARNINGS AND PRECAUTIONS

• Hypersensitivity

Hypersensitivity reactions including severe anaphylactic reactions have been observed. Monitor patients for infusion-related reactions. Permanently discontinue TRODELVY if severe or lifethreatening reactions occur.

• Nausea/vomiting

Use antiemetic preventive treatment and withhold TRODELVY for patients with Grade 3 nausea or Grade 3-4 vomiting at the time of scheduled treatment.

• Patients with Reduced UGT1A1 Activity

Individuals who are homozygous for the uridine diphosphate-glucuronosyl transferase 1A1 (UGT1A1)*28 allele are at increased risk for neutropenia following initiation of TRODELVY treatment.

• Embryo-fetal toxicity

TRODELVY can cause fetal harm. Advise patients of potential risk to a fetus and to use effective contraception.

ADVERSE REACTIONS

The most common adverse reactions (incidence >25%) in patients with mTNBC are nausea, neutropenia, diarrhea, fatigue, anemia, vomiting, alopecia, constipation, rash, decreased appetite, and abdominal pain. To report SUSPECTED ADVERSE REACTIONS, contact Immunomedics, Inc. at 1-888-983-4668 or FDA at 1-800-FDA-1088 or www.fda.gov/medwatch.

DRUG INTERACTIONS

• UGT1A1 inhibitors or inducers: Avoid concomitant use.

USE IN SPECIFIC POPULATIONS

• Lactation: advise not to breastfeed

FULL PRESCRIBING INFORMATION

WARNING: NEUTROPENIA AND DIARRHEA

• Severe neutropenia may occur. Withhold TRODELVY for absolute neutrophil count below 1500/mm^3 or neutropenic fever. Monitor blood cell counts periodically during treatment. Consider G-CSF for secondary prophylaxis. Initiate anti-infective treatment in patient with febrile neutropenia without delay

• Severe diarrhea may occur. Monitor patients with diarrhea and give fluid and electrolytes as needed. Administer atropine, if not contraindicated, for early diarrhea of any severity. At the onset of late diarrhea, evaluate for infectious causes and, if negative, promptly initiate loperamide. If severe diarrhea occurs, withhold TRODELVY until resolved to < Grade 1 and reduce subsequent doses.

INDICATIONS AND USAGE

TRODELVY is indicated for the treatment of adult patients with metastatic triple-negative breast cancer (mTNBC) who have received at least two prior therapies for metastatic disease. This indication is approved under accelerated approval based on tumor response rate and duration of response. Continued approval for this indication may be contingent upon verification and description of clinical benefit in confirmatory trials.

DOSAGE AND ADMINISTRATION

Important use information

Do NOT substitute TRODELVY for or use with other drugs containing irinotecan or its active metabolite SN-38.

Recommended dose and schedule

The recommended dose of TRODELVY is 10 mg/kg administered as an intravenous infusion once weekly on Days 1 and 8 of 21-day treatment cycles. Continue treatment until disease progression or unacceptable toxicity. Do not administer TRODELVY at doses greater than 10 mg/kg. Administer TRODELVY as an intravenous infusion only. Do not administer as an intravenous push or bolus.

First infusion: administer infusion over 3 hours. Observe patients during the infusion and for at least 30 minutes following the initial dose, for signs or symptoms of infusion-related reactions

Subsequent infusions: administer infusion over 1 to 2 hours if prior infusions were tolerated. Observe patients during the infusion and for at least 30 minutes after infusion.

Premedication prior to each dose of TRODELVY

Premedication for prevention of infusion reactions and prevention of chemotherapy-induced nausea and vomiting (CINV) is recommended.

• Premedicate with antipyretics, H1 and H2 blockers prior to infusion, and corticosteroids may be used for patients who had prior infusion reactions.

• Premedicate with a two or three drug combination regimen (e.g., dexamethasone with either a 5-HT3 receptor antagonist or an NK1 receptor antagonist, as well as other drugs as indicated).

Dose modifications for adverse reactions infusion-related reactions

Slow or interrupt the infusion rate of TRODELVY if the patient develops an infusion-related reaction. Permanently discontinue TRODELVY for life-threatening infusion-related reactions

Dose modifications for adverse reactions

Withhold or discontinue TRODELVY to manage adverse reactions as described in below Do not re-escalate the TRODELVY dose after a dose reduction for adverse reactions has been made.

Dose modifications for adverse reactions.

Adverse reaction	**Ocurrence**	**Dose modification**
Severe neutropenia		
Grade 4 neutropenia ≥7 days, OR Grade 3 febrile neutropenia (absolute neutrophil count < 1000/mm^3 and fever ≥38.5°C), OR At time of scheduled treatment, Grade 3-4 neutropenia which delays dosing by 2 or 3 weeks for	First	25% dose reduction and administer granulocytecolony stimulating factor (G-CSF)
	Second	50% dose reduction
	Third	Discontinue treatment
	First	Discontinue treatment

recovery to ≤ Grade 1 At time of scheduled treatment, Grade 3-4 neutropenia which delays dosing beyond 3 weeks for recovery to ≤ Grade 1		
Severe non-neutropenic toxicity		

Grade 4 non-hematologic toxicity of any duration, OR Any Grade 3-4 nausea, vomiting or diarrhea due to treatment that is not controlled with antiemetics and anti-diarrheal agents OR Other Grade 3-4 non-hematologic toxicity persisting >48 hours despite optimal medical management, OR At time of scheduled treatment, Grade 3-4 nonneutropenic hematologic or non-hematologic toxicity, which delays dose by 2 or 3 weeks for recovery to ≤ Grade 1	First	25% dose reduction
	Second	50% dose reduction
	Third	Discontinue treatment

CONTRAINDICATIONS

TRODELVY is contraindicated in patients who have experienced a severe hypersensitivity reaction to TRODELVY

Further information on **WARNINGS AND PRECAUTIONS**

Neutropenia

TRODELVY can cause severe or life-threatening neutropenia. Withhold TRODELVY for absolute neutrophil count below 1500/mm^3 on Day 1 of any cycle or neutrophil count below 1000/mm^3 on Day 8 of any cycle.

Withhold TRODELVY for neutropenic fever. Dose modifications may be required due to neutropenia. Febrile neutropenia occurred in 6% (24/408) patients treated with TRODELVY, including 8% (9/108) patients with mTNBC after at least two prior therapies. Less than 1% (1/408) of patients had febrile neutropenia leading to permanent discontinuation. The incidence of Grade 1-4 neutropenia was 64% in patients with mTNBC (n=108). In all patients treated with TRODELVY (n=408), the incidence of Grade1-4 neutropenia was 54%; Grade 4 neutropenia occurred in 13%. Less than 1% (2/408) of patients permanently discontinued treatment due to neutropenia. *(Figures 136, 137 and 138).*

Figure 136. Peripheral blood smear showing 4 normal multilobulated neutrophils against a background of red blood cells.

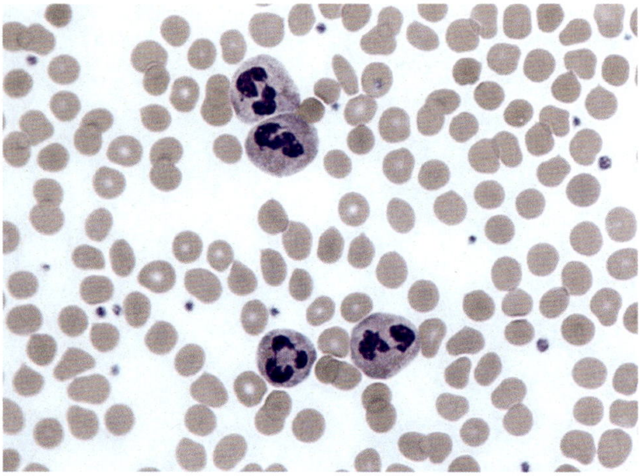

https://en.wikipedia.org/wiki/Neutrophil#/media/File:Neutrophils.jpg. This file is licensed under the Creative Commons Attribution-Share Alike 3.0 Unported license. No changes were madeto this image.

Figure 137. A neutrophil (aka neutrophil granulocyte) migrates from the blood vessel to the matrix, secreting proteolytic enzymes, to dissolve intercellular connections (to the improvement of its mobility) and envelop bacteria through phagocytosis.

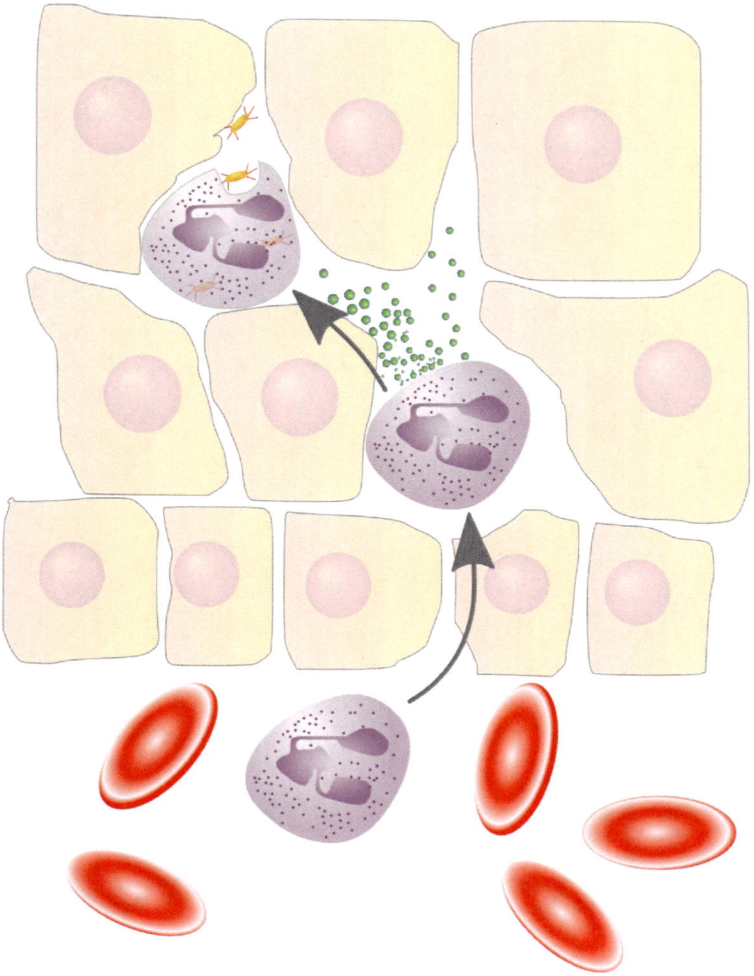

This image is by !Original: Dr. med. Mario Schubert, Heidelberg, GermanyVector: Mrmw - Own work based on: NeutrophilerAktion.png:, CC0, https://commons.wikimedia.org/w/index.php?curid=61571220. https://en.wikipedia.org/wiki/Neutrophil#/media/File:NeutrophilerAktion.svg. This file

is made available under the Creative Commons CC0 1.0 Universal Public Domain Dedication. No change were made to this image.

Figure 138. Scanning electron micrograph of a neutrophil (yellow) phagocytosing anthrax bacilli (orange). Scale bar is 5 µm.

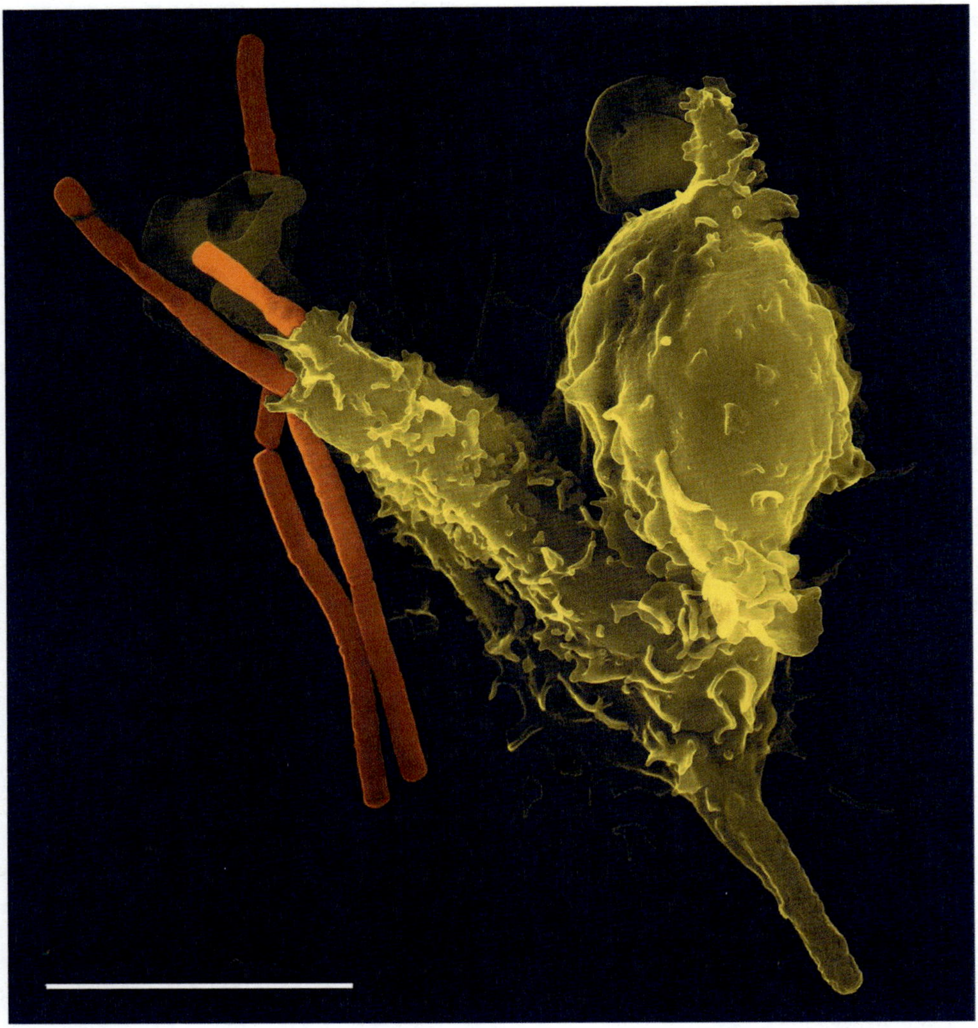

This image is by Volker Brinkmann - (November 2005). "Neutrophil engulfing Bacillus anthracis". PLoS Pathogens 1 (3): Cover page. DOI:10.1371. Retrieved on 2009-01-04., CC BY 2.5, https://commons.wikimedia.org/w/index.php?curid=2107792. https://en.wikipedia.org/wiki/Neutrophil#/media/File:Neutrophil_with_anthrax_copy.jp

g. This file is licensed under the Creative Commons Attribution 2.5 Generic license. No changes were made to this image.

CONTRAINDICATIONS

TRODELVY is contraindicated in patients who have experienced a severe hypersensitivity reaction to TRODELVY.

Diarrhea

TRODELVY can cause severe diarrhea. Withhold TRODELVY for Grade 3-4 diarrhea at the time of scheduled treatment administration and resume when resolved to ≤ Grade 1 [see Dosage and Administration (2.3)]. At the onset of diarrhea, evaluate for infectious causes and if negative, promptly initiate loperamide, 4 mg initially followed by 2 mg with every episode of diarrhea for a maximum of 16 mg daily. Discontinue loperamide 12 hours after diarrhea resolves. Additional supportive measures (e.g., fluid and electrolyte substitution) may also be employed as clinically indicated. Patients who exhibit an excessive cholinergic response to treatment with TRODELVY (e.g., abdominal cramping, diarrhea, salivation, etc.) can receive appropriate premedication (e.g., atropine) for subsequent treatments. Diarrhea occurred in 63% (68/108) of patients with mTNBC and 62% (254/408) of all patients treated with TRODELVY. In each population, events of Grade 3-4 occurred in 9% (10/108) of mTNBC patients and 9% (36/408) of all patients treated with TRODELVY. Four out of 408 patients (<1%) discontinued treatment because of diarrhea. Neutropenic colitis was observed in 2% (2/108) of patients in the mTNBC cohort and 1% of all patients treated with TRODELVY.

Neutropenic enterocolitis *is inflammation of the cecum (part of the large intestine) that may be associated with infection (Figure 139). It is particularly associated with neutropenia. Signs and symptoms of typhlitis may include diarrhea, a distended abdomen, fever, chills, nausea, vomiting, and abdominal pain or tenderness. The condition is usually caused by Gram-positive enteric commensal bacteria of the gut (gut flora). Clostridium difficile is a species of Gram-positive bacteria that commonly causes severe diarrhea and other intestinal diseases when competing bacteria are wiped out by antibiotics, causing pseudomembranous colitis, whereas Clostridium septicum is responsible for most cases of neutropenic enterocolitis. Typhlitis most commonly occurs in immunocompromised patients, such* as those undergoing chemotherapy, patients with AIDS, kidney transplant patients, or the elderly.

Figure 139. The human gastro-intestinal system.

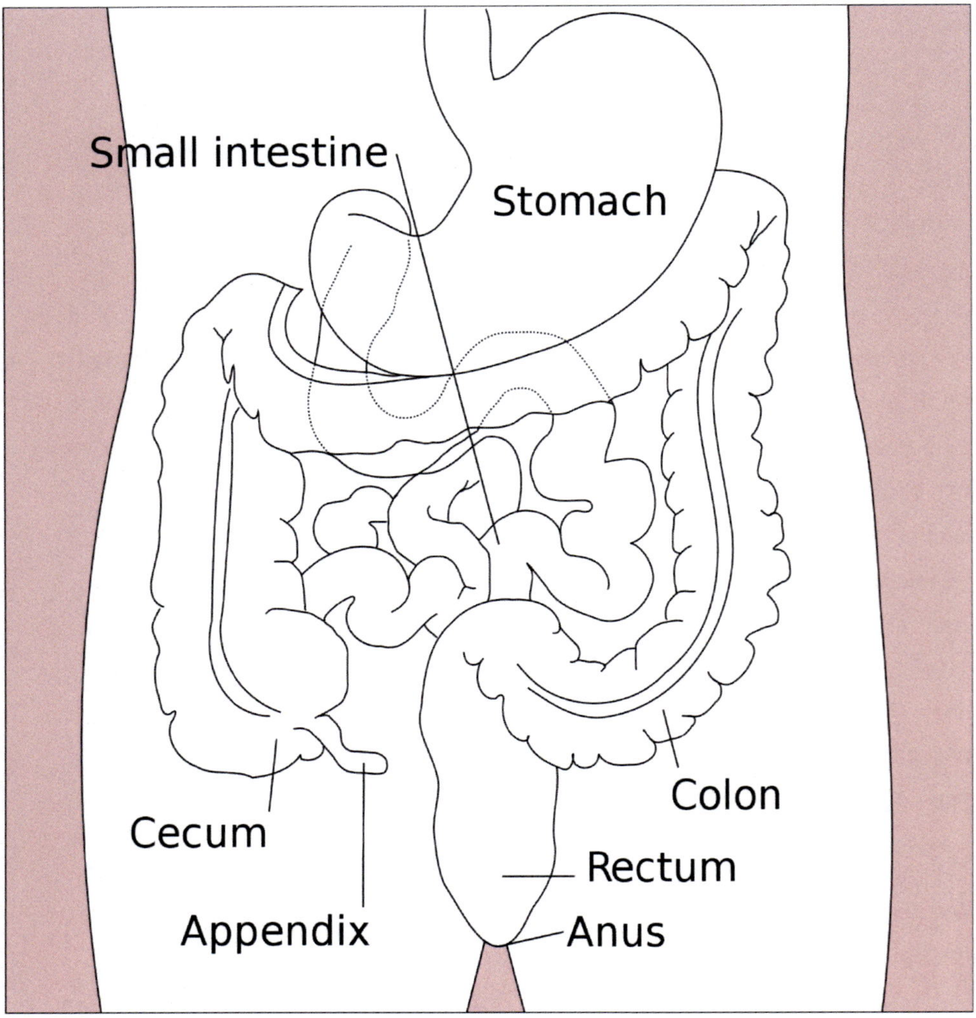

This image is by By Indolences created it on the English Wikipedia.This SVG image was created by Medium69.Cette image SVG a été créée par Medium69.Please credit this: William Crochot - US PD picture., Public Domain, https://commons.wikimedia.org/w/index.php?curid=1521879. https://en.wikipedia.org/wiki/Neutropenic_enterocolitis#/media/File:Stomach_colon_rectum_diagram-en.svg. This work has been released into the public domain by its author, Indolences at the Wikipedia project. This applies worldwide. This SVG image

was created by Medium69. Please credit this: William Crochot. No changes were made to this image.

Hypersensitivity

TRODELVY can cause severe and life-threatening hypersensitivity. Anaphylactic reactions have been observed in clinical trials with TRODELVY. Hypersensitivity reactions within 24 hours of dosing occurred in 37% (151/408) of patient treated with TRODELVY. Grade 3-4 hypersensitivity occurred in 1% (6/408) of patients treated with TRODELVY. The incidence of hypersensitivity reactions leading to permanent discontinuation of TRODELVY was 1% (3/408). Pre-infusion medication for patients receiving TRODELVY is recommended. Observe patients closely for infusion-related reactions during each TRODELVY infusion and for at least 30 minutes after completion of each infusion. Medication to treat such reactions, as well as emergency equipment, should be available for immediate use.

Nausea and vomiting

TRODELVY is emetogenic. Nausea occurred in 69% (74/108) of patients with mTNBC and 69% (281/408) of all patients treated with TRODELVY. Grade 3 nausea occurred in 6% (7/108) and 5% (22/408) of these populations, respectively. Vomiting occurred in 49% (53/108) of patients with mTNBC and 45% (183/408) of all patients treated with TRODELVY. Grade 3 vomiting occurred in 6% (7/108) and 4% (16/408) of these patients, respectively. Premedicate with a two or three drug combination regimen (e.g., dexamethasone with either a 5-HT3 receptor antagonist or an NK-1 receptor antagonist as well as other drugs as indicated) for prevention of chemotherapy-induced nausea and vomiting (CINV). Withhold TRODELVY doses for Grade 3 nausea or Grade 3-4 vomiting at the time of scheduled treatment administration and resume with additional supportive measures when resolved to Grade ≤ 1. Additional antiemetics and other supportive measures may also be employed as clinically indicated. All patients should be given take-home medications with clear instructions for prevention and treatment of nausea and vomiting.

Use in patients with reduced UGT1A1 activity

Individuals who are homozygous for the uridine diphosphate-glucuronosyl transferase 1A1 (UGT1A1)*28 allele are at increased risk for neutropenia and may be at increased risk for other adverse reactions following initiation of TRODELVY treatment. In 84% (343/408) of patients who received TRODELVY (up to 10 mg/kg on Days 1 and 8 of a 21-day cycle) and had retrospective UGT1A1 genotype results available, the incidence of Grade 4 neutropenia was 26% (10/39) in patients homozygous for the UGT1A1*28 allele, 13% (20/155) in patients heterozygous for the UGT1A1*28 allele and 11% (16/149) in patients homozygous for the wild-type allele. Closely monitor patients with reduced UGT1A1 activity for severe neutropenia. The appropriate dose for patients who are homozygous for UGT1A1*28 is not known and should be considered based on individual patient tolerance to treatment.

Embryo-fetal toxicity

Based on its mechanism of action, TRODELVY can cause teratogenicity and/or embryo-fetal lethality when administered to a pregnant woman. TRODELVY contains a genotoxic component, SN-38, and targets rapidly dividing cells. Advise pregnant women and females of reproductive potential of the potential risk to a fetus. Advise females of reproductive potential to use effective contraception during treatment with TRODELVY and for 6 months after the last dose. Advise male patients with female partners of reproductive potential to use effective contraception during treatment with TRODELVY and for 3 months after the last dose.

Immunogenicity

As with all therapeutic proteins, there is potential for immunogenicity. The detection of antibody formation is highly dependent on the sensitivity and specificity of the assay. Additionally, the observed incidence of antibody (including neutralizing antibody) positivity in an assay may be influenced by several factors including assay methodology, sample handling, timing of sample collection, concomitant medications, and underlying disease. For these reasons, comparison of the incidence of antibodies in the studies described below with the incidence of antibodies in other studies or to other sacituzumab govitecan products may be misleading. The analysis of immunogenicity of TRODELVY in serum samples from 106 patients with mTNBC was evaluated using an electrochemiluminescence (ECL)-based immunoassay to test for anti-sacituzumab govitecan-hziy antibodies. Detection of the anti-sacituzumab govitecan-hziy antibodies was done using a 3-tier approach: screen, confirm, and titer. Persistent anti-sacituzumab govitecan-hziy antibodies developed in 2% (2/106) of patients.

DRUG INTERACTIONS

Effect of Other Drugs on TRODELVY

UGT1A1 inhibitors

Concomitant administration of TRODELVY with inhibitors of UGT1A1 may increase the incidence of adverse reactions due to potential increase in systemic exposure to SN-38. Avoid administering UGT1A1 inhibitors with TRODELVY. UGT1A1 Inducers Exposure to SN-38 may be substantially reduced in patients concomitantly receiving UGT1A1 enzyme inducers. Avoid administering UGT1A1 inducers with TRODELVY.

USE IN SPECIFIC POPULATIONS

Pregnancy risk summary

Based on its mechanism of action, TRODELVY can cause teratogenicity and/or embryo-fetal lethality when administered to a pregnant woman. There are no available data in pregnant women to inform the drug-associated risk. TRODELVY contains a genotoxic component, SN-38, and is toxic to rapidly dividing cells. Advise pregnant women and females of reproductive potential of the potential risk to a fetus. The estimated background risk of major birth defects and miscarriage for the indicated population is unknown. In the U.S. general population, the estimated background risk of major birth defects and miscarriage in clinically recognized pregnancies is 2 – 4% and 15 – 20%, respectively.

Data

Animal data

There were no reproductive and developmental toxicology studies conducted with sacituzumab govitecan-hziy.

Lactation risk summary

There is no information regarding the presence of sacituzumab govitecan-hziy or SN-38 in human milk, the effects on the breastfed child, or the effects on milk production. Because of the potential for serious adverse reactions in a breastfed child, advise women not to breastfeed during treatment and for 1 month after the last dose of TRODELVY.

Females and males of reproductive potential

Pregnancy Testing

Verify the pregnancy status of females of reproductive potential prior to the initiation of TRODELVY.

Contraception

Females

TRODELVY can cause fetal harm when administered to a pregnant woman. Advise females of reproductive potential to use effective contraception during treatment with TRODELVY and for 6 months after the last dose.

Males

Because of the potential for genotoxicity, advise male patients with female partners of reproductive potential to use effective contraception during treatment with TRODELVY and for 3 months after the last dose.

Infertility

Females

Based on findings in animals, TRODELVY may impair fertility in females of reproductive potential.

Pediatric use

Safety and effectiveness of TRODELVY have not been established in pediatric patients.

Geriatric use

Of the patients who received TRODELVY, 19/108 (18%) patients with mTNBC and 144/408 (35%) of all patients were ≥ 65 years old. No overall differences in safety and effectiveness were observed between these patients and younger patients.

Hepatic impairment

No adjustment to the starting dose is required when administering TRODELVY to patients with mild hepatic impairment (bilirubin less than or equal to 1.5 ULN and AST/ALT < 3 ULN). The exposure of TRODELVY in patients with mild hepatic impairment (bilirubin less than or equal to ULN and AST greater than ULN, or bilirubin greater than 1.0 to 1.5 ULN and AST of any level; n=12) was similar to patients with normal hepatic function (bilirubin or AST less than ULN; n=45). The safety of TRODELVY in patients with moderate or severe hepatic impairment has not been established. TRODELVY has not been tested in patients with serum bilirubin > 1.5 ULN, or AST and ALT > 3 ULN, or AST and ALT > 5 ULN and associated with liver metastases. No dedicated trial was performed to investigate the tolerability of TRODELVY in patients with moderate or severe hepatic impairment. No recommendations can be made for the starting dose in these patients.

OVERDOSAGE

In a clinical trial, planned doses of up to 18 mg/kg (approximately 1.8 times the maximum recommended dose of 10 mg/kg) of TRODELVY were administered. In these patients, a higher incidence of severe neutropenia was observed.

Pharmacodynamics

Exposure-response relationships and the time course of pharmacodynamics response are unknown for sacituzumab govitecan-hziy.

Pharmacokinetics

The serum pharmacokinetics of sacituzumab govitecan-hziy and SN-38 were evaluated in a study in a population of mTNBC patients who received sacituzumab govitecan-hziy as a single agent at a dose of 10 mg/kg.

Distribution

The mean volume of distribution for sacituzumab govitecan-hziy was 0.045 L/kg.

Elimination

The mean half-life of sacituzumab govitecan-hziy and free SN-38 was 16 and 18 hours, respectively. The clearance of the sacituzumab govitecan-hziy was 0.002 L/h/kg.

Metabolism

No metabolism studies with sacituzumab govitecan-hziy have been conducted. SN-38 (the small molecule moiety of sacituzumab govitecan-hziy) is metabolized via UGT1A1. The glucuronide metabolite of SN-38 (SN-38G) was detectable in the serum of patients.

Specific populations

Pharmacokinetic analyses in a limited number of patients with mTNBC (n = 57) did not identify an effect of age or race on the pharmacokinetics of sacituzumab govitecan-hziy. Renal elimination is known to contribute minimally to the excretion of SN-38, the small molecule moiety of sacituzumab govitecan-hziy. There are no data on the pharmacokinetics of sacituzumab govitecan-hziy in patients with renal impairment or end-stage renal disease (CLcr ≤ 30 mL/min). The exposure of sacituzumab govitecan-hziy is similar in patients with mild hepatic impairment (bilirubin less than or equal to ULN and AST greater than ULN, or bilirubin greater than 1.0 to less than 1.5 ULN and AST of any level; n=12) to patients with normal hepatic function (bilirubin or AST less than ULN; n=45). Sacituzumab govitecan-hziy exposure is unknown in patients with moderate or severe hepatic impairment. SN-38 exposure may be elevated in such patients due to decreased hepatic UGT1A1 activity.

Drug interaction studies

No drug-drug interaction studies were conducted with sacituzumab govitecan-hziy or its components

Inhibitors or inducers of UGT1A1 are expected to increase or decrease SN-38 exposure, respectively.

Pharmacogenomics

SN-38 is metabolized via UGT1A1. Genetic variants of the UGT1A1 gene such as the UGT1A1*28 allele lead to reduced UGT1A1 enzyme activity. Individuals who are homozygous for the UGT1A1*28 allele are at increased risk for neutropenia from TRODELVY Approximately 20% of the Black or African American population, 10% of the White population, and 2% of the East Asian population are homozygous for the UGT1A1*28 allele. Decreased function alleles other than UGT1A1*28 may be present in certain populations.

Clinical efficacy of sacituzumab govitecan-hziy (TRODELVY) in the treatment of breast cancer

FDA NEWS RELEASE

FDA Approves New Therapy for Triple Negative Breast Cancer That Has Spread, Not Responded to Other Treatments

For Immediate Release:

April 22, 2020

Today, the U.S. Food and Drug Administration granted accelerated approval to Trodelvy (sacituzumab govitecan-hziy) for the treatment of adult patients with triple-negative breast cancer that has spread to other parts of the body. Patients must have received at least two prior therapies before taking Trodelvy.

"Metastatic triple-negative breast cancer is an aggressive form of breast cancer with limited treatment options. Chemotherapy has been the mainstay of treatment for triple-negative breast cancer. The approval of Trodelvy today represents a new targeted therapy for patients living with this aggressive malignancy," said Richard Pazdur, M.D., director of the FDA's Oncology Center of Excellence and acting director of the Office of Oncologic Diseases in the FDA's Center for Drug Evaluation and Research. "There is intense interest in finding new medications to help treat metastatic triple-negative breast cancer. Today's approval provides patients who've already tried two prior therapies with a new option."

9.19. TALAZOPARIB (TALZENNA)

TALZENNA™ (talazoparib) capsules, for oral use. Initial U.S. Approval: 2018

INDICATIONS AND USAGE

TALZENNA is a poly (ADP-ribose) polymerase (PARP) inhibitor indicated for the treatment of adult patients with deleterious or suspected deleterious germline BRCA-mutated (gBRCAm) HER2-negative locally advanced or metastatic breast cancer. Select patients for therapy based on an FDA-approved companion diagnostic for TALZENNA.

MECHANISM OF ACTION

Talazoparib is an inhibitor of poly (ADP-ribose) polymerase (PARP) enzymes, including PARP1 and PARP2, which play a role in DNA repair. In vitro studies with cancer cell lines that harbored defects in DNA repair genes, including BRCA 1 and 2 (*Figure 140),* have shown that talazoparib-induced cytotoxicity may involve inhibition of PARP enzymatic activity and increased formation of PARP-DNA complexes resulting in DNA damage, decreased cell proliferation, and apoptosis. Talazoparib anti-tumor activity was observed in human patient-derived xenograft breast cancer tumor models that expressed mutated or wild-type BRCA 1 and 2.

Figure 140. The BRCA genes are tumor suppressor genes pictured here on their respective chromosomes. BRCA 1 has the cytogenetic location 17q21 or the q arm of Chromosome 17 at position 21. BRCA 2 has the cytogenetic location 13q12.3 or the q arm of Chromosome 13 at position 12.3. Both genes produce proteins that help repair damaged DNA, keeping the genetic material of the cell stable. A damaged BRCA gene in either location can lead to increased risk of cancer, particularly breast or ovarian in women.

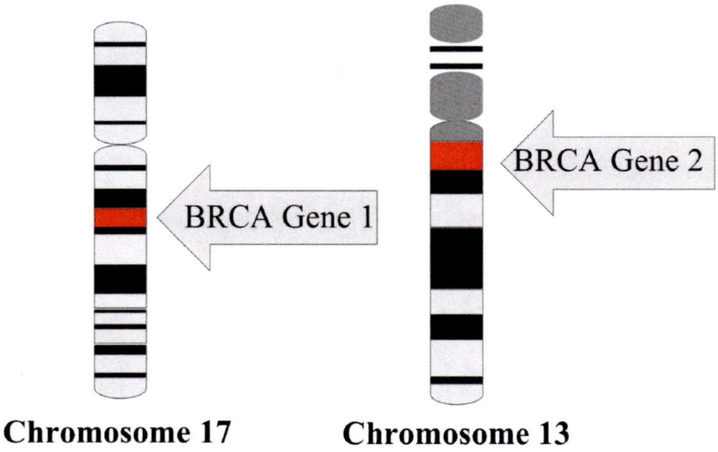

Figure 141. BRCA mutations are inherited in a genetically dominant fashion, from either parent.

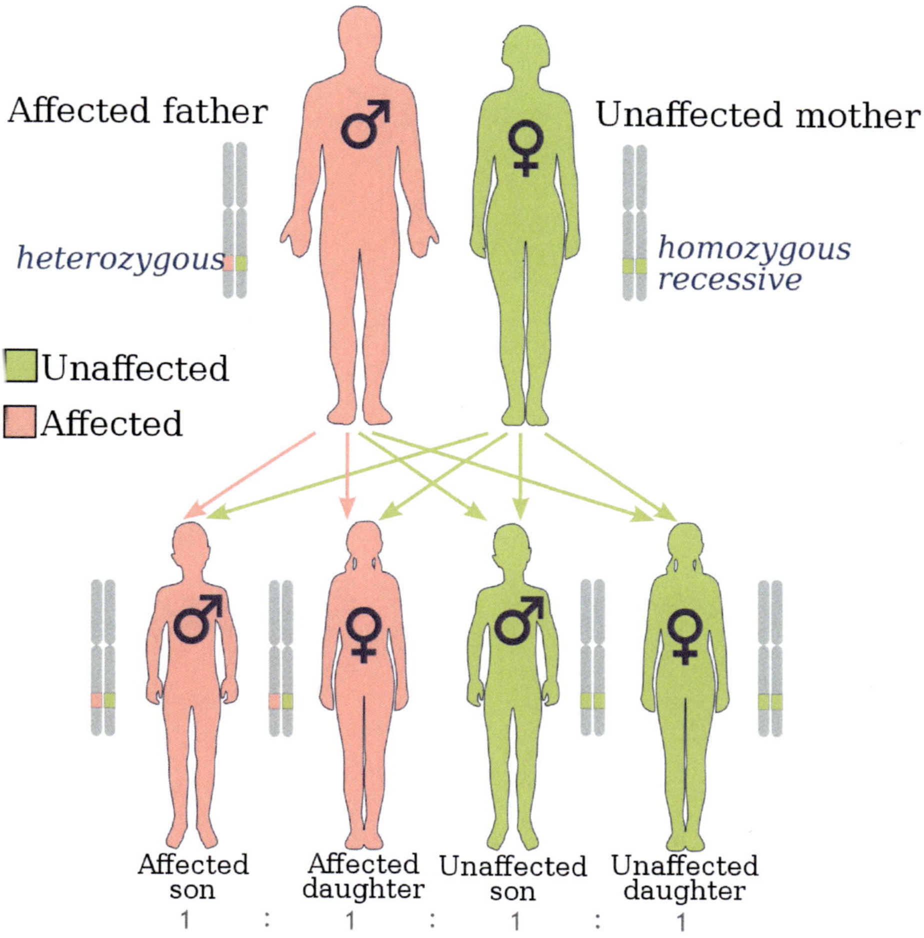

*This image is by Autodominant.svg: * Autodominant.svg, Public Domain, https://commons.wikimedia.org/w/index.php?curid=10784615. https://en.wikipedia.org/wiki/BRCA_mutation#/media/File:Autodominant_en.svg This image is a work of the National Institutes of Health, part of the United States Department of Health and Human Services. As a work of the U.S. federal government, the image is in the public domain. No changes were made to this work.*

Figure 142. The chemical structure of talazoparib

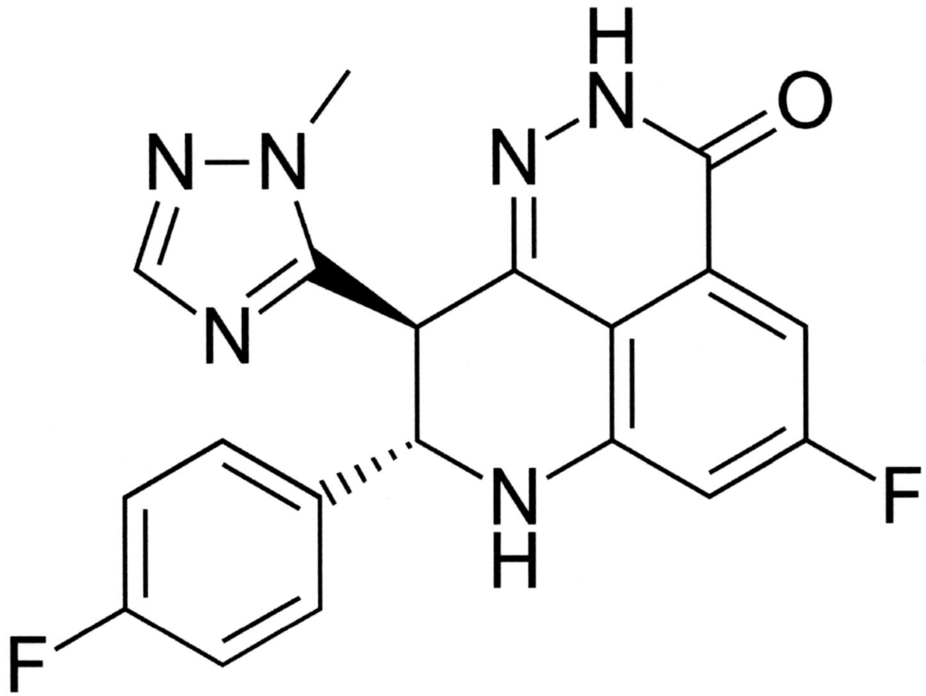

This image is by By Ed (Edgar181) - Own work, Public Domain, https://commons.wikimedia.org/w/index.php?curid=46375676. https://en.wikipedia.org/wiki/Talazoparib#/media/File:Talazoparib.svg. The copyright holder of this work has released it into the public domain. No changes were made to this image.

DESCRIPTION

Talazoparib is an inhibitor of mammalian polyadenosine 5'-diphosphoribose polymerase (PARP) enzyme. The chemical name of talazoparib tosylate is (8S,9R)-5-Fluoro-8-(4-fluorophenyl)-9-(1-methyl-1H-1,2,4-triazol5-yl)-2,7,8,9-tetrahydro-3H-pyrido[4,3,2-de]phthalazin-3-one 4-methylbenzenesulfonate. The chemical formula of talazoparib tosylate is C26H22F2N6O4S, and the relative molecular mass is 552.56 Daltons. The chemical structure of talazoparib tosylate is shown below: O HN F F N N N CH3 N NH CH3 O S O OH 8 9. Talazoparib tosylate is a white to yellow solid. TALZENNA capsules for oral use are available as a 0.25 mg hard hypromellose (HPMC) capsule that contains 0.363 mg talazoparib tosylate equivalent to 0.25 mg talazoparib free base or as a 1 mg HPMC capsule that contains 1.453 mg talazoparib tosylate equivalent to 1 mg talazoparib free base.

DOSAGE AND ADMINISTRATION

• The recommended dose of TALZENNA is 1 mg taken as a single oral daily dose, with or without food.

• Patients should be treated until disease progression or unacceptable toxicity occurs.

• For adverse reactions, consider dosing interruption or dose reduction.

• For patients with moderate renal impairment (CLcr 30 - 59 mL/min), the recommended dose of TALZENNA is 0.75 mg once daily.

DOSAGE FORMS AND STRENGTHS

Capsules: 0.25 mg, 1 mg

CONTRAINDICATIONS

None.

WARNINGS AND PRECAUTIONS

• **Myelodysplastic Syndrome/Acute Myeloid Leukemia (MDS/AML)**

MDS/AML has been reported in 2 out of 584 (0.3%) solid tumor patients treated with TALZENNA in clinical studies. Monitor patients for hematological toxicity at baseline and monthly thereafter. Discontinue if MDS/AML is confirmed.

• Myelosuppression

TALZENNA may affect hematopoiesis and can cause anemia, neutropenia, and/or thrombocytopenia.

Myelosuppression is the decrease in production of cells in the bone marrow responsible for providing immunity (white blood cells [leukocytes]), carrying oxygen (erythrocytes), and/or those responsible for normal blood clotting (platelets [thrombocytes]). Bone marrow suppression is a serious side effect of chemotherapy and certain drugs affecting the immune system such as azathioprine.

• Embryo-fetal toxicity

TALZENNA can cause fetal harm. Advise of the potential risk to the fetus and to use effective contraception.

ADVERSE REACTIONS

• The most common (≥20%) adverse reactions of any grade were: fatigue, anemia, nausea, neutropenia, headache, thrombocytopenia, vomiting, alopecia, diarrhea, decreased appetite.

• The most common laboratory abnormalities (≥25%) were: decreases in hemoglobin, platelets, neutrophils, lymphocytes, leukocytes, and calcium. Increases in glucose, alanine aminotransferase, aspartate aminotransferase, and alkaline phosphatase. To report SUSPECTED ADVERSE REACTIONS, contact Pfizer, Inc. at 1-800-438-1985 or FDA at 1-800-FDA-1088 or www.fda.gov/medwatch.

DRUG INTERACTIONS

• P-gp Inhibitors: reduce TALZENNA dose for certain P-gp inhibitors, and monitor for potential increased adverse reactions as appropriate.

• BCRP Inhibitors: Monitor for potential increased adverse reactions.

USE IN SPECIFIC POPULATIONS

Lactation

Advise women not to breastfeed.

FULL PRESCRIBING INFORMATION

INDICATIONS AND USAGE

TALZENNA is indicated for the treatment of adult patients with deleterious or suspected deleterious germline breast cancer susceptibility gene (BRCA)-mutated (gBRCAm) human epidermal growth factor receptor 2 (HER2)-negative locally advanced or metastatic breast cancer. Select patients for therapy based on an FDA-approved companion diagnostic for TALZENNA.

DOSAGE AND ADMINISTRATION

Patient selection

Select patients for the treatment of advanced breast cancer with TALZENNA based on the presence of germline BRCA mutations *(see Figures 140 and 141).* Information on the FDA-approved test for the detection of BRCA mutations is available at http://www.fda.gov/companiondiagnostics.

Recommended dosing

The recommended dose of TALZENNA is 1 mg taken orally once daily, with or without food. The 0.25 mg capsule is available for dose reduction. Patients should be treated until disease progression or unacceptable toxicity occurs. The hard capsules should be swallowed whole and must not be opened or dissolved. If the patient vomits or misses a dose, an additional dose should not be taken. The next prescribed dose should be taken at the usual time.

Dose modifications for adverse reactions

To manage adverse reactions, consider interruption of treatment with or without dose reduction based on severity and clinical presentation. Recommended dose reductions are indicated in below Treatment with TALZENNA should be discontinued if more than three dose reductions are required.

TDose reduction levels for adverse reactions

Dose level	**Dose**
Recommended starting dose	1 mg (one 1 mg capsule) once daily
First dose reduction	0.75 mg (three 0.25 mg capsules) once daily
Second dose reduction	0.5 mg (two 0.25 mg capsules) once daily
Third dose reduction	0.25 mg (one 0.25 mg capsule) once daily

Dose modification and management.

Monitor complete blood counts monthly and as clinically indicated.

Adverse Reactions	Withhold TALZENNA until levels resolve to	Resume TALZENNA
Hemoglobin <8g/dL	≥9 g/dL	Resume TALZENNA at a reduced dose
Platelet count <50,000/µL	≥75,000/µL	Resume TALZENNA at a reduced dose
Neutrophil count <1,000/µL	≥1500/µL	Resume TALZENNA at a reduced dose
Non-hematologic Grade 3 or Grade 4	Equal to, or less than, Grade 1	Consider resuming TALZENNA at a reduced dose or discontinue

Dose modifications for patients with renal impairment

For patients with moderate renal impairment (CLcr 30 - 59 mL/min), the recommended dose of TALZENNA is 0.75 mg once daily

Dose modifications for use with P-glycoprotein (P-gp) inhibitors

Reduce the TALZENNA dose to 0.75 mg once daily when coadministered with certain P-gp inhibitors. For additional information on interacting P-gp inhibitors. When the P-gp inhibitor is discontinued, increase the TALZENNA dose (after 3–5 half-lives of the P-gp inhibitor) to the dose used prior to the initiation of the P-gp inhibitor.

DOSAGE FORMS AND STRENGTHS

Capsules:

• 0.25 mg capsule with an ivory cap (printed with “Pfizer” in black) and a white body (printed with “TLZ 0.25” in black)

• 1 mg capsule with a light red cap (printed with “Pfizer” in black) and a white body (printed with “TLZ 1” in black)

CONTRAINDICATIONS: none.

WARNINGS AND PRECAUTIONS

Myelodysplastic syndrome/acute myeloid leukemia (MDS/AML) have been reported in patients who received TALZENNA. Overall, MDS/AML has been reported in 2 out of 584 (0.3%) solid tumor patients treated with TALZENNA in clinical studies. The duration of TALZENNA treatment in these two patients prior to developing MDS/AML was 4 months and 24 months, respectively. Both patients had received previous chemotherapy with platinum agents and/or other DNA damaging agents including radiotherapy. Do not start TALZENNA until patients have adequately recovered from hematological toxicity caused by previous chemotherapy. Monitor complete blood counts for cytopenia at baseline and monthly thereafter. For prolonged hematological toxicities, interrupt TALZENNA and monitor blood counts weekly until recovery. If the levels have not recovered after 4 weeks, refer the patient to a hematologist for further investigations, including bone marrow analysis and blood sample for cytogenetics. If MDS/AML is confirmed, discontinue TALZENNA.

Myelosuppression

Myelosuppression consisting of anemia, leukopenia/neutropenia, and/or thrombocytopenia, have been reported in patients treated with TALZENNA. Grade ≥3 anemia, neutropenia, and thrombocytopenia were reported, respectively, in 39%, 21%, and 15% of patients receiving TALZENNA. Discontinuation due to anemia, neutropenia, and thrombocytopenia occurred, respectively, in 0.7%, 0.3%, and 0.3% of patients. Monitor complete blood count for cytopenia at baseline and monthly thereafter. Do not start TALZENNA until patients have adequately recovered from hematological toxicity caused by previous therapy. If this occurs, dose modifications (dosing interruption with or without dose reduction) are recommended.

Embryo-fetal toxicity

Based on its mechanism of action and findings from animal data, TALZENNA can cause fetal harm when administered to a pregnant woman. In an animal reproduction study, administration of talazoparib to pregnant rats during the period of organogenesis caused fetal malformations and structural skeletal variations, and embryo-fetal death at exposures that were 0.24 times the area under the concentration-time curve (AUC) in patients receiving the recommended human dose of 1 mg daily. Apprise pregnant women and females of reproductive potential of the potential risk to a fetus. Advise females of reproductive potential to use effective contraception during treatment and for at least 7 months following the last dose of TALZENNA. Based on findings from genetic toxicity and animal reproduction studies, advise male patients with female partners of reproductive potential or who are pregnant to use effective contraception during treatment and for at least 4 months following the last dose of TALZENNA.

USE IN SPECIFIC POPULATIONS

Pregnancy risk summary

Based on findings from animal studies and its mechanism of action, TALZENNA can cause embryo-fetal harm when administered to a pregnant woman. There are no available data on TALZENNA use in pregnant women to inform a drug-associated risk. In an animal reproduction study, the administration of talazoparib to pregnant rats during the period of organogenesis caused fetal malformations and structural skeletal variations and embryo-fetal death at maternal exposures that were 0.24 times the AUC in patients receiving the recommended dose of 1 mg daily (see Data). Apprise pregnant women and females of reproductive potential of the potential risk to a fetus. The background risk of major birth defects and miscarriage for the indicated population is unknown. In the general U.S. population, the estimated background risks of major birth defects and miscarriage in clinically recognized pregnancies are 2% to 4% and 15% to 20%, respectively.

Data

Animal data

In an embryo-fetal development toxicity study, pregnant rats received oral doses of 0.015, 0.05, and 0.15 mg/kg/day talazoparib during the period of organogenesis. Talazoparib caused embryo-fetal death at doses ≥0.015 mg/kg/day (approximately 0.24 times the AUC in patients at the recommended dose). A dose of 0.015 mg/kg/day caused decreased fetal body weights and an increased incidence of fetal malformations (depressed eye bulge, small eye, split sternebra, and fused cervical vertebral arch) and structural variations including misshapen or incomplete ossification of the sternebra, skull, rib, and vertebra.

Lactation risk summary

There are no data on the presence of talazoparib in human milk, the effects of the drug on milk production, or the effects of the drug on the breastfed child. Because of the potential for serious adverse reactions in a breastfed child from talazoparib, advise lactating women not to breastfeed during treatment with TALZENNA and for at least 1 month after the final dose.

Females and males of reproductive potential

Pregnancy testing

A pregnancy test is recommended for females of reproductive potential prior to initiating TALZENNA treatment

Contraception

Females

TALZENNA can cause fetal harm when administered to pregnant women. Advise females of reproductive potential to use effective contraception during treatment and for at least 7 months following the last dose of TALZENNA.

Males

Based on genotoxicity and animal reproduction studies, advise male patients with female partners of reproductive potential and pregnant partners to use effective contraception during treatment with TALZENNA and for at least 4 months following the last dose

Infertility

Males

Based on animal studies, TALZENNA may impair fertility in males of reproductive potential.

Pediatric use

The safety and effectiveness of TALZENNA have not been established in pediatric patients.

Geriatric use

In clinical trials of TALZENNA enrolling 494 patients with advanced solid tumors who received TALZENNA 1 mg daily as monotherapy, 85 (17%) patients were ≥65 years of age, and this included 19 (4%) patients who were ≥75 years old. There were 5 patients ≥85 years old. No overall differences in safety or effectiveness of

TALZENNA were observed between these patients and younger patients, but greater sensitivity of some older individuals cannot be ruled out.

Renal impairment

Reduce the recommended dose of TALZENNA in patients with moderate renal impairment (CLcr 30 - 59 mL/min). No dose adjustment is required for patients with mild renal impairment (CLcr 60 - 89 mL/min). TALZENNA has not been studied in patients with severe renal impairment (CLcr < 30 mL/min) or patients requiring hemodialysis.

Hepatic impairment

TALZENNA has not been studied in patients with moderate hepatic impairment (total bilirubin >1.5 to 3.0 × upper limit of normal [ULN] and any aspartate aminotransferase [AST]) or severe hepatic impairment (total bilirubin >3.0 × ULN and any AST). No dose adjustment is required for patients with mild hepatic impairment (total bilirubin ≤1 × ULN and AST > ULN, or total bilirubin >1.0 to 1.5 × ULN and any AST).

OVERDOSAGE

There is no specific treatment in the event of TALZENNA overdose, and symptoms of overdose have not been established. In the event of overdose, discontinue treatment with TALZENNA, consider gastric decontamination, follow general supportive measures, and treat symptomatically.

Clinical efficacy of talozoparib (TALZENNA) in the treatment of breast cancer

Loss-of-function mutations in BRCA1 and BRCA2 are detected in at least 5% of unselected patients with breast cancer (BC). These BC susceptibility genes encode proteins critical for DNA homologous recombination repair (HRR). This review provides an update on oral poly (ADP-ribose) polymerase (PARP) inhibitors for the treatment of BC. Olaparib and talazoparib are PARP inhibitors approved as monotherapies for deleterious/suspected deleterious germline BRCA-mutated, HER2-negative BC. Olaparib is approved in the USA for metastatic BC and in Europe for locally advanced/metastatic BC. Talazoparib is approved for locally advanced/metastatic BC in the USA and Europe. In phase 3 trials, olaparib and talazoparib monotherapies demonstrated significant progression-free survival benefits compared with chemotherapy. Common toxicities were effectively managed by supportive treatment and dose interruptions/reductions. Veliparib combined with platinum-based chemotherapy has also shown promise for locally advanced/metastatic BC in a phase 3 trial. Differences in efficacy and safety across PARP inhibitors (olaparib, talazoparib, veliparib, niraparib, rucaparib) may relate to differences in potency of PARP trapping on DNA and cytotoxic specificity. PARP inhibitors are being investigated in early BC, in novel combinations, and in patients without germline BRCA mutations, including those with somatic BRCA mutations and other HRR gene mutations. Ongoing phase 2/3 studies include PARP inhibitors combined with immune checkpoint inhibitors for the treatment of triple-negative BC. Wider access to testing for BRCA and other mutations, and to genetic counseling, are required to identify patients who could benefit from PARP inhibitor therapy. The advent of PARP inhibitors has potential benefits for BC treatment beyond the locally advanced/metastatic setting.

Cortesi L, et al. An Overview of PARP Inhibitors for the Treatment of Breast Cancer. Target Oncol. 2021 May;16(3):255-282. doi: 10.1007/s11523-021-00796-4. Epub 2021 Mar 12. PMID: 33710534; PMCID: PMC8105250.

9.20. TUCATINIB (TUKYSA)

TUKYSA (tucatinib) tablets, for oral use. Initial U.S. Approval: 2020.

INDICATIONS AND USAGE

TUKYSA is a kinase inhibitor indicated in combination with trastuzumab and capecitabine for treatment of adult patients with advanced unresectable or metastatic HER2-positive breast cancer, including patients with brain metastases, who have received one or more prior anti-HER2-based regimens in the metastatic setting.

MECHANISM OF ACTION

Tucatinib is a tyrosine kinase inhibitor of HER2. In vitro, tucatinib inhibits phosphorylation of HER2 and HER3, resulting in inhibition of downstream MAPK and

AKT signaling and cell proliferation, and showed antitumor activity in HER2 expressing tumor cells *(Figure 143).*

Figure 143. A simplified representation of major signal transduction pathways in mammals. This image is reproduced here from Wikimedia Commons since permission has been granted by its creator, Cybertory, to copy, distribute and/or modify this document under the terms of the GNU Free Documentation License, Version 1.2 or any later version published by the Free Software Foundation; Author: By Cybertory - This file was derived from: Signal transduction v1.png, CC BY-SA 3.0, https://commons.wikimedia.org/w/index.php?curid=12081090. https://en.wikipedia.org/wiki/Creative_Commons_license. No change has been made to the image.

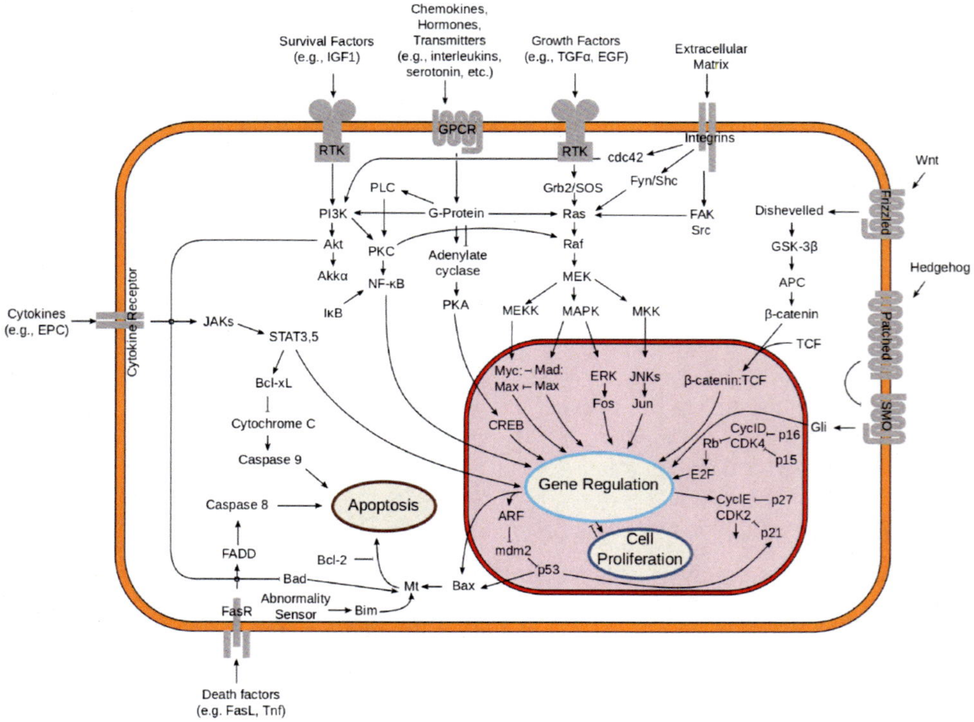

In vivo, tucatinib inhibited the growth of HER2 expressing tumors. The combination of tucatinib and trastuzumab showed increased anti-tumor activity in vitro and in vivo compared to either drug alone.

DESCRIPTION

Tucatinib is a kinase inhibitor. The chemical name is (N4-(4-([1,2,4]triazolo[1,5-a]pyridin-7-yloxy)-3 methylphenyl)-N6-(4,4-dimethyl-4,5-dihydrooxazol-2-yl)quinazoline-4,6-diamine. The molecular formula is C26H24N8O2, and the molecular weight is 480.52 g/mol. The chemical structure is as follows: O N N HN N H O N N N N.

TUKYSA (tucatinib) is supplied as 50 mg and 150 mg film-coated tablets for oral use and contain the following inactive ingredients: Tablet core: copovidone, crospovidone, sodium chloride, potassium chloride, sodium bicarbonate, colloidal silicon dioxide, magnesium stearate, and microcrystalline cellulose.

ADMINISTRATION

• Recommended dosage

300 mg taken orally twice daily with or without food.

• For patients with severe hepatic impairment, the recommended dosage is 200 mg orally twice daily.

DOSAGE FORMS AND STRENGTHS

Tablets: 50 mg and 150 mg.

CONTRAINDICATIONS

None.

WARNINGS AND PRECAUTIONS

• Diarrhea: severe diarrhea, including dehydration leading to acute kidney injury (Figure 144), and death, has been reported. Administer antidiarrheal treatment as clinically indicated. Interrupt dose, then dose reduce, or permanently discontinue TUKYSA based on severity.

Figure 144. Pathophysiology of acute kidney injury in the proximal renal tubule.

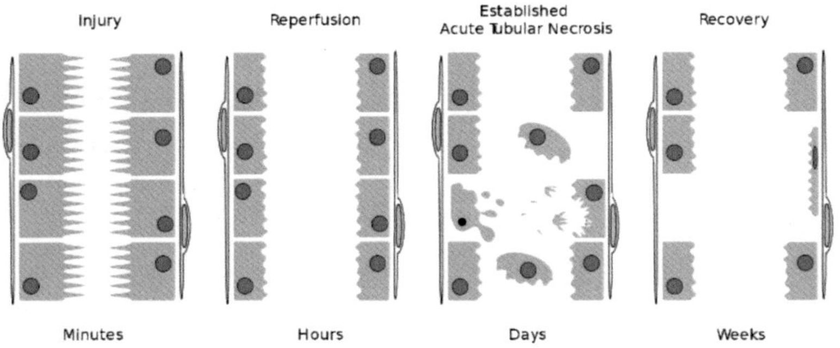

• Hepatotoxicity: Severe hepatotoxicity has been reported on TUKYSA. Monitor ALT, AST and bilirubin prior to starting TUKYSA, every 3 weeks during treatment and as clinically indicated. Interrupt dose, then dose reduce, or permanently discontinue TUKYSA based on severity.

Embryo-fetal toxicity

TUKYSA can cause fetal harm. Advise patients of potential risk to a fetus and to use effective contraception.

ADVERSE REACTIONS

The most common adverse reactions (≥20%) are diarrhea, palmar-plantar erythrodysesthesia, nausea, fatigue, hepatotoxicity, vomiting, stomatitis, decreased appetite, abdominal pain, headache, anemia, and rash. To report SUSPECTED

ADVERSE REACTIONS, contact Seattle Genetics at 1-855-4SEAGEN or FDA at 1-800-FDA-1088 or www.fda.gov/medwatch.

DRUG INTERACTIONS

• Strong CYP3A inducers or Moderate CYP2C8 Inducers

Avoid concomitant use.

• Strong CYP2C8 inhibitors

Avoid concomitant use; reduce TUKYSA dose if concomitant use cannot be avoided.

• CYP3A substrates

Avoid concomitant use with CYP3A substrates, where minimal concentration changes may lead to serious or life-threatening toxicities.

• P-gp substrates

Consider reducing the dose of P-gp substrates, where minimal concentration changes may lead to serious or life-threatening toxicities.

USE IN SPECIFIC POPULATIONS

Lactation: Advise not to breastfeed

FULL PRESCRIBING INFORMATION

INDICATIONS AND USAGE

TUKYSA is indicated in combination with trastuzumab and capecitabine for treatment of adult patients with advanced unresectable or metastatic HER2-positive breast cancer, including patients with brain metastases, who have received one or more prior anti-HER2-based regimens in the metastatic setting.

DOSAGE AND ADMINISTRATION

Recommended dosage

The recommended dosage of TUKYSA is 300 mg taken orally twice daily in combination with trastuzumab and capecitabine until disease progression or unacceptable toxicity. Advise patients to swallow TUKYSA tablets whole and not to chew, crush, or split prior to swallowing. Advise patients not to ingest tablet if it is broken, cracked, or not otherwise intact. Advise patients to take TUKYSA approximately 12 hours apart and at the same time each day with or without a meal. If the patient vomits or misses a dose of TUKYSA, instruct the patient to take the next dose at its usual scheduled time.

When given in combination with TUKYSA, the recommended dosage of capecitabine is 1000 mg/m^2 orally twice daily taken within 30 minutes after a meal. TUKYSA and capecitabine can be taken at the same time.

Dosage modifications for adverse reactions

The recommended TUKYSA dose reductions and dosage modifications for adverse reactions are provided in Tables 1 and 2. Refer to the Full Prescribing Information for trastuzumab and capecitabine for information about dosage modifications for these drugs.

Recommended TUKYSA dose reductions for adverse reactions

Dose reduction	**Recommended TUKYSA dosage**
First	250 mg orally twice daily
Second	200 mg orally twice daily
Third	150 mg orally twice daily

Permanently discontinue TUKYSA in patients unable to tolerate 150 mg orally twice daily.

Recommended TUKYSA dosage modifications for adverse reactions

Adverse Reaction[1]	Severity	TUKYSA dosage modification
Diarrhea	Grade 3 without anti-diarrheal treatment	Initiate or intensify appropriate medical therapy. Hold TUKYSA until recovery to ≤ Grade 1, then resume TUKYSA at the same dose level.
Diarrhea	Grade 3 with anti-diarrheal treatment	Initiate or intensify appropriate medical therapy. Hold TUKYSA until recovery to ≤ Grade 1, then resume TUKYSA

		at the next lower dose level.
Diarrhea	Grade 4	Permanently discontinue TUKYSA

Hepatoxicity[2]	Grade 2 bilirubin (>1.5 to 3 × ULN)	Hold TUKYSA until recovery to ≤ Grade 1, then resume TUKYSA at the same dose level.
Hepatoxicity	Grade 3 ALT or AST (> 5 to 20 × ULN) OR Grade 3 bilirubin (> 3 to 10 × ULN)	Hold TUKYSA until recovery to ≤ Grade 1, then resume TUKYSA at the next lower dose level.
Hepatoxicity	Grade 4 ALT or AST (> 20 × ULN) OR Grade 4 bilirubin (> 10 × ULN)	Permanently discontinue TUKYSA
Hepatoxicity2	ALT or AST > 3 × ULN AND Bilirubin > 2 × ULN	Permanently discontinue TUKYSA
Other adverse reactions	Grade 3	Hold TUKYSA until recovery to ≤ Grade 1, then resume TUKYSA at the next lower dose level.
Other adverse reactions	Grade 4	Permanently discontinue TUKYSA

[1] Grades based on National Cancer Institute Common Terminology Criteria for Adverse Events Version 4.03.

[2] Abbreviations: ULN = upper limit of normal; ALT = alanine aminotransferase; AST = aspartate aminotransferase.

Dosage modifications for severe hepatic impairment

For patients with severe hepatic impairment (Child-Pugh C), reduce the recommended dosage to 200 mg orally twice daily

Dosage modifications for concomitant use with strong CYP2C8 inhibitors

Avoid concomitant use of strong CYP2C8 inhibitors with TUKYSA. If concomitant use with a strong CYP2C8 inhibitor cannot be avoided, reduce the recommended dosage to 100 mg orally twice daily. After discontinuation of the strong CYP2C8 inhibitor for 3 elimination half-lives, resume the TUKYSA dose that was taken prior to initiating the inhibitor

DOSAGE FORMS AND STRENGTHS

Tablets

• 50 mg: round, yellow, film-coated, debossed with “TUC” on one side and “50” on the other side.

• 150 mg: oval-shaped, yellow, film-coated, debossed with “TUC” on one side and “150” on the other side.

CONTRAINDICATIONS

None.

DRUG INTERACTIONS

Effects of other drugs on TUKYSA

The following table summarizes the effect of other drugs on TUKYSA.

Strong CYP3A inducers or moderate CYP2C8 inducers

Clinical impact	Concomitant use of TUKYSA with a strong CYP3A or moderate CYP2C8 inducer decreased tucatinib plasma concentrations which may reduce TUKYSA activity.
Management	Avoid concomitant use of TUKYSA with a strong CYP3A inducer or a moderate CYP2C8 inducer.

Strong or moderate CYP2C8 inhibitors

Clinical impact	Concomitant use of TUKYSA with a strong CYP2C8 inhibitor increased tucatinib plasma concentrations which may increase the risk of TUKYSA toxicity.
Management	Avoid concomitant use of TUKYSA with a strong CYP2C8 inhibitor. Increase monitoring for TUKYSA toxicity with moderate CYP2C8 inhibitors.

The following table summarizes the effect of TUKYSA on other drugs.

CYP3A Substrates

Clinical impact	Concomitant use of TUKYSA with a CYP3A substrate increased the plasma concentrations of CYP3A substrate which may increase the toxicity associated with a CYP3A substrate.
Management	Avoid concomitant use of TUKYSA with CYP3A substrates, where minimal concentration changes may lead to serious or life-threatening toxicities. If concomitant use is unavoidable, decrease the CYP3A substrate dosage in accordance with approved product labeling.

P-glycoprotein (P-gp) substrates

Clinical impact	Concomitant use of TUKYSA with a P-gp substrate increased the plasma concentrations of P-gp substrate which may increase the toxicity associated with a P-gp substrate.
Management	Consider reducing the dosage of P-gp substrates, where minimal concentration changes may lead to serious or life-threatening toxicities

USE IN SPECIFIC POPULATIONS

Pregnancy risk summary

TUKYSA is used in combination with trastuzumab and capecitabine. Refer to the Full Prescribing Information of trastuzumab and capecitabine for pregnancy information. Based on findings in animals and its mechanism of action, TUKYSA can cause fetal harm when administered to a pregnant woman. There are no available human data on TUKYSA use in pregnant women to inform a drug-associated risk. In animal reproduction studies, administration of tucatinib to pregnant rats and rabbits during organogenesis resulted in embryo-fetal mortality, reduced fetal weight and fetal abnormalities at maternal exposures ≥ 1.3 times the human exposure (AUC) at the recommended dose (see Data). Advise pregnant women and females of reproductive potential of the potential risk to the fetus. The background risk of major birth defects and miscarriage for the indicated population is unknown. In the U.S. general population, the estimated background risk of major birth defects and miscarriage in clinically recognized pregnancies is 2%-4% and 15%-20%, respectively.

Data

Animal data

In pilot embryo-fetal development studies, pregnant rats and rabbits received oral doses of tucatinib up to 150 mg/kg/day during the period of organogenesis. In rats, oral administration of tucatinib resulted in maternal toxicity (body weight loss, reduced body weight gain, low food consumption) at doses ≥ 90 mg/kg/day. Fetal effects included reduced number of live fetuses, decreased fetal weight, and fetal abnormalities (increase in skeletal variations, incomplete ossification) at ≥ 90 mg/kg/day (approximately 3.5 times the human exposure at the recommended dose based on AUC). In rabbits, oral administration of tucatinib resulted in increased resorptions, decreased percentages of live fetuses, and skeletal, visceral, and external malformations in fetuses at doses ≥ 90 mg/kg/day (1.3 times the human exposure at the recommended dose based on AUC). Fetal abnormalities included domed head, brain dilation, incomplete ossification of frontal and parietal bones, and a hole in the parietal bone.

Lactation risk summary

TUKYSA is used in combination with trastuzumab and capecitabine. Refer to the Full Prescribing Information of trastuzumab and capecitabine for lactation information. There are no data on the presence of tucatinib or its metabolites in human or animal milk or its effects on the breastfed child or on milk production. Because of the potential for serious adverse reactions in a breastfed child, advise women not to breastfeed during treatment with TUKYSA and for at least 1 week after the last dose.

Females and males of reproductive potential

TUKYSA can cause fetal harm when administered to a pregnant woman. TUKYSA is used in combination with trastuzumab and capecitabine. Refer to the Full Prescribing Information of trastuzumab and capecitabine for contraception and infertility information.

Pregnancy testing

Verify the pregnancy status of females of reproductive potential prior to initiating treatment with TUKYSA.

Contraception

Females

Advise females of reproductive potential to use effective contraception during treatment with TUKYSA and for at least 1 week after the last dose.

Males

Advise male patients with female partners of reproductive potential to use effective contraception during treatment with TUKYSA and for at least 1 week after the last dose.

Infertility

Based on findings from animal studies, TUKYSA may impair male and female fertility

Pediatric use

The safety and effectiveness of TUKYSA in pediatric patients have not been established.

Geriatric use

In HER2CLIMB, 82 patients who received TUKYSA were ≥ 65 years, of whom 8 patients were ≥ 75 years. The incidence of serious adverse reactions in those receiving TUKYSA was 34% in patients ≥ 65 years compared to 24% in patients < 30 mL/min estimated by Cockcroft-Gault Equation), because capecitabine is contraindicated in patients with severe renal impairment. Refer to the Full Prescribing Information of capecitabine for additional information in severe renal impairment. No dose adjustment is recommended for patients with mild or moderate renal impairment (creatinine clearance [CLcr] 30 to 89 mL/min).

Hepatic impairment

Tucatinib exposure is increased in patients with severe hepatic impairment (Child-Pugh C). Reduce the dose of TUKYSA for patients with severe (Child-Pugh C)

hepatic impairment. No dose adjustment for TUKYSA is required for patients with mild (Child-Pugh A) or moderate (Child-Pugh B) hepatic impairment.

Pharmacodynamics

Exposure response relationship

Tucatinib exposure-response relationships and the time course of pharmacodynamics response have not been fully characterized.

Cardiac electrophysiology

No large mean increase in QTc (i.e., > 20 ms) was detected following treatment with TUKYSA at the recommended dose of 300 mg taken orally twice daily.

Pharmacokinetics

Tucatinib AUC0-INF and Cmax increases proportionally over a dosage range from 50 mg to 300 mg (0.17 to 1 times the approved recommended dosage). Tucatinib exhibited 1.7-fold accumulation for AUC and 1.5-fold accumulation for Cmax following administration of TUKYSA 300 mg twice daily for 14 days. Time to steady state was approximately 4 days.

Absorption

The median time to peak plasma concentration of tucatinib was approximately 2 hours (range 1 to 4 hours). Effects of Food Following administration of a single oral dose of TUKYSA in 11 subjects after a high-fat meal (approximately 58% fat, 26% carbohydrate, and 16% protein), the mean AUC0-INF increased by 1.5-fold, the Tmax shifted from 1.5 hours to 4 hours, and Cmax was unaltered. The effect of food on the pharmacokinetics of tucatinib was not clinically meaningful. Distribution The geometric mean (CV %) apparent volume of distribution of tucatinib was approximately 1670 L (66%). The plasma protein binding was 97.1% at clinically relevant concentrations.

Elimination

The geometric mean (CV %) half-life of tucatinib was approximately 8.5 (21%) hours and apparent clearance was 148 L/h (55%).

Metabolism

Tucatinib is metabolized primarily by CYP2C8 and to a lesser extent via CYP3A.

Excretion

Following a single oral dose of 300 mg radiolabeled tucatinib, approximately 86% of the total radiolabeled dose was recovered in feces (16% of the administered dose as unchanged tucatinib) and 4.1% in urine with an overall total recovery of 90% within 13 days post-dose. In plasma, approximately 76% of the plasma radioactivity was unchanged, 19% was attributed to identified metabolites, and approximately 5% was unassigned.

Specific populations

Age (< 65 (n =211); ≥ 65 (n = 27)), albumin (25 to 52 g/L), creatinine clearance (creatinine clearance [CLcr] 60 to 89 mL/min (n = 89); CLcr 30 to 59 mL/min (n = 5)), body weight (41 to 138 kg), and race (White (n=168), Black (n=53), or Asian (n=10)) did not have a clinically meaningful effect on tucatinib exposure.

Renal impairment

No clinically significant differences in the pharmacokinetics of tucatinib were observed in patients with mild to moderate renal impairment (creatinine clearance: 30 to 89 mL/min by Cockcroft-Gault). The effect of severe renal impairment (creatinine clearance: < 30 mL/min) on the pharmacokinetics of tucatinib is unknown.

Hepatic impairment

Mild (Child-Pugh A) and moderate (Child-Pugh B) hepatic impairment had no clinically relevant effect on tucatinib exposure. Tucatinib AUC0-INF was increased by 1.6 fold in subjects with severe (Child-Pugh C) hepatic impairment compared to subjects with normal hepatic function.

Drug interaction studies

The following table summarises the effects of other drugs on TUKYSA.

Concomitant rug (dose)	TUKYSA dose	Ratio (90% CI) of tucatinib exposure with and without concomitant drug	Ratio (90% ci) of tucatinib exposure with and without concomitant drug
		Cmax	AUC
CYP2C8 Substrate Repaglinide (0.5 mg single dose)	300 mg twice daily	1.7 (1.4, 2.1)	1.7 (1.5, 1.9)
CYP3A Substrate Midazolam (2 mg single dose)	300 mg twice daily	3.0 (2.6, 3.4)	5.7 (5.0, 6.5)
P-gp Substrate Digoxin (0.5 mg single dose)	300 mg twice daily	2.4 (1.9, 2.9)	1.5 (1.3, 1.7)
MATE1/2-K substratea Metformin[a] (850 mg single dose)	300 mg twice daily	1.1 (1.0, 1.2)	1.4 (1.2, 1.5)

[a]Tucatinib reduced the renal clearance of metformin without any effect on glomerular filtration rate (GFR) as measured by iohexol clearance and serum cystatin C. No clinically significant difference in the pharmacokinetics of tucatinib were observed when used concomitantly with omeprazole (proton pump inhibitor) or tolbutamide (sensitive CYP2C9 substrate).

In vitro studies

Cytochrome P450 (CYP) enzymes

Tucatinib is a reversible inhibitor of CYP2C8 and CYP3A and a time-dependent inhibitor of CYP3A, but is not an inhibitor of CYP1A2, CYP2B6, CYP2C9, CYP2C19, or CYP2D6.

Uridine diphosphate (UDP)-glucuronosyl transferase (UGT) enzymes

Tucatinib is not an inhibitor of UGT1A1.

Transporter systems

Tucatinib is a substrate of P-gp and BCRP, but is not a substrate of OAT1, OAT3, OCT1, OCT2, OATP1B1, OATP1B3, MATE1, MATE2-K, or BSEP. Tucatinib inhibits

MATE1/MATE2-K-mediated transport of metformin and OCT2/MATE1-mediated transport of creatinine. The observed serum creatinine increase in clinical studies with tucatinib is due to inhibition of tubular secretion of creatinine via OCT2 and MATE1.

Clinical efficacy of tucatinib in the treatment of breast cancer

In patients with HER2-positive breast cancer with brain metastases (BMs), the addition of tucatinib to trastuzumab and capecitabine doubled ORR-IC, reduced risk of intracranial progression or death by two thirds, and reduced risk of death by nearly half. To our knowledge, this is the first regimen to demonstrate improved antitumor activity against BMs in patients with HER2-positive breast cancer in a randomized, controlled trial.

Lin NU et al. J Clin Oncol 38:2610-2619.

10. Cytokine release syndrome (CRS)

CRS is a non-antigen specific toxicity that occurs as a result of an exaggerated immune response. It has been described following the the therapeutic administration of monoclonal antibodies including rituximab (Rituxan), muromonab (OKT3), alemtuzumab (Campath-1) as well as after the infusion genetically unmodifiedcytoxic T cells for EBV-associated lymphoma and after the infusion of genetically modified chimeric antigen receptor (CAR) T cell therapy. Onset typically occurs minutes to hours after the infusion. Clinical features include fever, rash, tachycardia, and hypotension. Some patients have required transfer to an intensive care unit for management of respiratory distress and renal dysfunction. Large numbers of lymphocytes (B cells,T cell and/or natural killer cells), and/or myeloid cells (macrophages, dendritic cells and monocytes) become activated and release inflammatory cytokines including TNF-alpha, interferon-gamma, IL-1beta, IL-2, IL-6, IL-8 and IL-10. Uncontrolled studies have suggested that the use of the anti-IL-6receptor antibody, tocilizumab (Actrema), with or without corticosteroids, can reverse the syndrome.

11. CONCLUSIONS: THE IMPACT OF THESE NEW DRUGS ON THE CLINICAL MANAGEMENT OF BREAST CANCER IN AUSTRALIA – A PEER REVIEW OF CURRENT PRACTICE

Detailed understanding of how normal cells and malignant cells work at the molecular level has provided many new targets for the development of new therapeutic agents. Medical oncology has been the biggest beneficiary of these todate, with many new drugs now available to treat both the four most common carcinomas – lung, breast, colo-rectal and prostate – as well as new drugs for less common malignancies such as renal cell carcinoma. These new agents target specific proteins on the surface of the malignant cell or enzymes that catalyze reactions inside the cell essential for normal cell function. Before the introduction of trastuzumab in 1998, HER2+ breast cancer had a very poor prognosis. For patients whose primary breast cancer is HER2+, HER2-directed therapy should be incorporated in their first-line treatment. Herceptin is also effective for metastatic HER2+ breast cancer. Now trastuzumab has been linked to hyaluronic acid (HERCEPTIN HYLECTA) to allow subcutaneous administration by a health professional in the patient's home, thus obviating the need for a hospital outpatient visit to receive the drug as an intravenous infusion (especially useful during pandemics such as that due to Covid-19). Additionally, trastuzumab has been linked with specific toxins (antibody-drug conjugates), so that the antibody delivers the toxin to appropriate cells (ie those over-expressing HER2. Two examples are Fam-trastuzumab-derluxican-nhxi (ENHERTU) and Ado-trastuzumab emtansine (KADCYCLA).

For patients with metastatic, HER2-negative breast cancer
with germline BRCA mutations who have previously been treated with chemotherapy an oral inhibitor of poly (ADP-ribose) polymerase (PARP) can be added.

New small molecules have been developed including cyclin-dependent kinase (CDK) inhibiors such as tucatinib. Women who progress ≥12 months from the end of adjuvant endocrine therapy (ET) and patients who present with de novo metastatic breast cancer can be offered first-line ET or ET in combination with a cyclin-dependent kinase (CDK) 4/6 inhibitor. Other acceptable options include single-agent fulvestrant or anastrozole, or fulvestrant in combination with an AI or ribociclib.

This drug can treat brain metastases from breast cancer, an area treatable previously only by palliative irradiation to the brain. Other small molecules include P13K inhibitors such as alpelesib, the kinase inhibitor everolimus and PARP inhibitors such as olaparib. For patients who have previously experienced progression on an aromatase inhibitor (AI) and CDK 4/6 inhibitor, one approach should consider the patient's tumor phosphatidylinositol-4,5-bisphosphate 3-kinase catalytic subunit alpha (PIK3CA) status: for those with PIK3CA-mutant cancers progressive on the combination of AIs and CDK 4/6 inhibitors, the combination of fulvestrant with the alpha isoform-specific phosphoinositide 3-kinase (PI3K) inhibitor alpelisib can be used. For those with PIK3CA-mutant cancers progressive on the combination of AIs and CDK 4/6 inhibitors, options include fulvestrant monotherapy or everolimus-based combinations, with a choice between them driven by side-effect profiles.

The pharmacopeia for breast cancer has thus expanded enormously and medical oncologists will need to have very specific guidelines for when to use what option. Medical school, pharmacy and nursing classes will need updated curricula. It is already necessary to have a detailed knowledge of both the cellular and molecular biology of human cells in order to practice medicine with excellence. To really understand how these drugs work at the molecular level it would be worth undertaking a Master's degree, or a PhD, in molecular biology. Soon, if not now, it will be difficult for medical oncologists to be general medical oncologists managing each type of cancer – there are simply too many new drugs, many of which have signicant side-effects. Medical oncologists will need to subspecialize in, say, one of the big four carcinomas. This is already happening. This trajectory of new knowledge is only going to increase.

In this review of Australian peer practice in the management of breast cancer it should be noted that, of the 20 biological targeted agents that are FDA-approved for the treatment of breast cancer in the USA, 12 are available in Australia on on the PBS, six have not yet been approved (ENHERTU, HERCEPTIN HYLECTA, Margetuximab-cmkb, neratinib (Nerlynx), Phesgo and Trodelvy), and two have been submitted for approval (alpelisib and tucatinib)

13. Abbreviations used (other than those explained in Table1, Table 2 and in the FDA-derived text). This list includes abbreviations used in other books in the series Medicine 2020 and the series Modern Medicine 2021.

AC, adriamycin and cyclophosphamide (combination chemotherapy)

ACE, angiotensin-converting-enzyme

ADC, antibody-drug conjugate

ADCC, antibody-dependent cellular cytotoxicity

ADCC, antibody directed enzyme prodrug therapy

AGEP, acute generalized exanthematous pustulosis

AI, aromatase inhibitor

ALK, anaplastic lymphoma kinase

ALL, acute lymphoblastic leukemia

ALT, alanine aminotransferase

AML, acute myeloid leukemia

aPTT, activated partial thromboplastin time

ARR, administration-related reaction

AS, adverse reaction

AS, ankylosing spondylitis

ASCT, autologous stem cell transplant

AST, aspartate aminotransferase

ATA, anti-therapeutic antibody

ATM, ataxia telangiectasia mutated (gene)

AUC, Area Under the Concentration – time curve

AUC (0-inf): AUC curve to infinite time. As we cannot get the assays to go to infinity, we have to extrapolate to infinity. This can be calculated from the AUC(0-t) by the addition of a constant (Clast/λz), where Clast is the last observed quantifiable concentration and λz is the terminal phase rate constant.

BCG, Bacille Calmain-Guerin

BCR-ABL, breakpoint cluster region/Abelson

BCRP, breast cancer resistance protein

b DMARD, biologic disease-modifying anti-rheumatic drug

BRACA1, breast cancer susceptibility gene 1

BTK, Bruton's tyrosine kinase

CAT, cyclophosphamide, adriamycin and taxane (combination chemotherapy)

CDC, complement-dependent cytotoxicity

CDK, cyclin-dependent kinase

C-G, Cockoft-Gault (formula)

cHL, classical Hodgkin Lymphoma

CINV, chemotherapy-induced nausea and vomiting

CIS, carcinoma in situ

CLL, chronic lymphocytic leukemia

Clcr, creatinine clearance rate

CMF, cyclophosphamide, methotrexate, and fluorouracil (combination chemotherapy

CML, chronic myelogenous leukemia (also known as chronic myeloid leukemia)

CPS, combine positive score

CR, complete remission

CRC, colorectal carcinoma

CRS, cytokine release syndrome

CS, cytokine storm

csDMARD, synthetic disease-modifying anti-rheumatic drug

CSF1R, colony-stimulating factor receptor 1

CT, computed tomography

CTCAE, Common Terminology Criteria for Adverse Events

DCIS, ductal carcinoma in situ

DFS, disease-free survival

dMMR, deficient mismatch repair

DPP4, dipeptidyl peptidase-4

DRESS, drug reaction with eosinophilia and systemic symptoms. DRESS syndrome is classified as one form of severe cutaneous adverse reactions (SCARs). In addition to DRESS, SCARs includes four other drug-induced skin reactions, the Stevens–

Johnson syndrome (SJS); Toxic epidermal necrolysis (TEN), Stevens–Johnson/toxic epidermal necrolysis overlap syndrome (SJS/TEN)

EBC, early breast cancer

ECG or EKG, electrocardiogram

EFS, event-free durvival

EGF, epidermal growth factor

EGFR, epidermal growth factor receptor

EN, erythema nodosum

ER, estrogen receptor

ET, endocrine therapy

ErbB, derived from erythroblastic leukemia viral oncogene

FBG, fasting blood glucose

FEC, fluorouracil, epirubicin and cyclophosphamide (combination chemotherapy)

FGF, fibroblast growth factor

FGFR, fibroblast growth factor receptor

FISH, fluorescence in situ hybridization

FKBP12/mTOR, FK Binding Protein-12/mammalian target of rapamycin

Flt3, fms like tyrosine kinase 3

FPG, fasting plams glucose

FSH, follicle-stimulating hormone

FU, fluouracil

gBRCAm, BRCA mutated

GD, gestational day

GI, gastro-intestinal

GIST, gastrointestinal stromal tumor

GFR, glomerular filtration rate

GMR, geometric mean ratio

HCC, hepatocellular carcinoma

HER, human epidermal receptor

HER2, human epidermal growth factor receptor 2

HNSCC, head and neck squamous carcinoma

HR, hormone receptor

HRR, homologous recombination repair

HSCT, hematopoietic stem cell transplant

JAK, Janus kinase

KLIFS-3, kinase-ligand interaction fingerprint and structure residue-3

IBC, inflammatory breast cancer

IC, immune cell

IFN, interferon

IL, interleukin

ILD, interstitial lung disease

ILN, interstitial lung disease

IRR, infusion-related reaction

ITP, idiopathic thrombocytopenic purpura

LCIS, lobular carcinoma in situ

LFT, liver function test

LH, luteinizing hormone

LLN, lower limit of normal

LVEF, left ventricular ejection fraction

Mab, monoclonal antibody

MATE, multi-antimicrobial extrusion protein

MBC, metastatic breast cancer

MCC, Merkel cell carcinoma

mCRPC, metastatic castrate resistant prostate cancer

MEK, mitogen-activated protein kinase

MRI, magnetic resonance imaging

MSI-H, microsatellite instability – high

MUGA, multigated acquisition

NCI-CTC, National Cancer Institute – Clinical Toxicity Criteria

Nib, small **i**n**hib**itory molecule

NMIBC, non-muscle invasive bladder cancer

NRH, nodular regenerative hyperplasia (of the liver)

NSCLC, non-small cell lung cancer

OS, overall survival

PARP, poly(ADP-ribose) polymerase

PDGF, platelet-derived growth factor

PDGFR, platelet-derived growth factor receptor

PFS, progression-free survival

Ph+, Philadelphia chromosome positive

PI3K, phosphatidylinositol 3-kinase

PI3KA, phosphatidylinositol-4,5-bisphosphate 3-kinase catalytic subunit alpha

PJIA, polyarticular juvenile idiopathic arthritis in patients aged 2 years or older

PJP, *Pneumocystis jiroveci* pneumonia

PK, pharmacokinetic analysis

PKA, protein kinase A

PMBCL, primary mediastinal B cell lymphoma

PNET, progressive neuroendocrine tumor (of the pancreasP

PR, progesterone receptor

pRb, retinoblastoma protein

PsA, psoriatic arthritis

PsO, plaque psoriasis

RA, rheumatoid arthritis

RAF, rapidly accelerated fibrosarcoma

RCC, renal cell carcinoma

RET, "rearranged during transfection"

ROCK, Rho-associated protein kinase

ROS, 'orphan' receptor tyrosine kinase

rb, retinoblastoma (gene or protein)

scFv, single-chain Fv fragment

SCARS, severe cutaneous adverse reactions

SCLC, small cell lung cancer

SERD, selective estrogen receptor degrader

SEGA, subependymal giant cell astrocytoma

SLAM, signalling lymphocytic activation molecule family (CD319)

SJS, Stevens–Johnson syndrome

SLL, small lymphocytic lymphoma

SYK, spleen tyrosine kinase

SWFI, sterile water for injection

TBC.tuberose sclerosid complex

TCH, docetaxel, carboplatin, and trastuzumab (combination chemotherapy)

TEN, toxic epidermal necrolysis

TNBC, triple negative breast cancer

TMB- high, tunor mutational burden - high

TNF, tumor necrosis factor

TRK, tropomyosin receptor kinase

ts DMARD, targeted synthetic disease-modifying anti-rheumatic drug

Tyk, tyrosine-protein kinase

UGT1A1, uridine diphosphate-glucuronosyl transferase 1A1

ULN, upper limit of normal

VEGF, vascular endothelial growth factor

VEGFR, vascular endothelial growth factor receptor